# Introduction to Therapeutic Counseling
## Voices from the Field

5th Edition

Jeffrey A. Kottler
*California State University, Fullerton*

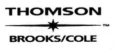

**THOMSON**
**BROOKS/COLE**

Australia • Canada • Mexico • Singapore • Spain • United Kingdom • United States

*Dedicated to the memory of Robert W. Brown*

**THOMSON**

**BROOKS/COLE**

Editor: *Julie Martinez*
Assistant Editor: *Shelley Gesicki*
Editorial Assistant: *Amy Lam*
Technology Project Manager: *Barry Connolly*
Marketing Manager: *Caroline Concilla*
Marketing Assistant: *Mary Ho*
Advertising Project Manager: *Tami Strang*
Project Manager, Editorial
   Production: *Ellen Brownstein*

Print/Media Buyer: *Rebecca Cross*
Permissions Editor: *Bob Kauser*
Production Service: *Pre-Press Co., Inc.*
Copy Editor: *Cheryl Hauser*
Cover Designer: *Didona Design*
Compositor: *Pre-Press Co., Inc.*
Printer: *Transcontinental-Louiseville*

Cover images:
*Mel Curtis/Getty Images; Corbis; Eyewire
Collection/Getty Images; Ryan McVay/
Getty Images; Ryan McVay/Getty Images;
Bruce Ayres/Stone/Getty Images;
Comstock Images, Inc.*

Printed in Canada
2  3  4  5  6  7  06  05  04

Library of Congress Control Number: 2002115947

For more information about our products,
contact us at:

**Thomson Learning Academic Resource Center
1-800-423-0563**

For permission to use material from this text,
contact us by:
**Phone:** 1-800-730-2214  **Fax:** 1-800-730-2215
**Web:** http://www.thomsonrights.com

Student Edition with InfoTrac College Edition:
ISBN 0-534-52339-0

Student Edition without InfoTrac College Edition:
ISBN 0-534-52343-9

**Brooks/Cole–Thomson Learning**
511 Forest Lodge Road
Pacific Grove, CA 93950
USA

**Asia**
Thomson Learning
5 Shenton Way #01-01
UIC Building
Singapore 068808

**Australia/New Zealand**
Thomson Learning
102 Dodds Street
Southbank, Victoria 3006
Australia

**Canada**
Nelson
1120 Birchmount Road
Toronto, Ontario M1K 5G4
Canada

**Europe/Middle East/Africa**
50/51 Bedford Row
London WC1R 4LR
United Kingdom

# CONTENTS

# PREFACE

This text was originally created out of a very personal need to create a student-centered introduction to our field. I felt frustrated at times because the personalized warmth and sensitivity that are the basis of our profession have not been reflected in academic experiences. Too often, education emphasizes theoretical knowledge and scholarly inquiry to the exclusion of student involvement. It has been my intention that this book would not only meet the stringent demands of scholarship but also provide a lively and dynamic overview of the counseling profession in which the student is fully engaged in this process.

This text speaks directly to you, the student, challenging you to explore your personal motives for choosing counseling as an area of interest, as well as helping you to personally integrate much of the research and theoretical concepts. More than ever before, the voices of beginning and experienced counselors are used to reflect the realities of practice, to make the ideas come alive, and to help you personalize the content in ways that it becomes immediately applicable to your life. In fact, there is no other profession that not only allows you to personalize concepts to your own life, but encourages you to do so; almost everything you read about in this text has implications and applications to what you do on a daily basis. You will find innumerable ways not only to improve immediately your therapeutic skills but also your personal relationships.

# WHAT YOU CAN DO

One of the distinguishing features of this text, which makes it unique in the field, is its student-oriented focus on the realities of counseling practice. In addition to presenting the major historical, theoretical, and research foundations in a highly readable style, I try to engage you in a dialogue about the counseling profession and its underlying concepts, as well as personal goals for the future.

It is so often the relationships we develop with people that become the foundation for a meaningful effort to change. This is as true in relationships between an author and readers as it is between a counselor and clients, or an instructor and students. More than ever before, I strive to connect with readers in such a way that they are likely to explore the process of counseling as well as its content.

In order to make the complex conceptual ideas of counseling come alive, the "Voices from the Field" have been expanded. In these excerpts from interviews, beginning and experienced practitioners speak openly and honestly about the challenges they face and the ways they have resolved difficulties. They present practical advice based on their experiences. When these voices are added to those of the author, readers are exposed to the realities of counseling practice in such a way that they can make informed choices about where and how to practice new skills and knowledge. You would be well advised to use this material as a springboard for your own interviews with practitioners.

One of the assignments I routinely give when I teach this class is to ask students to interview a minimum of six to ten counselors in the field, representing at least three different specialty areas. I can think of few other learning experiences that are more revealing than talking to people who are doing what you someday hope to do yourself. Ask them for advice. Find out what they love and hate about their work. It is not unusual that you will even make contacts that may someday turn into an internship placement or even a job offer.

The end of each chapter contains a series of experiential and reflective exercises that will further help you to personalize material. These introspective activities are useful as a structured journal for you to apply concepts discussed in class and in the text to your own life. In addition, they may be helpful as questions to be explored in cooperative learning groups in class. Whether you use the exercises or not, you will find it helpful to use a journal throughout the semester to keep track of important ideas, dialogue with me and your instructor, make sense of complex ideas, and personalize material in a way that is useful to you.

# WHAT TO EXPECT

*Introduction to Therapeutic Counseling: Voices From the Field* is designed for initial courses in human service programs with titles such as "Principles of Counseling," "Professional Orientation," "Counseling Theory and Practice," "Introduction to Helping," and "Human Resource Development." The book emphasizes the development of a professional identity, ethical standards for practice, basic process skills, the therapeutic relationship, personal theory building, and understanding of meaningful research. I am also especially concerned with presenting a contemporary "cutting-edge" focus on the practical realities of counseling. Too often students complain that their courses and texts did not prepare them for the daily grit and grind of what it means to be a counselor.

Particular attention is devoted to the major specialties and diverse settings in which counseling takes place, such as schools and clinics and medical, industrial, mental health, community agency, and private practice settings. I quite deliberately made the size of the book realistic for a semester's work and planned the number and length of chapters to be manageable for the student struggling to digest a new world of terminology and concepts.

The book is organized into four broad focus areas: professional identity factors, theoretical and research foundations, counseling applications, and issues in therapeutic practice. Whereas the first two sections (Chapters 1 through 8) help you to learn the foundations of therapeutic counseling, the latter two sections (Chapters 9 through 15) apply these concepts to the various specialties within the field. You are thus encouraged to master the basic theory and research of the field and become familiar with the generic therapeutic skills, as well as to begin thinking about the realities of developing a flexible specialty, making yourself marketable, finding suitable employment, and staying passionately committed to the profession.

## WHAT'S NEW?

One of the most exciting and disorienting aspects of counseling is how rapidly the field changes. This evolution in theory and research parallels the changes that practitioners experience so often. More than once I've had the fleeting fantasy of sending "recall notices" to all the clients I've seen in the past, notifying them that however I once helped them is now obsolete and that they should return for new, improved methods that no longer resemble the ways I once operated. Indeed, when I read the things I wrote in previous editions of this text, I'm stunned by the ways I've changed.

Consistent with the mood of our times, I continue to emphasize a philosophy of counselor education and training that my friend and coauthor, Bob Brown (now deceased) and I first proposed a number of years ago—one that is integrative and pragmatic and that seeks to combine the best of existing approaches. The text has also been expanded considerably to include more detailed discussion on today's major issues: multicultural sensitivity, historical roots of our profession, licensure and credentialing, constructivist thinking, family violence, sexism and age discrimination, computer applications, managed care and brief therapies, legal and ethical conflicts, and gender issues, to name a few. Because I have spent so much time working in other countries, and within other cultures, this book has a much more international flavor that includes diverse examples of counseling practice.

I have added the following new features:

- The text is synchronized with its own website that contains online quizzes for each chapter. This allows students to check their own comprehension of the reading assignments, as well as to prepare for the exams.

- Infotrac is incorporated into the text, making it easier for students to use and understand research and the literature.
- The practical exercise at the end of each chapter provide instructors with structures that can be used in a variety of ways: 1) take-home exam questions, 2) homework assignments, 3) extra credit assignments, 4) in-class activities, 5) opportunities for student further self-study.
- The "voices from the field" provide a real-life, practical context for the complex ideas and theories presented. Students not only read about the concepts, but actually experience them vicariously through the narratives of practicing counselors who speak frankly and authentically about what it's really like to do this job.
- Case examples and personal stories make the material come alive, maintain the student's interest, and make it easier for instructors to lead spirited discussions about the ideas.
- Key Concepts and Key Names have been added to the beginning of each chapter, making it easier for students to organize their study of important material.

I have added and expanded sections on counseling specialties that have blossomed in recent years: pastoral counseling, marriage and family counseling, sex counseling, conflict mediation, rehabilitation counseling, counseling in private practice, higher education, and industry. I have also added material on the diagnostic process in counseling, as well as the counselor functioning as a consultant and personal coach. Sections on managed care and technology have also been considerably expanded.

I have followed the advice offered by many of the students and faculty who valued the previous editions of this text: I have continued the effort to distill the common factors that operate in all effective helping efforts, seeking to integrate and simplify the essence of our profession. I have also retained a personal narrative voice that engages the reader with humor and case examples, keeping this text accessible for students struggling to find their way through the complex maze of this wonderful field. Finally, I hope that you will find the "Voices from the Field" boxes and end of chapter exercises useful in articulating your own reactions to what you've experienced.

## ACKNOWLEDGMENTS

I want to thank the "voices from the field" who agreed to be interviewed for this book and who were willing to be so honest and open about their experiences in the trenches. More than anything else in this text, it is your stories that give life and realism to the theory, research, and concepts presented.

Robert Brown, my friend and officemate, coauthored the first three editions of this text and died during the process of writing the 4th edition. Over the course of almost two decades we taught and counseled together, consulted on difficult cases, and shared confidences. Just before Bob died, he dictated to me his last thoughts about his life and words of advice for future readers. This is part of what he had to say: "Don't take yourself too seriously, but take yourself measurably. Don't take yourself in a manner that is cavalier, but take yourself in a manner that has sincerity and thoughtfulness about it."

I hope, Bob, that this book still retains the playfulness, the sincerity, and the thoughtfulness that you considered so important.

I would like to thank the following individuals who served as reviewers for this text:

Cathie Barret-Kruse, University of Texas, Permian Basin
Pat Bellomo, Lourdes College
Jinni Leigh Blalack, Union University
Korinne Cilanek, University of Minnesota
Dona Kennealley, University of South Dakota
Miriam Stark Parent, Trinity Evangelical Divinity School
Kenny Paris, Northeastern State University
Conni Sharp, Pittsburgh State University
Jan Wertz, Kentucky Wesleyan College

I would like to thank Julie Martinez for helping to guide the development of this 5th edition. I am also grateful for the assistance of Gerri McDaniel and Lisa Hayes who helped with the research for the latest edition.

*Jeffrey A. Kottler*

## ABOUT THE AUTHOR

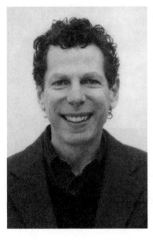

Jeffrey A. Kottler has authored over 40 books in the field for counselors, therapists, teachers, and the public, including *Compassionate Therapy: Working With Difficult Clients* (1992), *On Being a Therapist* (1993), *The Language of Tears* (1996), *The Last Victim* (1999), *Doing Good: Passion and Commitment For Helping Others* (2000), *Theories in Counseling and Therapy: An Experiential Approach* (2002), *Counselors Finding Their Way* (2002), and *Making Changes Last* (2002).

Jeffrey has worked as a teacher, counselor, and therapist in a preschool, middle school, mental health center, crisis center, university, community college, and private practice. He has served as a Fulbright Scholar and Senior Lecturer in Peru (1980) and Iceland (2000), teaching counseling theory and practice. He has also served as a visiting professor in New Zealand, Australia, Hong Kong, and Nepal. He is currently Chair of the Counseling Department at California State University, Fullerton.

# THE PROFESSIONAL
# COUNSELOR

# I

# WHAT COUNSELING IS AND HOW IT WORKS

KEY CONCEPTS

Personal motives

Making a difference

Commitment to professional helping

Countertransference

Informed consent

Living with anxiety

Neutral posture

Tolerance for ambiguity

Subjugating personal needs

Process definition of counseling

Movement toward integration

Common factors

Significance of self

Professional organizations (ACA, AAMFT, APA)

# WHAT COUNSELING IS AND HOW IT WORKS

# CHAPTER I

## WHY BE A COUNSELOR?

It is both interesting and useful to begin the systematic study of the counseling profession by exploring your own motives for entering the profession. The decision to become a counselor is as complex and multifaceted as any concern with which our clients might wish help. You will expect—even demand—that your clients be completely honest with themselves, that they confront their self-deceptions, ambivalence, and motives behind actions. It is only fair that you attempt to be honest with yourself as well.

Students enter the counseling field, as they do any other profession, for a variety of reasons. Some people genuinely wish to save the world; others, more modestly, wish to save themselves. Many deliberately choose this field because there are so many opportunities to apply classroom and book studies to their own lives. Others quite unabashedly admit that it was a toss-up for them between going to see a counselor for their own problems and becoming one.

The personal motives behind career decisions are indeed important to examine as this introduction to therapeutic counseling begins. Such an understanding will permit a more thoughtful and clear-headed approach to the material presented. A typical class often includes students who see themselves as missionaries. They choose to study counseling because they have a strong desire to help others: to make a difference in the lives of those who are suffering. They frequently have a kind of empathy that comes from personal experience. They suffered and were saved; now the roles can be reversed. They wish to make the world a bit more civilized. Perhaps this reason belongs, even slightly, to any of us who select this path; after all, it can't be for the liberal financial rewards, lack of stress, and guaranteed job for life.

Altruism and idealism certainly play a huge role in people's decisions to become a helping professional. You might be enrolled in this program for a variety of reasons, all related to making a difference in the world (Kottler, 2000):

1. You have some natural talent or proclivity toward helping others. Maybe you have served that role throughout your life.
2. You enjoy touching others' lives, knowing that you have influenced or impacted someone.
3. You derive tremendous satisfaction from the kind of close, intimate relationships that take place in helping encounters.
4. Your own problems seem diminished in comparison to those of your clients.
5. You are able to gain broadened perspectives on the meaning of life as a result of your searching conversations with others.
6. You are able to give something back to your community, to use your own learning experiences to benefit others.
7. You pass on a legacy to others as part of your commitment and dedication to service.
8. You help yourself by helping others.

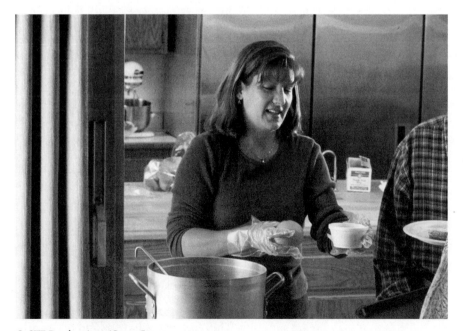

© SW Productions/Getty Images.

## VOICE FROM THE FIELD

I always knew that I wanted to help people, though I thought originally about a medical career. It wasn't until I faced the realities of what was involved in getting into and graduating from medical school that I began considering alternatives. You see, ever since I was a kid my worth was measured by what I could do for others. You might consider this part of my family culture. It is just understood that each of us will do something that involves helping others.

I would not be altogether truthful if I didn't mention that being a counselor means a heck of a lot more to me than helping people. That is important and all, but so are some other reasons that I don't ordinarily admit. For instance, I have this thing about being in control. I have often felt that way in most of my relationships, so I am excited about learning ways to build trust with people. This will help me in my work but I know it will also help me with my friends and my boyfriend. I quite like the idea that after I graduate I will be much better at getting people to like and respect me.

I am also somewhat of a busybody, meaning I like to know what other people are up to. When I find out that somebody else is having problems or doing strange things, in a perverse way it makes me feel better, that maybe I'm not so strange myself. I think it is really exciting that we get to hear about people's most intimate secrets.

Yet there are many other reasons people choose counseling as a profession. The selection could be pragmatic: grades or test scores may prevent a move into more highly competitive programs. Or the time commitments required by some disciplines may seem excessive or overwhelming. Counseling seems a reasonable compromise; the program can be completed in a few years and then the credentials will permit practice in many attractive settings.

As the student above reluctantly admits, some people have a strong personal motivation for entering the helping professions. The counselor is able to satisfy unfulfilled nurturing needs by rescuing people with problems—as well as to participate in intimate relationships—while always maintaining control (Herron & Rouslin, 1984; Kottler, 1995; Robertiello, 1978). Some people are attracted to counseling because they enjoy the power they can wield in influencing other people's lives. Counselors and other therapeutic practitioners are, in fact, the real power brokers in our society. They have become the oracles, the witch doctors, the gurus, the wizards, the mentors. They listen with compassion and speak with authority. They have the answers and, although they often won't reveal them directly, if clients behave and do what they are supposed to, they will be gently prodded to discover truth for themselves.

Students also select counseling for many of the same practical reasons that lead to any other career. They need the degree for a pay raise or promotion. They are after prestige and status. The courses are offered at convenient times. Tests are infrequent or the program doesn't appear too demanding. And, indeed, counseling does not at first glance seem as rigorous as training in engineering, nuclear physics, or neurosurgery.

## VOICE FROM THE FIELD

I had a lot of grief at a young age. Since then I've felt drawn to those who are hurting, especially those who are dying. I know this sounds morbid, but I really do like working at the hospice with cancer patients and their families. I'm so impressed with the ones who die with dignity and good humor.

Early on, I thought my motivations were purely altruistic. Hah! I know better now. I'm more realistic and honest about what drives me and also what pushes my buttons. The truth is that this work makes me feel needed. This is especially true with my dying patients. If this work ever stops meeting my needs, I'll stop doing it.

---

But don't be fooled. A counseling program is about the most challenging emotional experience a student can undertake. Although some counseling programs do not create intense academic pressure, all emphasize skill mastery and performance competencies. Counseling programs are not only interested in your ability to succeed at academic tasks but also your ability to translate book and classroom learning into action. The bottom line for success in a counseling program is what you can do and what you can deliver.

Another large part of the work you do will involve addressing your own personal reactions to your work, often called *countertransference* reactions. This refers to the phenomenon, originally described by Sigmund Freud (1912), in which clinicians lost their objectivity and clarity because of their own personal issues that interfered with their work. Their perceptions of their clients become distorted and their interpretations polluted by their own personal stuff. While countertransference is often not addressed nearly as much in training as it should be, it is absolutely critical that you have a handle on your own biases, unresolved issues, and strong emotional reactions that may interfere with your ability to think clearly and respond helpfully to clients (Bemak & Epp, 2001; DeLucia-Waack, 1999).

Just consider, for example, some of the opinions or values you hold as most sacred. How do you feel about the death penalty, or abortion, or gun control, or even your deepest religious (or nonreligious) convictions. Now imagine that someone walks in your door and presents a point of view that is the direct opposite of what you believe. Will you be able to respond to this person with compassion and caring, freed from your own personal biases that may be clouding your judgments?

The pressure and inward journeys necessary for growth and counseling skill development are well worth the effort. This profession offers the student more advantages on both a personal and a professional level than almost any other field. Where else can all life experiences—books, films, travels, relationships, fantasies, jobs, losses, disasters, and triumphs—help the professional to be more effective? Everything and everyone teaches a counselor to understand the human world better, to have more compassion, to be a better communica-

## VOICE FROM THE FIELD

I don't have kids, and I don't think I ever will. But there are hundreds, probably thousands of children who I have worked with during the past years. I'd like to think some of them will remember me for a very long time. Maybe until the day they die.

I know that there are several mentors and teachers who influenced me in ways that I'll never forget. They live inside me. Their words still echo in my mind. At times I even smile when I catch myself saying something just the way that they would.

It gives me chills to think that others might someday feel so grateful for my efforts to help them. Maybe long after I'm not around anymore I will still live inside the children I worked with.

tor, to comprehend more completely the intricate complexities of behavior. Every experience allows you to teach from what you know.

What other profession teaches skills and competencies applicable to work that can be so easily applied to your personal world? Counseling trains people to be more passionate consumers of life. Intensive training in observing nonverbal behavior, analyzing motives, handling confrontations, and reflecting feelings helps counselors to be more attractive human beings, experts at efficiently developing trusting, productive relationships. If counselors can do that in their offices, they can certainly do it with their friends, children, spouses, and parents.

Counseling inspires the student to be a knowledgeable generalist, a Renaissance scholar, a devourer of truth in any palatable form. We are not restricted to our texts for learning. We read literature, history, anthropology, sociology, biology, biochemistry, education, psychology, and philosophy, and they are all beneficial—even necessary—if we are truly to understand this abstract thing called the human mind.

Counseling permits practitioners to make a difference in people's lives and to see the results in their own lifetimes. One of the ways in which we attempt to confront our own mortality is by preserving our spirit long after physical death. Certainly the principal reward for a dedicated teacher, counselor, or therapist is the knowledge that a generation of clients will remember and use the help that was offered. Our profession allows us to productively face our own fears of death by leaving behind those who, because of our efforts, feel less pain.

Counselors become more wise and self-aware with every client they see. Each presented concern forces us to consider introspectively our own degree of stability. Every discussed problem reminds us of those issues that we still have not fully resolved. A client complains of periodic urges to break out of the mold and run away, while the counselor silently considers his or her own rebellious impulses. A boring relationship, fear of failure, career stagnation, sexual frustrations, loneliness, parental dependence—all subjects that are commonly presented—force the counselor to resolve them, once and for all, in his or her own life. The profession thus continually encourages its practitioners to upgrade their personal effectiveness.

At this very moment you may want to examine your personal motives for studying counseling. (Note: This is one of several reflective questions that you may wish to address in your journal). Better yet, talk to other students about what motivates them as well—not just the socially acceptable and politically correct reasons, but also the deeper, more personal drives. Although you may never fully understand all the factors, needs, interests, values, and unconscious processes that are influencing your decision, the quest is nevertheless valuable. It is likely that only years after graduation—and perhaps after your own experiences as a client—will you have a focused picture of your honest motives. This process of self-inquiry, once begun, is self-perpetuating because of the growth it fosters. And the beginning is *now*.

## TO BE A COUNSELOR

Choosing counseling as a career sets into motion a chain of events and leads to a series of direct and indirect consequences, the impact of which is often initially unclear. The choice to be a counselor, for example, not only dramatically affects the education, training, and molding of the student who made the decision but also affects that individual's family and friends. Imagine, for example, that you simply studied the impact of birth order on personality development. How can you *not* look at your life and your relationships with family members differently after that? Or consider the very real possibility that, in any given week in your professional life, you will listen to clients struggle with fears of dying, infidelity, loneliness, dependency, boredom, suicidal thoughts, and a hundred other issues that have haunted you throughout your life.

I have always thought that if we were to present you with fully disclosing "informed consent" (an ethical concept you will learn about later that refers to disclosure of risks so you can make knowledgeable decisions about your participation), we would have to tell you that deciding to be a counselor has huge implications for your life in a number of ways. For one thing, *all* your relationships will change. You will develop new expectations and standards for intimacy. You will learn skills that enable you to develop closer levels of intimacy with others, and you will want to use that newfound ability to enrich your family and work relationships. In a sense, you will be ruined—forever dissatisfied with superficial encounters. After all, how can you settle for rather inane interactions when daily you talk to people about their most intimate secrets, their most powerful insights, and their most meaningful feelings? The truth is that your love relationships may very well change forever and many of your friendships may be outgrown. You are not only choosing a new profession but a new way of being, a new way of relating to yourself, to others, and to the world.

Choosing to be a counselor means opening yourself up to intense self-scrutiny and personal growth. It means examining your strengths and limitations as a human being, exploring your vulnerabilities, and identifying those aspects of your functioning that you need to improve. All these changes emerge as the consequence of simply selecting studies in counseling. A number of other implications flow from choosing to be a counselor.

## VOICE FROM THE FIELD

I was filled with so much anxiety almost every moment of my beginning years as a counselor. First, I wondered constantly if I had whatever it took to be good at this job. I compared myself to others and usually found myself wanting in some way. I wasn't smart enough. I couldn't express myself as well as others. I didn't have nearly the same life experiences or academic background as those who seemed so far ahead of me.

And then when I started seeing clients, I felt so anxious that I wouldn't be able to help them. I didn't know if I'd say or do the right thing. I had this vision that even though I was pretending to know what I was doing, the client would see right through me and know I was clueless.

Even after all these years I still feel anxious every time a new client walks in. I wonder if I can help him or her. I worry about whether I know enough, or whether someone else might do a better job. So you see, the anxiety lessens a bit but it never goes away.

## Dealing with Anxiety

I am not referring yet to the anxiety of your clients but rather your own internal pressure and apprehensions about this work. Anxiety is not only an expected condition for life as a counseling student but a normal one (Christensen & Kline, 2001). You will feel anxious about so many aspects of your training:

- Are you smart enough, or capable enough, to make it in this field?
- Is this the right job for you? Are you wasting your time?
- Will you ever know enough to be able to help someone?
- Will others find out how inadequate you really feel inside?
- Will your personal issues interfere with your ability to help people?
- Will you hurt someone because of some lapse or mistake?
- Will you be forced to look at things that you would rather avoid?

The answers to these questions cannot be addressed in a single sitting. You will likely continue to struggle with them your whole career.

## Making a Commitment

To be a counselor means making a commitment to a profession and a lifestyle. For every spectacular success there are also failures. Counselors must learn not only to temper their exhilaration after witnessing phenomenal change, but also to cope with the frustrations of resistant clients, rigid institutional policies, overworked administrators, irate parents, and confusing laws. Although there are few greater feelings of victory than knowing that a person has been helped as a direct result of our efforts, often clients do not accommodate our wishes or cooperate with our interventions. They may stubbornly insist on staying miserable in spite of our best attempts at helping them to find another way.

## VOICE FROM THE FIELD

One risk of being a counselor that I never considered was how my skills would change all my relationships. At first, I was so proud of what I learned and could do. But it's a mixed blessing. For instance, with my spouse sometimes when we aren't connecting, I lapse into one-upsmanship stuff. I critique her relationship clumsiness compared to what I've been trained to do.

I've benefited enormously from what I've learned but sometimes it all seems to get in the way for me. I find it hard to let go of my counselor role and just be a person. I'm always analyzing everything, and frankly, that pisses people off.

---

At times a counselor will do everything perfectly: Patiently build a trusting relationship with a client and gently lead her through the successive counseling stages—exploring, reflecting, analyzing, interpreting, and confronting—and then, finally, the time comes for action. Let's say the client agrees that a divorce is imminent. The marriage has become destructive; her husband abusive. She realizes she cannot grow further while handcuffed. She has worked through her guilt over deserting him, her fear of disapproval by mutual friends, and her fear of making it on her own without a man to lean on. She is ready—or so she says. But time is up for this week's session. She will do her homework and be prepared by next week to make the commitment to beginning her new life as a single woman.

Eagerly, the counselor awaits the report next week. He tries hard not to pat himself on the back because he does feel proud. He has done good work. The next week arrives. The counselor waits in his office—and waits. The client doesn't show. She doesn't return!

The counselor calls her, only to receive the cold announcement, without any explanation, that she will no longer be coming back for sessions. That's it. Before the counselor can sort out the mess, there is a knock on the door. His next client is waiting impatiently for the session.

## Striving for Excellence

To be a counselor means taking responsibility for your own growth and striving for excellence in your personal behavior.

Every client presents a novel challenge. Five people who are depressed will act differently as a result of the symptoms they may call depression. One person is lethargic and drained, whereas another appears agitated and emotionally overwrought. One client has lost 14 pounds and reports being able to sleep only fitfully; another has gained considerable weight and seems to sleep all the time. One person talks constantly about suicidal fantasies, whereas an-

## VOICE FROM THE FIELD

The other day I was helping someone sort out the reasons why she was so isolated and lonely in her life. I was giving her feedback on what she does to create barriers in her relationships and keep others at a distance. I was specifically highlighting what behaviors she favors that are most annoying and I was telling her all this stuff in the most gentle way that I could.

This happens more often than I'd like to admit but the woman was hardly listening to me. What I was saying was too threatening for her to hear. Or maybe she wasn't ready to hear it yet. I don't know.

But the really weird thing is that I realized I was talking to myself as much as I was talking to her. I happen to have a similar problem of keeping myself isolated. I use my work to do that. I blame my schedule. But damn, I realized at that moment that my frustration towards my client for not listening was really directed towards myself: I wasn't listening either!

---

other is incensed that you would even bring up self-destructive behavior. Yet among these diverse experiences, depression is the central theme.

Even though depression is but one of a dozen major problems that frequently present themselves to a counselor, there are endless variations on those themes. To be optimally helpful to each client, you will have to understand the issues thoroughly and have had some experience in handling them. Although much of this expertise will come from class lectures and readings, your own personal experiences will prove invaluable.

Whereas a male counselor cannot directly relate to the struggle of a female client considering an abortion and can never have worked through it himself, it is likely that this counselor has accumulated rich personal experiences in resolving similar value conflicts. And although a female counselor can never know the shame that her impotent male client feels, she does know the awful dread of being unable to perform adequately.

The consensus among many counselors is that each client provides them an opportunity after the session to look inward, personalize the material, and ask the question, "To what extent is this a concern of mine?" When a client complains of stagnation in life, of too many predictable routines and boring people, how can the counselor not examine this pattern in his or her own life? Fears of growing old, of failure, of rejection, of loving, of hating—all hit a familiar chord. And the degree to which the counselor has successfully struggled with any of these themes will determine, to some extent, his or her capacity for understanding the client's fears and resolving them.

A client complains of a bad temper and uncontrolled explosive outbursts. But the counselor knows, not just theoretically but personally, the value of a bad temper—how it provides an instant excuse for abusing others: "Sorry. I couldn't help it. I have a bad temper." Beyond such insight, the counselor also knows personally just how to control his or her own anger.

In one study, master therapists who were nominated by their peers as being at the top of their profession were found to have a number of characteristics that went beyond mere professional competence (Jennings & Skovholt, 1999). Of course they had excellent relationship skills, but they were also very committed to working on their own emotional health. They were voracious learners, driven to excel in as many facets of life as they could.

Counselors, then, are constantly striving for more mastery in their lives, applying the technology of psychological helping to themselves. At any moment in time the counselor ought to be able to articulate three or four specific personal areas in need of upgrading—and be actively involved in the process.

## Adopting a Neutral Posture

To be a counselor implies a dedication to helping other people without having a vested interest in the particular directions that they may choose.

Based on his or her particular religious beliefs, lifestyle preferences, and value system, every counselor has a notion about what is generally good for people, whether it be brown rice, plenty of fresh air, a God-fearing home, or good loving. Clients, therefore, present the counselor with the dilemma of which way to influence them: in a way that is consistent with the counselor's own beliefs or in quite another direction—one that the client may genuinely prefer.

In the social world, people are quite liberal in dispensing their opinions on a variety of issues; in the counseling session, such casually stated advice can be harmful. Counselors are interested in creating neither disciples nor dependents. They will understand that, by answering the client's persistent question, "What should I do?" they fall into one of two traps. Either they offer poor advice, which then teaches the client to resent the professional forever and not to take responsibility for the negative outcome, or—worse—they offer sound advice, giving the client the clear message that the thing to do with a difficult question is just to run back to the counselor for help.

Yet a counselor often has strong personal opinions on whether clients should join the Army or go back to school, get a divorce or endure the marriage, tell off nosy parents or buy them a present, turn themselves in to the authorities or learn to be more discreet, punt or go for a touchdown. Counselors are hardly all-knowing experts, creative problem solvers, or detached, objective professionals; we bring our own biases, our own unique histories, our own personal stories to the relationship. As such, the counseling relationship is a moral and political enterprise rather than a strictly neutral one, in spite of our best interests to rein in our biases (Bacaigalupe, 2002).

It is first necessary for the counselor to be aware of his or her own values and then, as far as is humanly possible, to block their effects on a client's decisions. Neutrality is the catchword of a therapeutic relationship. Although counselors may feel strongly about choices that clients make, they must accept the consequences of communicating those preferences. This caution does not mean that counselors attempt to hide their true feelings from clients, using the

Hey, I know that I'm supposed to be paying attention to what clients are saying during sessions. I learned a long time ago how important listening skills are and how critical it is that clients feel heard and understood. Maybe even once upon a time, I did focus almost all the time.

But here's a secret: In my experience, no matter how much I concentrate and how hard I try, I don't think I'm really giving full attention more than half the time. Furthermore, I think this is better than what most counselors do.

Of course, my clients don't know how much my mind wanders and how often my attention drifts. There is just so much to think about, and so much to do, and so many buttons that are pushed in any session, that it's almost impossible to stay on track all the time. I think what makes a really exceptional counselor, though, is someone who works harder and harder to control personal stuff and give clients as much as we can.

---

mask of professional distance and neutrality. Rather, counselors work toward conquering the need for an investment in client decisions beyond a professional responsibility.

## Subjugating Personal Needs

To be a counselor involves controlling your own needs, desires, and preferences in favor of the best interests of the client.

One reason counseling is such difficult work is that the professional makes a deliberate decision to suspend all distractions—both internal and external—while in session. Whether the phone rings in another room or a siren blares through the streets, the counselor blocks out all stimuli that are extraneous to the task at hand.

Even more difficult to banish are internal distractions. To be most helpful to the client, to focus all of your energy therapeutically, you must immerse yourself totally in the helping role. Attention to a grumbling stomach or an ingrown toenail will reduce your concentration. To daydream or indulge in fantasy while pretending to listen is obviously counterproductive. And to permit yourself the luxury of liking or disliking clients during a session will only further reduce effectiveness. The counselor therefore becomes quite adept in the meditation-type skills of gently pushing aside distracting thoughts, indulgent feelings, and any other internal behavior that reduces concentration, without sacrificing the genuineness of being human.

A rationale for the necessity to receive some compensation in exchange for delivering a therapeutic service is that it does require such extraordinary effort to stifle your natural urges. It is for this reason that counseling is an activity that is far from "natural." It is highly unnatural to push aside your urges of attraction, indulgence, and selfishness.

## VOICE FROM THE FIELD

I was leading a group and the members were all playing the game, "Is it safe here?" Each person was testing things, trying to decide if it was safe enough to risk sharing themselves in an authentic way. We'd been going on like this for some time. One person was saying, "I'll do it if you will," and another was responding with, "Well, if you go first then I'll follow," and a third was saying, "Maybe I'll go later, but only if you guys go first."

I had this choice to let this go on, or really push them to a deeper level. I've got to tell you: it would have been a heck of a lot easier to just let things stay on the surface. I knew that if I challenged them I'd get some flack. And sure enough, it took a lot of work to confront their caution. But that's my job, that's why I get paid to do this stuff. I know that if they stay comfy and chatty not much useful is going to happen.

## Coping with Discomfort

To be a counselor requires that you learn to become comfortable in the presence of others' discomfort.

One goal of counseling is often to make people squirm. Until clients become dissatisfied with themselves, disgusted by their self-sabotaging behaviors, they will rarely change. Counselors often help to intensify this discomfort as a means of encouraging continued flight toward mental health. Confrontation is intended to force the client to face discrepancies, incongruence, and inconsistency. And the counselor must get used to despair. The one place in the world where people feel safe to cry and honestly express their pain is in the counselor's office. Often the feelings of desperation are even exaggerated because the therapeutic environment is so nurturing and accepting. Clients will complain and show rage and hurt. They will cry and scream and stamp their feet. And counselors take the full force of this emotional energy.

Counselors need to become proficient at facing outbursts calmly. Often they must reinterpret psychological discomfort as a sign that things are going according to plan rather than as a signal to retreat. Only when clients are uncomfortable may we be certain they are seriously working on themselves. They do not come for a good time.

## Dealing with Ambiguity

To be a counselor requires that you function well with abstract ideas and ambiguous circumstances.

Counselors inhabit a professional world characterized by uncertainty and ambiguity. Clients are often not fully aware of their real problems. They report discomfort, vague and abstract, but circle relentlessly when the counselor attempts to help them focus. Very often clients want counseling because they are experiencing a true dilemma wherein no answer or response is truly satisfactory. Consider, for example, the man who has met a woman he deeply loves

## VOICE FROM THE FIELD

One of the biggest mistakes I ever made was when a client came back beaming, obviously helped by our sessions together. He went on at some length about the ways his life was now different. I sat there preening, just feeling so good about my skills and ability.

As I listened to him make his report, I reviewed in my mind all the things I thought might have helped him. The previous week, for instance, I tried a new kind of interpretation in which I reframed his problem differently. Pretty cool, I thought at the time.

And sure enough, I was confident this was what made the difference.

Almost as an afterthought, as he was about out the door, I asked him, "By the way, what did I do that you found so helpful?" Imagine my surprise, and disappointment, when he recited some obscure thing that I never remember saying in the first place. How humbling to realize that I often don't know what I do that matters most.

---

and with whom he wishes to spend his life. But she has a child, and he—after some traumatic past experiences—has realized that he is not comfortable in the parenting role. He wants to be with her yet is unable to share her role as a parent. The dilemma is real, and no alternative is completely satisfying. He comes for counseling, and your job is to help him resolve this thorny issue.

Counselors must develop empathy for clients who seem unfocused, who vacillate daily, and who seem unhappy but don't know why. In a sense, counselors (and other social scientists) must abandon their search for cause and effect and come to terms with ambiguity and uncertainty, which reflect the reality of the individual. Counselors must relinquish the quest for answers and instead relish the challenge of helping clients with their abstractions and the uncertainty inherent in reality. To be a counselor means dedicating oneself to the resolution of conflicts that are often irreconcilable, solving problems that have no right answers, and mediating disputes among parties who enjoy fighting.

## DEFINITIONS OF COUNSELING

Counseling is indeed an ambiguous enterprise. It is done by persons who can't agree on what to call themselves, what credentials are necessary to practice, or even what the best way is to practice—whether to deal with feelings, thoughts, or behaviors; whether to be primarily supportive or confrontational; whether to focus on the past or the present. Further, the consumers of counseling services can't exactly articulate what their concerns are, what counseling can and can't do for them, or what they want when it's over.

Practitioners, as well, sometimes struggle with trying to articulate what counseling is and how and why it works. The truth is that in spite of our best intentions and our solid grounding in theory, research, and technique, we don't always know what makes the greatest difference with our clients.

As a beginner, it is very important for you to realize that proper training and education will prepare you to do a number of things that research has indicated are consistently useful with some clients, presenting some complaints, in some situations. Nevertheless, you must also be prepared to live with a certain amount of ambiguity and uncertainty, not only about what is going on with your clients but also what is going on within the counseling process. In time, good counselors do have a way of sorting things out. Such positive outcomes begin with the way you set the stage for treatment.

At several points in his or her professional life—if not on comprehensive examinations, then certainly with every astute client—the practitioner will be asked to define what it is she or he does. This definition ought to be as specific as possible, describing in detail what counselors do, why they do it, and how it works.

This definition, like counseling itself, should be a process—one designed to stimulate thinking so that ideas can ferment, evolve, and grow into a personal conception. Textbook definitions, although elegant, incisive, and comprehensive, almost always lack one essential ingredient: personalized meaning. As a beginner to this complex field who is already somewhat confused regarding what counseling is, the last thing in the world you need is another academic-sounding description of something that you don't really understand but that nevertheless sounds good to others (who may not understand it either). One definition of counseling is presented in a way that most people in the field could live with—regardless of differences in their personalities, work settings, and preferred approaches. Further, this definition is offered in such a way that, after you have studied it a bit, you can actually describe to someone else what counseling is and give a fairly intelligible explanation of why and how it works. (I would even suggest you try this to boost your confidence.)

Counseling is:

- A profession with a history and set of standards, distinct from other related disciplines such as social work, psychology, and psychiatry.
- An activity that is designed to work with relatively normally functioning individuals who are experiencing developmental or adjustment problems.
- A relationship, whether in a group, family, or individual format, that is constructed in a way to promote trust, safety, and change.
- Multidimensional, dealing with human feelings, thoughts, and behaviors, as well as with the past, present, and future.

Counseling is a process that has a series of sequential steps:

- Helping people to articulate why they are seeking help.
- Formulating goals and expectations for treatment.
- Teaching clients how to get the most from the counseling experience.
- Developing a high degree of trust and favorable expectations for change.
- Diagnosing those concerns and dysfunctional areas in need of upgrading.
- Exploring the client's world, including past and present functioning.
- Discussing underlying issues and concerns.
- Supporting and accepting the client as a person while selectively reinforcing those behaviors that are most fully functioning.
- Confronting inconsistencies in the client's thoughts, language, and behavior.

- Challenging assumptions that are inappropriate, self-destructive, or irrational.
- Uncovering hidden and unconscious motives behind actions.
- Encouraging people to accept more responsibility for their choices and actions.
- Helping clients to develop more options for their lives and to narrow alternatives to those that are most suitable.
- Providing constructive feedback.
- Structuring opportunities for practicing new ways of acting and being.
- Facilitating greater independence in the client so that counseling ends in the most efficient period of time.

Yes, this definition *is* long—and certainly too cumbersome to memorize and spit back exactly as you read it. But remember that the objective is for you to be able to describe this wonderful and complex process in your own unique way. The following example illustrates how a counselor would actually use this definition in his or her work.

CLIENT: My mom thinks I should come to see you, but I don't really know what you can do. (This confusion is not unusual in a first interview.)

COUNSELOR: What is it that your mother thinks I can do? (Rule number one in counseling is: When you don't know what else to do, put the ball back in the client's court to buy time until you can think of something else to say.)

CLIENT: I don't know. She mentioned that maybe you could hear my problem and then fix it for me. (Again, it is pretty typical that clients believe we have magic wands.)

COUNSELOR: Without knowing exactly what problem you are referring to, maybe it would be helpful for you if I could explain a bit about what I do. The people that I see want to learn about themselves, about why they do the things they do; they want to understand better why they keep repeating the same mistakes over and over. (The client looks perplexed. I'd better bring this more down to earth.)

People come to see me because they feel safe here. They can talk about anything they want and know that I will listen carefully and I won't ever criticize them. I will keep whatever we talk about private, unless they seem inclined to hurt themselves or someone else. Most people also appreciate the fact that I am completely honest. (Aha. This seems to be hitting home.)

But just as important as being a good and safe listener, my job is to help you identify changes you want and need to make in your life and then help you get there. Ultimately, this experience will be useful to the extent that it helps you reach your desired goals.

Although this definition-in-action is hardly as specific and clear an explanation of counseling as a client (or you) might like, this still illustrates the value of being able to describe the process in a personal way. It also raises other questions, notably how and why counseling works in the first place.

## VOICE FROM THE FIELD

I'm an elementary school counselor and it's often challenging to explain to younger kids what counseling is all about and how it all works. I usually say something like this when someone new comes in:

"I have a way cool job! I'm a person who gets to talk to kids like you! When you come here you get to talk about whatever is on your mind, whether it's happy stuff or sad stuff. I have a playroom. I give them a little personal show-and-tell tour and when you come to visit me we can play and talk about what's going on with you. This isn't like going to the doctor. When you come here, I won't stick you with anything or make you do anything you don't want to do. And what we talk about in here is just between you and me, unless someone is hurting you or something like that."

## WHY DOES THERAPEUTIC COUNSELING WORK?

Although at this juncture the jury has not yet returned to deliver its final verdict, we do know that therapeutic counseling probably works as a combination of factors that many theorists find significant. You will learn in later chapters about how client-centered theorists believe that the nurturing relationship between counselor and client plays the biggest role in facilitating change; the behaviorists have evidence to indicate that reinforcement, modeling, and structured practice make the greatest difference; the psychoanalytic practitioners prefer to emphasize unconscious desires; the constructivists emphasize different perceptions of reality; and the cognitive clinicians claim that counseling works by teaching people to think more rationally, and so on. By now it must have occurred to you that in this first chapter (or in a beginning course), it is not likely that you are going to get a completely acceptable answer to the question, "Why does counseling work?" Have patience.

On a more optimistic note, the field of counseling is currently driven by a movement toward synthesis and integration of existing knowledge. This is true of research, which is applying new methodologies such as meta-analysis, as well as synthesizing what is known. For example, whereas the methodology of a huge study in *Consumer Reports* was somewhat flawed, the researchers sought to identify the extent and circumstances under which therapy and counseling are useful. The results of this ambitious survey were that indeed counseling does work, that it is cost-effective, and that it does improve the quality of life (Seligman, 1998).

Somewhat less definitive, however, is specifying which factors in counseling have the most positive impact. One predictor of success may be largely determined by variables related to clients, such as their motivation, severity of symptoms, and personal attitudes (Tallman & Bohart, 1999). That isn't to say that what we do and how we act as counselors aren't important, merely that our best efforts should be directed toward matching our approach to the specific circumstances of each client.

In counselor training as well, there is a strong movement toward standardization of curricula through accreditation and the development of generic training models across the nation. Professional organizations such as the American Counseling Association (ACA), American Association for Marriage and Family Therapy (AAMFT), National Association of Social Work (NASW), and the American Psychological Association (APA) have been instrumental in developing relatively universal principles and content that should be included in the preparation of any clinician. These organizations have been so proactive and effective in their efforts, that licensure laws have been passed in almost every state and province making it possible for counselors and therapists to practice independently (or under supervision) and receive third-party reimbursement for their services.

In the case of theory development as well, efforts are directed toward finding common factors that operate in all helping systems as well as toward combining the advantages of several therapeutic approaches into a unified model (Capuzzi & Gross, 2001; Corey, 2000; Goldfried, 1982; Kleinke, 1994; Kottler, 1991; Lazarus, 1995; Young, 1992). More recently, efforts have been directed towards finding common variables associated with constructive therapeutic change (Maione & Chenail, 1999; Tryon, 2002). These can be sorted according to factors related to the client (expectations, personality, symptoms), factors related to the counselor (experience, training, skills, personality), administrative factors (waiting list, length of treatment, setting), and those related to the quality of the relationship that is established).

Eclecticism, pragmatism, and integrationism have become the watchwords of the profession. Many years ago, several writers such as French (1933), Kubie (1934), Rosenzweig (1936), Dollard and Miller (1950), Thorne (1950), Frank (1973), Strupp (1973), Truax and Carkhuff (1967), and Wachtel (1977) began to look at the common elements of various helping approaches in an effort to find the essence of what makes counseling and therapy most helpful. You must understand that prior to these years and even up to the present, there have been furious debates—even outright wars—among various theoretical camps, each convinced that they have cornered the market on what is "truth." You may even sense conflicts within your own department in which each instructor may present a different version of what constitutes "good counseling."

Perhaps of all the attempts to sort out this confusion, the classic book by Brammer, Abrego, and Shostrum (1998) entitled *Therapeutic Counseling and Psychotherapy* (now in its seventh edition) became most influential in its effort to bring diverse elements together into a unified model of helping. It is in this very tradition and spirit that we attempt to integrate many of the factors that various schools of thought find significant. Every practitioner's style of practice is different and depends on such factors as personality, theoretical preferences, and the setting in which one works. But research does support that certain elements, such as an effective counseling relationship, collaboratively structured roles, and positive expectations on the part of the client, consistently lead to constructive changes. And then your own use of the "self,"

## VOICE FROM THE FIELD

I do different things on different days. On some days I'm a farmer—I till soil within people so that their own seeds of wisdom can grow. Some days, I'm a one-man rescue operation, carefully moving someone back from the brink of self-destruction. Some days, I'm a one-man band, playing accompaniment for someone who walks to the beat of a different drum. At times I'm a mirror, trying to reflect what I understand. I'm at my best when I'm a sponge—being present, listening, and soaking up the essence of another person and the hurt inside. I am frequently privileged to be a traveler—a visitor to exotic lands in the client's worlds. But on most days, I'm a struggler, trying to find my way, and trying to help others do the same.

---

that is your intuition, creativity, personality, interpersonal style, and yes, personal issues, also have a huge impact on what you do and how it is received by others (Kottler & Markos, 1997; Lum, 2002).

Counseling is less likely to be effective when the counselor is inexperienced, self-indulgent, and rigid and forces compliance to a personal agenda. Similarly, counseling is more likely to be helpful when the clinician's role is flexible, genuine, and accepting. This means that you can keep your "self" sufficiently clear, stable, open, and receptive in order to hear and understand those you are trying to help.

## Significance of the Self

What counseling is and how it works are important concepts that can be defined and illustrated. But any explanation of counseling, however precise, exists only in a static sense. Life can be given to a definition, vitality breathed into a process, only in the context of a person—the self of the counselor.

You would only have to consider the power of the self with respect to your own learning processes. Think about the times in your life you were most impacted by a class. Certainly the content was interesting and the subject appealing, but just as important, it was the person of the teacher that made the material come alive. It was the essential self of this mentor or instructor that captivated your interest and motivated you to learn. It was the connection you felt to this person, this essential self, that led you to work hard, to study and practice, to become devoted to the subject. The same is no less true in counseling: It is through the self as an instrument that we are able to understand and influence others (Combs & Gonzalez, 1994).

According to this perspective, the most effective counselors are able to perceive primarily from an internal rather than an external frame of reference. They tend to perceive others as being capable, as internally motivated, and in positive but realistic terms. They identify themselves strongly with others and feel an affinity with the human race. Additionally, they perceive their mission as altruistic rather than self-indulgent, as freeing rather than controlling, and as self-revealing rather than self-concealing.

Each of these characteristics aids in organizing personal reality and serves as a foundation from which the counselor's self mediates the counseling process. In a classic study, Fiedler (1950) illustrated the importance of the self in the counseling process by comparing the quality of the therapeutic relationships in psychoanalytic, nondirective, and Adlerian therapies. He found that the style and personal relationships of the experts in each of the three approaches were more similar than different. He also found that the non-experts were more different from one another in relationship style than were the experts and, further, that the non-experts tended to be less similar than the experts in their own orientation. He therefore concluded that theoretical orientation was not the distinguishing variable separating expert from non-expert therapists; rather, the difference was more related to personal style independent of conceptual affiliation. A common thread unified the expert therapists, particularly with regard to relationship variables. In those instances in which there is a difficulty creating an alliance in counseling, it is due more often to the counselor's personality than to the client's motivation.

Effective counselors, regardless of their setting, culture, and preferred approach, demonstrate certain human qualities that make them attractive and influential to others. Those counselors who are expert at using the self as an instrument—and who are powerful models with the capacity for influencing others—tend to cross theoretical boundaries. In spite of how they label themselves—as behaviorists, humanists, constructivists, Adlerians, Gestaltists, or Rational-Emotivists—the most dynamic practitioners are intensely aware of the potential influence their selves can wield: as modelers of personal expertness, as reinforcers of appropriate behavior, and as nurturers of warmth and support.

Thus the self is the most significant dimension in therapeutic counseling; what counseling is and how it works depend to a large extent on the personal characteristics of the counselor. Quite a number of writers (Corey & Corey, 1998; Gladding, 2000; Jennings & Skovholt, 1999; Kottler & Hazler, 1997) have compiled lists of those qualities they feel are necessary for the counselor's self to be in proper operating condition. A composite of these personality characteristics includes self-confidence, high energy level, sense of humor, neutrality, flexibility, emotional stability, experience in risk taking, analytic thinking, creativity, enthusiasm, honesty, and compassion.

In reviewing these personal attributes, you cannot help but evaluate the extent to which you possess them and reflect on how much personal growth lies ahead. Yet in counselor training, the development of self as a more effective person parallels the evolution of therapeutic skills. The self becomes refined and nurtured as a sensitive and operative component of the counseling process. As the self evolves, the counselor becomes more aware of personal assets and limitations, biases, and areas in need of upgrading. Actually, this opportunity to examine your own personal functioning is the greatest benefit in joining the counseling profession. On a daily basis, you not only have the opportunity to make a difference in other people's lives, but you can also continue to work on improving the quality of your own existence.

## SUMMARY

In this chapter you have explored the decision to enter the field of counseling from a personal perspective. Honesty and self-awareness are themes that you will encounter again in this book and throughout your daily practice as a counselor; in this field, there is simply no place to hide. Your personal awareness and understanding of the motives and payoffs for choosing counseling as a career objective will affect the energy, vitality, and commitment you bring to this introductory course and, ultimately, to the field.

In this relatively young profession there are many opportunities for creative individuals to make an impact. But this flexibility of roles also results in confusion among people as to exactly what counseling is, how and why it works, and how it differs from other mental health disciplines. It is therefore necessary for the beginning counselor to define the counseling process and profession assertively, both to carve out a useful identity and to provide a realistic and explicit portrait for clients who wish to know what services can and will be delivered.

## SELF-GUIDED EXPLORATIONS

1. The choice to be a counselor, or even to take a course on the subject, sets in motion a number of consequences that may affect your relationships, financial situation, sleep and lifestyle habits, family life, and self-image. Mention several ways that you are already aware of in which aspects of your life are changing as a result of your decision to study counseling.

2. Even from your limited experiences thus far in learning about the profession of counseling, you already have the barest glimmering of how and why counseling works. It may be quite interesting for you, some years in the future, to look back on your definition of counseling, as articulated in the beginning of your training. What would you say to a friend who asks you: "You're studying to be a counselor? I've always wondered how that works. What is counseling, anyway?"

3. List some of your fears and apprehensions about training to be a counselor. Describe some of your self-doubts. Talk to classmates you trust about your anxiety and share common themes in your experiences.

4. a. If you are completely honest with yourself, what are the *real* reasons you are considering counseling as a career? Apart from helping others, what aspects of your motivation have to do with helping yourself in some ways? Within a group, or on your own, brainstorm as many personal motives as you can think of to explain why you are interested in this work.

   b. Take all your reasons and organize them into three main categories that make sense to you. Give each grouping a name.

   c. What do you conclude based on this analysis of motives?

5. A composite of some personal qualities associated with effective counselors is listed below. For each of these characteristics that you believe are

crucial to successful professional functioning, rate where you see yourself now versus where you would like to be.

| Personal Quality | Where I Am Now | Where I Want to Be |
|---|---|---|
| Self-confidence | 1 2 3 4 5 6 7 | 1 2 3 4 5 6 7 |
| High energy | 1 2 3 4 5 6 7 | 1 2 3 4 5 6 7 |
| Sense of humor | 1 2 3 4 5 6 7 | 1 2 3 4 5 6 7 |
| Flexibility | 1 2 3 4 5 6 7 | 1 2 3 4 5 6 7 |
| Risk-taking | 1 2 3 4 5 6 7 | 1 2 3 4 5 6 7 |
| Emotional stability | 1 2 3 4 5 6 7 | 1 2 3 4 5 6 7 |
| Honesty | 1 2 3 4 5 6 7 | 1 2 3 4 5 6 7 |
| Compassion | 1 2 3 4 5 6 7 | 1 2 3 4 5 6 7 |
| Dependability | 1 2 3 4 5 6 7 | 1 2 3 4 5 6 7 |

How are you going to move from where you are now to where you would like to be?

## For Homework:

Interview several counselors in the field who work in different settings and specialty areas. Ask them about: (1) what they like most and least about their work, (2) how their training best and least prepared them for the realities of what they do, (3) what they face as their greatest frustrations and challenges, and (4) what advice they would offer you as a beginner to the field.

## SUGGESTED READINGS

Corey, M. S., & Corey, G. (1998). *Becoming a helper* (3rd ed.). Pacific Grove, CA: Brooks/Cole.

Gladding, S. T. (2001). *Becoming a counselor: The light, the bright, and the serious.* Alexandria, VA: American Counseling Association.

Kottler, J. A. (2000). *Doing good: Passion and commitment for helping others.* New York: Brunner/Routledge.

Kottler, J. A. (2002). *Counselors finding their way.* Alexandria, VA: American Counseling Association.

Lee, C. C., & Walz, G. R. (1998). *Social action: A mandate for counselors.* Alexandria, VA: American Counseling Association.

Ram Dass & Gorman, P. (1985). *How can I help? Stories and reflections on service.* New York: Knopf.

Welch, I. D. (1998). *The path of psychotherapy: Matters of the heart.* Pacific Grove, CA: Brooks/Cole.

Yalom, I. (1989). *Love's executioner and other tales of psychotherapy.* New York: Basic Books.

# FOUNDATIONS OF COUNSELING

KEY CONCEPTS

Professional identity

Mental health professions

Counseling and therapy

Cathartic method

Pragmatism

Guidance movement

Medical model

Core conditions

Managed care

Scientific method

# FOUNDATIONS OF COUNSELING

# CHAPTER 2

## BASICS OF HISTORY AND RESEARCH

In most disciplines, history and research are often relegated to those requirements that everyone thinks are necessary but very few students relish studying. Who cares, after all, about what some obscure philosopher or educator said a hundred years ago? You just want to help people. Of what value is some research study with a bunch of charts and numbers when all you want to do is figure out how to help some poor kid stop trying to kill himself?

Yet the past is the basis for the present and future, and research is the foundation for everything we know. One of the first tasks that occurs in every counseling endeavor, regardless of the practitioner's theoretical preferences, is taking a thorough client history and collecting systematic research on the nature of the presenting problem. We explore childhood experiences, medical history, and family lineage. We track every aspect of the client's social, emotional, physical, religious, educational, and vocational background in order to develop a complete portrait of functioning.

After this personal history is initiated, next begins a research process to familiarize yourself with the literature related to your client's concerns, cultural background, and particular life circumstances. In order to formulate some sort of treatment plan, you also review the research in your own work setting related to the issues presented. Whether you're aware of it or not, you've also been doing your own research, systematically keeping

## VOICE FROM THE FIELD

I've been so confused about what the differences are between one kind of counselor or another. In one place you're called an LPC [Licensed Professional Counselor], then you cross the state line and the license they have is an MFT [Marriage and Family Therapist]. I've got one friend who has the same degree I have but because she lives in another part of the country, she's called an LLP [Limited Licensed Psychologist]. I mean, give me a break!

Then, to make matters worse, each of the different specialties have different exams you have to pass, different theories they like, and even a different scope of practice. They're supposed to specialize in different areas, but really they all fight for the same clients. And I don't think anyone could watch a counselor or therapist in action and be able to figure out what kind they were. It sure makes it difficult for someone to figure out what the best kind of training is to help people.

---

track of what has worked in the past, under which circumstances, with which clients. All of this review of the past helps you to gain some sort of grasp on what is happening in the present.

And if personal history is important to understand and help the client, then a knowledge of the profession's history is necessary for you to function as a literate professional—even to understand how counseling fits within the context of other helping professions.

## THE IDENTITY OF COUNSELING

As you may already be aware, there are tremendous disagreements regarding professional identity and who is the rightful heir to the title "helper." Psychiatrists, social workers, psychiatric nurses, psychologists, marriage and family therapists, counselors, pastoral care workers, and human service specialists all claim that their training and abilities are superior to those of their colleagues. Various titles are used to describe the work of helping others depending on the school attended or the state of the established practice. Yet among these divergences there is a central core, an essence of effective practice, regardless of how it is labeled.

Whether it takes place in schools, community agencies, or private practice, the act of helping clients work through personal issues is best called *therapeutic counseling*, a hybrid term that distinguishes *counseling* as the professional identity and *therapeutic* as the modality. This practitioner is thus distinguished from some of the predecessors in the evolution of our field, such as "guidance counselor" or "career education consultant." This is not to say that therapeutic counselors (especially those in schools) don't regularly provide the services of career guidance among their other functions. But the therapeutic aspect has to do with far more than merely providing information or facilitating decision making. It involves helping clients to personalize their decisions in such a way that they become part of them—that their underlying feelings and thoughts are dealt with as well.

The "Voice from the Field" on the previous page is not far wrong in expressing her confusion over the identity of counseling as distinct from other disciplines. While there is considerable overlap between the various mental health groups—and certainly commonality in their history and research base—there are also some distinct differences.

Among the various groups in Table 2.1, matters are made more complex by the different degrees that are offered. In some parts of North America, depending on the state or province and rural or urban setting, a clinician may need a doctoral degree to practice; in others a master's degree, bachelor's degree, or even associate's degree is sufficient. Which type of program you are enrolled in and which type of degree you are seeking will depend not only on the state or province you reside in, but also your career aspirations.

There are estimated to be something over a half million mental health care providers (counselors, family therapists, social workers, and psychologists) in the United States (American Counseling Association, 2001). When pastoral workers and clergy who practice counseling are also included in the professional group, that figure doubles in size. Some states are dominated by marriage and family therapists (California), others by social workers (Alabama, Illinois, Iowa, New York, Wisconsin, and Nevada), others by psychologists (Tennessee), and still others by counselors (Ohio, Texas, and Florida). Although in theory, each of these professions has a unique and distinct heritage and style of training, in practice they may do very similar things, depending on how licensure defines the scope of practice.

Depending on which type of program you are currently enrolled in, it would be helpful for you to understand some of the unique facets of or your own professional identity even if we all share common theoretical frameworks, ethical concepts, and standards of practice. Nevertheless, whether I have been licensed as a psychologist, family therapist, or counselor (I am currently licensed as all three in various states), I have always appreciated and preferred thinking of the work I do as "counseling."

Many people use the term counseling interchangeably with "therapy," and in many ways the two words do refer to essentially the same sort of professional helping activity. Yet using the term counseling has allowed me to emphasize the particular nature of my work that specializes in:

1. Preventing rather than only fixing problems
2. Using a developmental rather than psychopathological model of diagnosis
3. Focusing on adjustment issues and developmental concerns rather than more severe psychopathology
4. Doing relatively short-term rather than long-term work
5. Practicing in community rather than medical settings

These sort of generalizations are misleading and, to some extent, inaccurate. Psychiatrists and psychologists are often known to prefer working with relatively normal people who present adjustment disorders—such individuals

TABLE 2.1 | ALLIED MENTAL HEALTH PROFESSIONAL GROUPS

| Professional Group | Specialization |
| --- | --- |
| Counselors | Therapeutic interventions with relatively normal-functioning clients who are experiencing adjustment reactions, developmental issues, and problems of daily living including career, education, family, personal, and esteem issues. |
| Psychologists | Diagnosis, treatment, and clinical management of persons with psychopathological symptoms and other severe mental disturbances. |
| Psychiatrists | Medical management of patients with clinically significant psychological problems; use of medication, hospitalization, and therapy to restore normal functioning. |
| Social Workers | Social casework and therapy to mediate relationships with social structures like schools, agencies, and health care facilities. |
| Family Therapists | Systemic approach to diagnosing and treating problems in a family context. Extensive use of more active/directive interventions to realign family structures. |
| Pastoral Care | An approach to helping that is embedded in religious, spiritual, or ministerial work, combining theology with community service. |

are more verbal, articulate, grateful, and they pay their bills on time. Likewise, although the focus of training in most counseling, human service, and family therapy programs is on doing relatively brief interventions with moderate- to high-functioning people, many graduates end up working with severely disturbed, dual-diagnosed populations. To complicate matters further, some specialties, such as "counseling psychology," combine features of both disciplines, emphasizing more cultural diversity, career development, and community involvement than traditional clinical psychology (Goodyear et al., 2000).

I don't wish to confuse you about some of the similarities and differences between counseling and therapy, or between any of the mental health professions, but just to alert you that such distinctions exist. For the purposes of this textbook, I will use the term counseling, and speak about the profession of counseling, but you will find that many of the concepts apply equally well to other disciplines.

Counselor education will provide a solid grounding in developmentally based theory and interventions, as well as training in skills related to building effective therapeutic relationships, whether in individual, group, or family settings. This training makes you ideally qualified to work with a wide range of people, especially those who are suffering from adjustment reactions to daily life. In fact, you are far better prepared than those in any other mental health

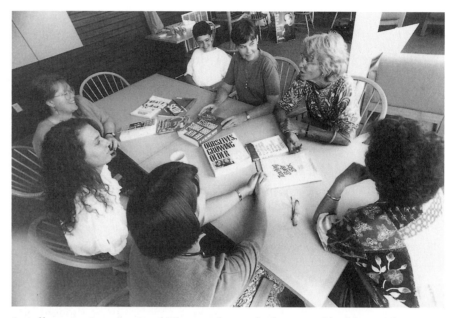

A staff meeting in action in which counselors and other mental health specialists collaborate in case planning and treatment. In ideal settings, professional competition and jealousies are put aside for the sake of client welfare and staff morale. © Gale Zucker/Stock Boston.

specialty to work through such issues. Counseling is the only helping discipline that has both a preventive/developmental orientation and a remedial model that makes use of diagnosis and treatment (Altekruse, Harris, & Brandt, 2001). This focus means that we are trained to prevent problems as much as we can by intervening within an early developmental context, as well as to assess and treat problems that have already arisen.

Counselors are not in competition with allied professional groups; each discipline reflects specialized skills and various professional competencies that overlap yet have distinctive components. For example, although clinical psychologists do counseling, their area of training and expertise is more centered on psychodiagnosis—psychotherapy with patients demonstrating psychopathological disorders—and the management of clinically significant mental illness. They also are highly trained in the administration and interpretation of psychological testing. Counselors do not generally develop expertise in these areas as much as they specialize in brief treatment modalities with less disturbed individuals. These distinctions, however, become even more muddled when we consider that in recent years the specialties of "clinical counseling" and "mental health counseling" have been geared toward work with client populations that previously had been restricted to social workers, psychologists, and psychiatrists. In some settings, in fact, such as community mental health centers and hospitals, various practitioners do essentially the same things regardless of their professional identity.

## VOICE FROM THE FIELD

I ended up doing an internship at the Salvation Army. Here I was seeing people who are dual diagnosed—they are both mentally ill and addicted to one or more substances. I know that I was told that my training would not prepare me for this job. Practically all the people I worked with in role plays, and then in my practicum, were supposedly relatively high-functioning clients with adjustment reactions. I saw a lot of mild depression, career indecision, that sort of thing.

In the area in which I live there is just nobody else who can see these people. I suppose psychologists, or better yet psychiatrists, would be far better trained than me to work with these people. But where are they? Probably in the suburbs seeing people who are better educated, who are articulate, and who can pay their bills. I don't mean to be cynical but I know a lot of people like me who end up doing jobs that are way out of our league. Don't get me wrong: I love this work. But it seems to me that the supposed specialties between professions are not as divided as some people think they are.

---

The allied professional groups can be thought of as forming a mental health treatment team that responds to various clients who experience problems within their areas of specialization. The team concept recognizes the responsibility of professionals to provide relevant services within their respective areas of competence and, further, demands effective communication and cooperation among professionals.

## HISTORY OF THERAPEUTIC COUNSELING

A unique aspect of counseling as a profession is that its foundation is grounded in so many other disciplines; it is a hybrid of knowledge from philosophy, education, psychology, psychiatry, sociology, and family studies. Even today, programs that train counselors are found in academic units as diverse as colleges of education or health sciences, departments of psychology or family studies, schools of human services, and religious institutions.

Therapeutic counseling and its related disciplines of psychiatry, psychology, social work, and guidance have experienced an uneven progression of development. In the days of our Paleolithic ancestors, the first mental health professionals were fond of drilling holes in a client's head to permit demons to escape. Through the days of ancient Mesopotamia and Persia, the classical Greek and Roman eras, and into modern times, early therapeutic counselors were primarily philosophers, physicians, or priests.

The primitive days of the nineteenth century spawned the first real counselors, the experts who attempted to heal by talking (even if they did so in ways we now find a bit bizarre). It is incredible to think that one hundred years ago, therapeutic counseling as we know it did not exist. And it has been only in the past fifty years that counseling has emerged as a distinct field apart from its related mental health disciplines.

The "talking cure" is a concept that we take for granted today, yet a century ago it was a revolutionary idea that was not only unaccepted but held in disrepute, smacking of witchcraft and the occult. The cathartic method of talking out problems was pioneered by Sigmund Freud at the turn of the century as a method for treating persons with psychological problems. Although the concept had existed for many years, it took Freud to build credibility for the technique. Today most people agree that talking over problems is helpful, sharing feelings and concerns is useful, and professional helpers are reasonable alternatives for those faced with problems or difficult situations. Interpersonal communication and verbal interaction form the heart of therapeutic counseling, albeit in a substantially different format from what Freud envisioned. Counselors, clients, and the person in the street all believe that constructive change can occur when a counselor and a client work together toward identified, realistic goals.

## The Ancient Philosophers

The first counselors were leaders of the community who attempted to provide inspiration for others through their teachings. They were religious leaders such as Moses (1200 B.C.), Mohammed (600 B.C.), and Buddha (500 B.C.). They were also philosophers such as Lao-tzu (600 B.C.), Confucius (500 B.C.), Socrates (450 B.C.), Plato (400 B.C.), and Aristotle (350 B.C.).

Many of these philosophers and religious leaders functioned as "counselors" in that they worked with a group of disciples, trying to impart wisdom to stimulate emotional, spiritual, and intellectual growth. Although their approaches to helping are considerably different from those of most contemporary counselors, we have inherited a few of their basic tenets:

- There is no single right answer to any question worth asking.
- There are many possible interpretations of the same experience.
- Any philosophy is worthless if it is not personalized and made relevant to everyday life.

These same principles, spoken in the forums of Rome, Athens, and Mesopotamia, are very much a part of what today's counselors work with on a daily basis—helping clients to find their own path to inner peace.

## The First Psychiatrists

Besides those who sought to "heal" others' suffering through educational and spiritual paths, other pragmatic practitioners tried to combine philosophy with what they observed about human behavior. Foremost among these medical philosophers was Hippocrates (400 B.C.), who introduced many ideas that we now take for granted, including the concepts of *homeostasis* (the natural balance of the body) and *prognosis* (the prediction of outcomes).

Hippocrates emphasized the importance of a complete life history before undertaking any treatment (which unfortunately was usually bloodletting) and devised the first comprehensive classification of mental disorders. He is

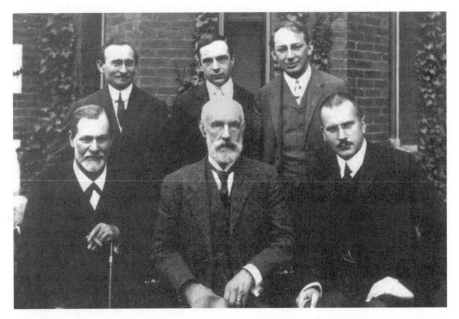

In September 1909, Sigmund Freud was invited to the United States to give a series of lectures on his theories. He is pictured here (bottom left) sitting next to the American psychologist G. Stanley Hall and colleague Carl Jung. In the top row (from left to right) are three of Freud's disciples: A. A. Brill, Ernest Jones, and Sandor Ferencsi.

Archives of the History of American psychology, the University of Akron/Seymour Wapner gift/Permission Clark University Archives.

also credited with developing—over two thousand years ago—the first counseling interventions, relying on many techniques that are still in use today: systematic diagnostic interviews, detailed history taking, trust building in a therapeutic relationship, and even dream interpretation and acknowledgment of repressed feelings.

There really were not many improvements on Hippocrates' theories until the last century or two. (Remember, the favored "treatment" in the Middle Ages for those suffering from emotional problems was being burned at the stake.) But when Sigmund Freud and his colleague Joseph Breuer evolved their "talking cure" of healing through catharsis, the professions of counseling and psychotherapy were truly born. Freud was not only a talented physician, writer, teacher, thinker, and astute observer of the human condition, but he was also remarkably persuasive as an influencer of others. He recruited into his camp a flock of followers from all over the world to spread the word about his newfound cure for emotional suffering. Many of their names may be familiar to you: Carl Jung, Alfred Adler, Wilhelm Reich, and even his own daughter, Anna Freud.

The nineteenth century produced a number of great philosophers who had a significant impact on the development of Freud and his students. Such thinkers as Søren Kierkegaard, G. W. F. Hegel, and Friedrich Nietzsche were just as influential on this new profession as were Freud's own colleagues in medicine. In addition, a number of brilliant mentors had instructed Freud in the intricacies of the brain as well as introduced him to the technique of hypnosis as a means of accessing the mind's inner secrets. Add to that training Freud's own penchant for philosophy, literature, and archaeology, and he was ideally suited to pull all this knowledge together into the first comprehensive model for understanding and changing human behavior.

Throughout his prolific life, churning out volume after volume of meticulously documented theories on the human condition, Freud accomplished several remarkable feats, including:

- Plotting the anatomy of the human nervous system
- Developing the first form of local anesthesia for eye surgery
- Adapting the technique of hypnosis for studying the inner world
- Formulating models of personality development and psychopathology
- Emphasizing unconscious motives behind human behavior
- Suggesting that dreams have meanings that can be uncovered and interpreted
- Studying the underlying structure of society
- Developing the first formal methodology of therapeutic counseling

Although it is popular nowadays to ridicule many of Freud's ideas, to call him obsolete, sexist, controlling, sexually obsessed, neurotic, and a host of other names, it must be remembered that he was the primary mentor of the first generation of therapeutic counselors. Many of the most famous names in the field, representing quite diverse approaches—Albert Ellis, Murray Bowen, Fritz Perls, Alfred Adler, Carl Rogers, Eric Berne—were all at one time practicing Freudian analysts. It would be difficult, therefore, to underestimate Freud's importance in the development of counseling, even if contemporary practitioners no longer employ his methods the way they were originally intended. (But then, how many techniques in *any* profession remain intact after a hundred years?)

## Influences from Psychology

About the same time that Freud was laying the foundation for psychiatric counseling, another discipline was making its own contribution: the burgeoning field of psychology. As was the case with the first psychiatrists and counselors, all the first psychologists were philosophers. Beginning with René Descartes (1596–1650), who was among the first to study the mind as distinct from the body and soul, and continuing through the British empirical philosophers such as John Locke (1632–1704), George Berkeley (1685–1753), David Hume (1711–1776), and John Stuart Mill (1806–1873), who analyzed human experience in terms of its basic elements, the discipline of philosophy gave rise to the new science of psychology.

Every undergraduate psychology major memorizes the fact that the discipline was born when Wilhelm Wundt (1832–1920) founded the first

## VOICE FROM THE FIELD

Okay. Enough is enough! This is just about all the history I can take. What's with all these names and dates? Am I supposed to be able to remember all this stuff? Is this going to be on the test?

I mean, give us a break! I'm trying to sort all this stuff out, figure out who is really important and which of these dead, white guys you just stuck in to impress us. I'm all for history and all, but I've got my limit. This is just overwhelming.

I guess the big picture isn't the specifics but just that counseling comes from a lot of different places. I can see that what we do is like philosophers. Doctors too. It's interesting that all these names you're throwing at us are familiar, but I've never thought of them as being part of this profession.

---

experimental laboratory in 1879. However, it was really the American philosopher William James (1842–1910) who was the first to be awarded the title "Professor of Psychology." For our purposes, James' ideas are more relevant to the development of therapeutic counseling as a separate discipline. He was intensely interested in the concepts of free will, consciousness, and adaptive functioning and believed humans to be creatures of emotion and action as well as thought and reason. He was also instrumental in developing the philosophy of "pragmatism," which is very much alive today in the spirit of flexibility and integration that permeates the development of new helping models. According to James (1907), the pursuit of knowledge is best directed toward finding useful tools that can be both applied to practical situations and scientifically validated. You will find that almost a hundred years later, after his treatise on the subject, that pragmatism is still a guiding force for what we do.

Of course, many other names are associated with the development of psychology, such as G. Stanley Hall, who received the first doctorate in psychology and became the bridge between this new science and the field of education. Certainly the behaviorists, led by John Watson and B. F. Skinner, also made significant contributions to the understanding and management of human behavior through their experimental studies of reinforcement. A number of other experimental psychologists, such as Max Wertheimer and Wolfgang Kohler, approached things from quite a different perspective. From their studies of how apes solve problems, they concluded that learning does not necessarily follow an orderly progression; sometimes sudden insights play a part, whereby a person conceptualizes the whole as greater than the sum of its elemental parts.

## The Guidance Era

In the early part of the twentieth century, a completely different movement was taking place. It was a time of significant social reform, and there was an emerging recognition that social forces and individual development could be assisted, directed, and—more important—guided. This awareness was especially evident in the field of education and the specialty of career guidance.

The industrial age was then flourishing; technical training and skilled workers were becoming necessary, and new programs in vocational guidance attempted to respond to these needs. Although there were a number of pioneers who took the initiative in this field, Frank Parsons is often credited as the founder of the vocational guidance movement. In his book *Choosing a Vocation* (Parsons, 1909), he described a three-part model for career counseling: (1) an analysis of one's own personal interests, abilities, and aptitudes; (2) an exploration of available occupations; and (3) the application of a systematic reasoning process to find a good match between the two. This procedure, Parsons believed, would place individuals in work settings most appropriate to their skills and education.

Parsons and several colleagues applied their new technology of testing and interviewing to help Boston's unemployed youth identify interests and abilities and find suitable work. Thus the vocational guidance field became respectable, enabling counselors to specialize in a particular aspect of human conflict. It carved a niche for guidance personnel in educational settings; however, it also prevented the integration of the structured teaching model of vocational guidance into the mainstream of therapeutic counseling. For the next sixty years counselors were seen primarily as school specialists who helped children make educational and occupational decisions.

In addition to the school guidance movement, several other influences during this time contributed to the development of counseling as a profession (Gladding, 2000; Glossoff, 2001; Nugent, 2000). These included:

1. The development of standardized testing during World War I as a means to measure aptitudes, abilities, and even personality traits
2. The birth of the Veterans' Administration after World War II, recruiting professionals to help aid the adjustment of soldiers
3. The passage of the National Defense Education Act to channel more youth into the sciences after the Soviet Union launched Sputnik, demonstrating they were ahead in the space race
4. The evolution of vocational rehabilitation as a specialty to work with those who are disabled
5. The creation of the first counseling services on college campuses
6. The establishment of a comprehensive mental health system
7. The launching of the American Personnel and Guidance Association as the first professional organization for counselors
8. Federal legislation such as the Americans with Disabilities Act, Vocational Educational Act, and Work Incentives Improvement Act that mandated assistance to those with disabilities
9. Influence of accreditation by the Council for the Accreditation of Counseling and Related Educational Programs (CACREP) to parallel actions by the American Association for Marital and Family Therapy (AAMFT), Council on Rehabilitation Education (CORE), and the American Psychological Association (APA)

10. Spread of licensure laws across states and provinces providing greater legitimacy to counselors and family therapists
11. Increased cultural diversity in population through immigration requiring expertise in fostering greater harmony and adjustment
12. Managed care movement recognizing cost efficiency of using nonmedical practitioners to treat mental health problems

## The Counseling Era

Not all of the contributors to the mental health movement were philosophers, psychiatrists, psychologists, or educators. One of the most influential figures in the early part of the twentieth century was an abused mental patient. In *A Mind That Found Itself*, Clifford Beers (1945) described his harrowing experiences at the hands of an insensitive system that treated him as a lunatic rather than as a human being. In this classic work (which eventually led to the establishment of the National Association for Mental Health), Beers proposed that what the emotionally disturbed person needs most of all is a compassionate friend. It was the field of therapeutic counseling that finally responded to his plea.

The prevailing "medical model" espoused by psychiatrists and some psychologists had reigned supreme. This framework emphasized the diagnosis of psychopathology. Patients who sought therapeutic services were viewed as afflicted with a form of mental illness that could be treated by a number of medical options—electroconvulsive shock treatment, psychosurgery (frontal lobotomies), psychopharmacology, and, as a last resort, medical psychotherapy, which usually took the form of long-term psychoanalysis with sessions three to four times a week for a half-dozen years or more. To this day, the medical model is still at the core of many diagnostic systems, such as those used in a variety of clinical settings.

At the midpoint of the twentieth century, a lone voice was heard above the throng of psychiatrists and psychologists. Carl Rogers (1902–1987) began to argue persuasively that the traditional doctor/patient pattern of interaction proposed by the medical model was not appropriate for working with the vast majority of human beings. According to Rogers, people with emotional problems are not "sick" or "mentally ill"; most people simply need a safe environment in which to work out their difficulties. He maintained that the most effective vehicle to accomplish this task was within the context of a therapeutic relationship.

In spite of the initially cool reception to the ideas in client-centered theory, Carl Rogers emerged as a significant force in the field of counseling, changing previous thinking about the nature of the healing alliance. In retrospect, it seems difficult to imagine counseling today without the impact of Rogers and his ideas about the importance of relationship variables.

Client-centered counseling became the theoretical focus of many counselor education programs during the 1950s and early 1960s. On the whole, Rogers was enthusiastically embraced and legions of counselors were trained in nondirective, client-centered techniques. But in spite of the general acceptance of client-centered counseling, some concerns were emerging that questioned the nature of this approach and criticized its relevance for many client populations. Additionally, the operational difficulties involved in defining the tasks of the counselor and the difficulties in gathering empirical evidence to support the client-centered approach caused further questioning and exploring.

The 1960s and early 1970s saw much change and refocusing in the counseling field. The wide acceptance of the Rogerian approach came under increased scrutiny. Carkhuff and Berenson (1977) and Krumboltz (1966) wrote books that were quite influential in challenging the field to move toward a more behavioral slant, whereas Ellis (1962) and other cognitive therapists emphasized the role of thinking in the counseling process. Other theorists joined the defection with their ideas: Gestalt therapy, transactional analysis (TA), values clarification strategies, reality therapy, and others all clamored for attention and vied for influence.

From this rich inquiry and challenge there seemed to emerge a focus that gained wide credibility in counselor education. Robert Carkhuff and several collaborators (Carkhuff & Berenson, 1977; Truax & Carkhuff, 1967) imposed a systematic and generalist approach to the task of helping. Carkhuff suggested that counselors must be skilled, reliable, and capable of delivering effective levels of core counseling skills. He defined the skills and developed methods of assessing effectiveness. The work of Carkhuff is widely accepted, with much counselor training emphasizing the development of generic skills that provide a base for effective helping relationships. In a class on techniques of counseling you are likely to follow one of several systematic skills models (Cormier & Cormier, 1998; De Jong & Berg, 2002; Doyle, 1998; Egan, 2002; Murphy & Dillon, 1998; Young, 2001) that were patterned after Carkhuff's identified "core conditions." Today, therapeutic counseling is built on the work of Carkhuff, who has developed a base for the skill-development process; Rogers, who emphasized the importance of the relationship dimension in counseling; and Freud, who gave credibility to the idea of treatment through talking.

In a sense, this represents the generic foundation for training in therapeutic counseling. To achieve maturity as a professional, it is necessary to integrate the various approaches to counseling within the generic model used in most training. It is a mistake to assume that minimal generic skills will prepare a person to function as a counselor. Therefore, in your training you will first learn the basic skills of reflecting, confronting, summarizing, attending, and goal setting and will then expand on this base from the diverse sources of theory and technique available to therapeutic counselors.

Table 2.2 summarizes the contributions of many individuals to the field of therapeutic counseling. These are included not to overwhelm you with a bunch of names you will quickly forget but to impress you with the long and distinguished list of notable figures who have contributed to contemporary practice. I also wish to stress how truly interdisciplinary the profession of therapeutic counseling really is, encompassing the work of medicine, philosophy, education, and the social sciences, as well as more recent contributions from the various mental health specialties.

TABLE 2.2 | SUMMARY OF HISTORICAL FIGURES IN THERAPEUTIC COUNSELING WITH CONTRIBUTIONS FROM PHILOSOPHY, EDUCATION, MEDICINE, LITERATURE, AND SOCIAL SCIENCE

| | | |
|---|---|---|
| 400 B.C. | Hippocrates | Classified types of mental illness and personality disorders |
| 400 B.C. | Socrates | Encouraged self-awareness as purest form of knowledge |
| 350 B.C. | Plato | Postulated human behavior in terms of internal states |
| 350 B.C. | Aristotle | Designed first rational psychology to manage emotions |
| 400 | St. Augustine | Prescribed introspection to master emotions |
| 1500 | Niccolo Machiavelli | Brought attention to group dynamics and social interaction |
| 1550 | Johann Weyer | Documented case histories of depression |
| 1600 | William Shakespeare | Created a literature of psychologically complex characters |
| 1625 | René Descartes | Attempted to resolve dualism of mind and body |
| 1675 | John Locke | Theorized that all knowledge originates from experience |
| 1675 | Baruch Spinoza | Developed an integrative personality theory |
| 1800 | Johannes Muller | Plotted the physiology of the nervous system |
| 1800 | Philippe Pinel | Described various forms of neurosis and psychosis |
| 1800 | Anton Mesmer | Used hypnotic suggestion to cure psychological symptoms |
| 1850 | Charles Darwin | Set forth an evolutionary theory of individual differences |
| 1850 | Jean Charcot | Scientifically studied hypnosis to give it respectability |
| 1850 | Søren Kierkegaard | Developed existential philosophy of creating meaning |
| 1880 | G. Stanley Hall | Began first child guidance clinic |
| 1890 | James Cattell | Coined the term *mental tests* |
| 1890 | Jesse Davis | Became first school counselor |
| 1900 | Emil Kraepelin | Systematized the classification of mental disorders |
| 1900 | William James | Postulated comprehensive theory of emotions |
| 1900 | Ivan Pavlov | Described behavioral theory of conditioned reflexes |
| 1900 | Sigmund Freud | Devised first systematic form of therapeutic counseling |
| 1905 | Alfred Binet | Invented first intelligence test |
| 1910 | Frank Parsons | Established field of vocational guidance |
| 1910 | Clifford Beers | Published autobiography of experiences as a mental patient |
| 1920 | Carl Jung | Proposed theory of collective unconscious |
| 1920 | Alfred Adler | Authored theory of individual psychology |
| 1920 | J. L. Moreno | Invented psychodrama |
| 1920 | John Watson | Developed notions of prediction and control of behavior |
| 1930 | Robert Hoppock | Studied levels of job satisfaction |
| 1940 | B. F. Skinner | Formulated theory of operant conditioning |

*(continued)*

TABLE 2.2 | SUMMARY OF HISTORICAL FIGURES IN THERAPEUTIC COUNSELING (CONTINUED)

| 1940 | E. G. Williamson | Published standard text on school counseling |
|------|------------------|----------------------------------------------|
| 1945 | Gregory Bateson | Emphasized family influences in mental problems |
| 1945 | Kurt Lewin | Used training-group format for personal development |
| 1950 | Viktor Frankl | Emphasized search for meaning in human experience |
| 1950 | Milton Erickson | Focused on linguistic aspects of therapeutic encounter |
| 1950 | Carl Rogers | Emphasized importance of relationship in counseling |
| 1955 | Rollo May | Developed framework for existential therapy |
| 1955 | Abraham Maslow | Researched what makes people most healthy |
| 1955 | Donald Super | Introduced theory of vocational decision making |
| 1955 | Rudoph Dreikurs | Developed Adlerian theory into popular treatment |
| 1960 | Joseph Wolpe | Devised systematic theory of behavior therapy |
| 1960 | Jay Haley | Began strategic family therapy |
| 1960 | Albert Ellis | Developed cognitive-based therapy |
| 1960 | Jean Piaget | Studied children's unique moral and cognitive patterns |
| 1960 | Frederick Thorne | Created integrative theory of helping |
| 1965 | William Glasser | Developed reality therapy |
| 1965 | Fritz Perls | Popularized Gestalt therapy |
| 1965 | Robert Carkhuff | Organized and researched the skills of helping |
| 1965 | John Krumboltz | Published theory of behavioral counseling |
| 1965 | Murray Bowen | Brought attention to family-of-origin issues |
| 1965 | Virginia Satir | Described communication theory in family therapy |
| 1970 | Jerome Frank | Authored seminal work on persuasion in healing |
| 1970 | Salvador Minuchin | Developed structural basis for family therapy |
| 1970 | Aaron Beck | Developed cognitive therapy for depression |
| 1975 | Allen Bergin | Edited first comprehensive handbook on therapy |
| 1975 | Heinz Kohut | Contributor to development of self-psychology |
| 1975 | Helen Kaplan | Published classic work on sex counseling |
| 1980 | Paul Pederson | Championed cause of diversity issues |
| 1980 | John Norcross | Represented new movement toward integration of theories |
| 1980 | Irvin Yalom | Synthesized current theory on existential counseling |
| 1980 | Carol Gilligan | Pioneered research on gender differences in development |
| 1980 | Arnold Lazarus | Developed multi-modal therapy |
| 1985 | Rachel Hare-Mustin | Represented feminist approaches to counseling |
| 1985 | Paul Watzlawick | Shifted emphasis from objectivism to social constructivism |

*(continued)*

TABLE 2.2 | SUMMARY OF HISTORICAL FIGURES IN THERAPEUTIC COUNSELING (CONTINUED)

| 1985 | Steve de Shazer | Promoted brief forms of intervention |
| 1985 | Allen Ivey | Devised developmental/multicultural model for practice |
| 1985 | Norman Gysbers | Created developmental guidance program for schools |
| 1990 | Michael White | Developed narrative approaches to counseling |
| 1990 | Francine Shapiro | Developed method for treating traumatic stress |
| 1990 | John Gottman | Developed research base for doing marital counseling |
| 1990 | Monica McGoldrick | Plotted role of family life cycle in counseling |
| 1990 | Derald Sue | Spearheaded multicultural counseling competencies |
| 1990 | Jeffrey Zeig | Organized conferences to promote synthesis of approaches |

## The Era of Therapeutic Counseling

At one time, 80 percent of all students enrolled in counseling programs were following a school-based employment track. Now that trend has shifted, and the majority of new counselors are targeting themselves for employment in various agencies as community counselors, clinical counselors, mental health counselors, or marital and family counselors. Clearly, the focus of counseling is now less educational and more therapeutic. This fact is reflected in the progressive name changes of the American Counseling Association (ACA), which a few years ago was called the American Association for Counseling and Development (AACD) and a few years before that was known as the American Personnel and Guidance Association (APGA). It is evident in the rapid growth of organizations like the American Mental Health Counselors Association and the International Association of Marriage and Family Counselors. And it is certainly obvious from the emergence of licensing and credentialing for professional counselors.

In today's climate of "managed care," in which health insurance agencies and large employers are attempting to control costs associated with mental health treatment, counselors are playing a bigger role in many regions because of our emphasis on brief treatment and our cost effectiveness when compared to other professionals. In spite of these changes, there are still considerable doubts about whether such a movement will ultimately be good for our profession and consumers of our services. Regardless of our preferences, the counseling profession has now become strongly influenced (and controlled) by the values associated with managing costs. We are now asked not only to help people but to do so in the most efficient and cost-effective way possible, as well as to document these outcomes. While this does compromise a certain degree of independence and freedom in how we practice, there have also been several positive effects that have led to increased accountability and the development of more efficient methods (Frager, 2000; Hoyt, 2000).

This cadre of new counselors is still using the core skills of practice that have been identified for some time but is also drawing heavily from other fields while researching, developing, and expanding the intervention base. The emphasis is on approaches that are developmentally oriented and that use relatively short-term strategies designed to reduce symptoms, eliminate self-defeating behaviors, and increase self-esteem, self-efficacy, and self-management skills. Therapeutic counselors focus on developing a solid relationship, identifying core issues, understanding them from a developmental perspective, and employing interventions best suited to the particular client and clinical situation.

The latest movement within the helping professions has been a drive toward greater integration of existing research and theory into a coherent model that most practitioners can follow. As a result, counselor training programs are becoming more standardized across North America as current theorists attempt to reconcile the conflicts and differences among competing schools of thought. Another movement that is growing in its influence is the application of therapeutic counseling to diverse populations, with special emphasis on increasing our responsiveness to underserved groups such as oppressed minorities, the aged, and the disabled.

# LICENSING AND REGULATION IN COUNSELING

The best evidence for how far we have developed in our history is found in the progress made in the credentialing of counselors across the country. There was a time, just a few decades ago, when there were no standards for the preparation of counselors, no licensure laws, no certifications for specialties in any area. As a result, therapeutic counselors did not enjoy the professional autonomy and respect granted to our colleagues in social work, psychology, and psychiatry.

Efforts to standardize counselor training and to regulate the practice of clinicians began in 1973, when the Association for Counselor Education and Supervision developed a knowledge base to provide the foundation for future licensing efforts (Brooks & Gerstein, 1990). Before we could decide who should be allowed to practice counseling, we needed to establish minimum standards of training and education. Soon after this report was created, a number of states in succession, beginning with Virginia, passed licensing laws. Since that time, the field has enacted a number of different licensure, certification, and regulatory bodies, many of which are in direct competition with one another and present a confusing array of options for practitioners. As I have remarked earlier, depending on the jurisdiction in which you live, you could very well become licensed as a counselor, family therapist, or psychologist.

The licensure initiative must be understood in the context of two other attempts to legitimize counseling as a profession that evolved simultaneously. In 1981, the American Counseling Association established an independent agency to accredit training programs in the field. This Council for the Accreditation of Counseling and Related Educational Programs (CACREP) developed minimum requirements for graduate programs at the master's and doctoral levels, including specialties in mental health, school counseling, student personnel, community/agency counseling, and marriage and family counseling. Other professional organizations such as the American Psychological Association (APA) and American Association for Marriage and Family Therapy (AAMFT) have developed similar standards in which certain core content and curricular experiences are required.

More and more counselor preparation programs are structuring their curricula around content areas and clinical experiences that may seem familiar to you in your own program. Although the core requirements can be met in different ways, generally the following content areas are either represented as separate courses or infused into several classes throughout the program:

1. Professional orientation, introducing you to the identity of your profession and specialty
2. Human growth and development, concentrating on the background you will need to understand how people learn and grow
3. Social and cultural foundations, providing much of the theoretical background necessary for functioning effectively with diverse populations
4. Therapeutic relationships, covering the process and skills involved in developing alliances that are likely to lead to constructive learning and change
5. Group work, preparing you to understand the dynamics, stages, and processes of counseling in groups
6. Career development, focusing on the theory and practice of vocational decision making
7. Assessment, including methods of gathering information, formulating diagnoses and treatment plans, and administering and interpreting tests
8. Research and evaluation, helping you to make sense of the professional literature, to read studies critically, and to construct legitimate evaluation methods in your work
9. Family systems theory and practice that prepares you to work with couples and families.

In addition to this general preparation, there are also various specialty areas such as marital and family therapy, school counseling, rehabilitation counseling, student personnel, and substance abuse counseling. Finally, depending on program accreditation and jurisdictional licensure requirements, you are expected to have certain supervised clinical experiences, including documented hours in practica and internships.

As a result of this standardization of training, counselors are earning greater respect and recognition from colleagues in other fields, and from clients who prefer to work with practitioners employing a developmental rather than a medical model. Our legitimacy is even attested to by our eligibility for third-party reimbursement from clients' insurance companies. Although at one time, being able to participate in managed care, employee assistance, and preferred provider programs was seen as a major victory, now many practitioners are beginning to wonder whether we are increasingly losing control over our case management decisions because of third-party intrusions.

## VOICE FROM THE FIELD

It really amazes me how much things have changed in the past several years. Becoming licensed as a counselor is a big deal in my state. I can do so many things now that just weren't possible in earlier years.

Yeah, it means a lot to be eligible for third-party reimbursement, so I can compete in the marketplace with other professionals, but more than that, licensure means that I'm taken so much more seriously.

I just wish the laws were standardized from one place to another; it makes things kind of difficult when you want to relocate. That's why accreditation is becoming more and more important.

It is probably a very good idea, even this early in your program, to begin researching the licensing requirements in your own area as well as the certification options that will be available to you on graduation. For example, neighboring states may have quite different licenses available to practitioners at the master's level. Those you will see most frequently include (1) Licensed Professional Counselor (LPC), (2) Marital and Family Counselor (MFC), and (3) Limited Licensed Psychologist (LLP). Almost every region has a unique professional climate, each specialty you consider—whether in schools, agencies, rehabilitation settings, religious organizations, private practices, universities, or industry—will have different requirements in course content, internships, and supervision.

# RESEARCH FOUNDATIONS OF COUNSELING

The foundations of the counseling profession are certainly built on a history of ideas. Yet the origins of this knowledge, and almost everything we know and understand about how counseling works, have been constructed primarily from a systematic investigation process known as research.

Research and the practice of counseling have typically been seen as two discrete functions within the same profession. Practitioners and scientists are generally viewed as approaching a common problem from different directions. The practitioner actually works with clients and learns from the clients. The practitioner bases decisions about treatment on his or her experience and knowledge about what has been effective in previous clinical work. The scientist often has little or no involvement with direct service but studies human behavior in controlled experimental situations. In actuality, one of the most dominant models of effective practice in the field is one in which both research and clinical work are linked closely together.

## Counselors as Scientist-Practitioners

The scientist-practitioner model suggests that counselors engage in research while delivering direct services to clients (Claiborn, 1987; Hoshmand &

## VOICE FROM THE FIELD

I'm completing my internship hours for licensure, so I still see myself as a student at this point. Researching new ideas, client problems, psychotropic drugs, or a new technique is perfectly natural for someone like me in a learner's role. What's changed for me, though, since I left school, is that this is no longer an academic activity; research has become for me a practical extension of what I do as a good counselor.

I don't want this to sound like I keep my nose to some researcher's grindstone all the time. I'm not just a counselor. I'm a busy mom and wife, a committee chair, and a dozen other things. I have a life! But I do adopt a mindset and an active learning approach to my work. I'm pretty good at what I do but the only way that I can get better is to keep asking questions, digging for answers, learning new things, and trying out new things. That's what research is all about.

Polkinghorne, 1992; Tryon, 2002). Many practicing counselors see value in this concept because they are often faced with questions about the counseling process that can only be answered by research. This helps them to determine which interventions work with individual clients or particular client populations. Eldridge (1982) and Strupp (1989) have noted that the roles of the counselor and researcher can fit together effectively, making it possible for the practitioner to become literate in both areas.

Counseling is a process of helping clients change ineffective and maladaptive behaviors. For this to work well, the counselor must be able to assess the impact of any intervention; otherwise you will have no way to know if what you are doing is helpful or harmful. Imagine, for example, that a client with whom you have been working for some time has not been responding to your best intentions. You have tried your favorite method, in this case a low-key relationship-oriented approach, but to no avail. At what point do you abandon your strategy and try something else? If you are to move on to a different treatment plan, which path is most likely to prove successful, at least based on the prior experience of others who have worked in this area?

In order to function effectively, you will want to know precisely the effects of any given theory, attitude, or action so that you may reliably duplicate the intervention in the future. Knowing which counseling skills are most likely to produce desirable results is critical, especially if you want to make a positive difference in people's lives on a consistent basis.

## Counseling and Research Processes

It may appear at first as if the process of helping clients and the process of conducting research are as different as night and day. Yet they are actually more alike than you would imagine, especially considering the systematic, intentional ways they go about making sense of a phenomenon and then designing interventions to reach desired goals. In both counseling and research processes, you would recognize the following steps:

1. Awareness of a problem and the need for a solution
2. Systematic study of the context and background of the problem
3. Summary of what is known about the problem and what has been tried before to solve it
4. Functional definition of the problem so that it may be solved
5. Generalization from the study of particular instances to a similar class of events
6. Prediction of outcome and selection of actions based on their probability of success
7. Testing of hypotheses in a plan of action
8. Evaluation of results
9. Inferences drawn and generalizations made to other situations

Researchers and counselors are both systematic in their efforts to understand the world and how it works so they can determine the most effective ways to implement changes. Consider, for example, the scientific method outlined above as it is applied to a particular case in counseling.

1. *Awareness of problem:* A young woman sought professional help because of anxiety, an inability to sleep, and panic attacks that left her feeling dizzy and wobbly.
2. *Relevant background:* The woman was employed as a medical assistant and worked in the same office as her husband and father, who are both physicians. Prior to the onset of her symptoms she had been a person in remarkable control of her body, her mind, and her life. She was generally happy but discussed some career dissatisfaction. Exploration of her past revealed that she felt much resentment toward her parents for showing favoritism to a younger, rebellious sister and for forcing her into a medical career she never liked.
3. *Prior attempts at resolution:* Antianxiety medication, psychoanalytic therapy, and a variety of neurological tests produced no further insight into the problem and no alleviation of the symptoms.
4. *Functional definition:* Her symptoms were defined by the counselor as her body's attempt to break through her overcontrolled exterior and let her know she was not living her own life. Further, the symptoms gave her an excuse to quit her job, put distance between herself and her parents, and at the same time create more intimacy with her husband without the added work strain. The problem was defined as career-induced anxiety that was exaggerated by irrational thinking processes, repressed feelings, and a tendency toward overcontrol.
5. *Generalizations:* A series of affective and cognitive-based interventions were used to explore the connections between her specific symptoms and her life history. The counselor discovered that it had always been difficult for her to ask for help or initiate life changes; generally some dramatic event precipitated action in such a way that she didn't have to make decisions.

Insights into her relationships with family members were also generated, and she was helped to explore her feelings.

6. *Predictions:* It was predicted that, if she quit her job, reduced the unnecessary pressures in her life, began an exercise regime, confronted her parents with denied feelings, and worked toward being her own person within the nurturing environment of the counseling relationship, her symptoms would significantly diminish.

7. *Hypothesis testing:* The prediction was tested as a hypothesis by implementing the plan of action within the context of the supportive counseling relationship.

8. *Evaluation:* Within days after she quit her job, the woman's symptoms reduced in frequency and intensity. However, as weeks progressed and the woman was forced to deal with issues of boredom, structuring her time, and confronting her family members, the anxiety returned. As successive parts of the treatment program continued and she dealt more constructively with her need for control, the anxious and panicky feelings as well as psychosomatic complaints eventually diminished. A 90-day follow-up visit indicated that although her symptoms occasionally returned, she was able to deal successfully with them by applying rehearsed strategies.

9. *Inferences:* The client was able to generalize the work she did on these few aspects of her life to other components. She learned to relinquish complete control in other relationships and situations and to live a more spontaneous and flexible life. The counselor was able to draw inferences from this case to other therapeutic situations. His own theory of counseling was broadened to include the knowledge acquired through this counseling experience. It is likely that future therapeutic efforts will be even more effective as the practitioner incorporates the lessons of this case into his counseling approach.

This case study illustrates the research process in action as the counselor systematically identifies and defines the underlying complaints, intervenes, and assesses the impact of treatment. As you become more comfortable with the language and strategies involved in interpreting research literature as well as conducting meaningful evaluation projects, it will become easier to apply the skills of helping in a more intentional and consistent manner.

## Research for the Counselor

Three aspects of research are important for students of therapeutic counseling to learn. First is the terminology and language of the research field, by which communication is possible with other professionals. Many terms such as *hypothesis*, *variance*, and *extraneous variable* are used in everyday discussions.

Second is knowledge of the classic studies of the field and their implications for clinical work (see Table 2.3). Counselors who are knowledgeable about the research that supports the process of counseling are able to engage in relevant conversations with other professionals and are able to understand

TABLE 2.3 | A SAMPLING OF CLASSIC RESEARCH IN THERAPEUTIC COUNSELING

| Date | Author(s) | Title | Contribution |
|------|-----------|-------|--------------|
| 1920 | Watson & Rayner | Conditioned Emotional Reactions | Demonstrated that emotional reactions to stimuli can be conditioned or learned |
| 1938 | Skinner | The Behavior of Organisms | Demonstrated the principles of instrumental conditioning |
| 1950 | Dollard & Miller | Personality and Psychotherapy | Applied learning theory to the therapy process |
| 1950 | Fiedler | A Comparison of Therapeutic Relationships | Suggested that personal variables other than the therapists' theoretical orientation determine counseling effectiveness |
| 1952 | Eysenck | Effects of Psychotherapy | Suggested that persons receiving therapy did not improve more than persons not receiving therapy |
| 1956 | Bateson & others | Toward a Theory of Schizophrenia | Brought attention to the influence of families on psychological conditions |
| 1963 | Truax | Effective Ingredients in Psychotherapy | Suggested that therapist-offered conditions would result in either improvement or deterioration |
| 1966 | Holland | The Psychology of Vocational Choice | Presented the hexagonal model to describe the relationship between personality and occupational interests |
| 1968 | Strong | Counseling: An Interpersonal Influence Process | Suggested that counselors promote personal change through social forces |
| 1969 | Bandura | Principles of Behavior Modification | Clarified the effects and empirical base of behavior modification |
| 1969 | Carkhuff | Helping and Human Relations | Summarized research on core conditions of counseling |
| 1971 | Ivey | Microcounseling | Presented a training system for interviewers based on giving skills and feedback |
| 1977 | Smith & Glass | Meta-Analysis of Psychotherapy Outcome Studies | Used meta-analysis techniques to describe the effectiveness of psychotherapy |

*(continued)*

TABLE 2.1 | A SAMPLING OF CLASSIC RESEARCH IN THERAPEUTIC COUNSELING (CONTINUED)

| Date | Author(s) | Title | Contribution |
|------|-----------|-------|--------------|
| 1985 | Gelso & Carter | The Relationship in Counseling and Psychotherapy | Definitively reviewed literature related to components and processes of the relationship in counseling |
| 1989 | Heppner & Claiborn | Social Influence Research | Reviewed and critiqued studies dealing with power in counseling |
| 1992 | McNamee & Gergen | Therapy as Social Construction | Compiled major contributions to constructivist approach to counseling |
| 1994 | Dawes | House of Cards | Challenged clinical assumptions and treatment methods currently in use |
| 1995 | Rennie | Clients' Deference in Psychotherapy | Representative of "grounded theory" in qualitative research to study client experience |
| 1997 | Hill & others | A Guide to Conducting Consensual Qualitative Research | Provided methodological standards for gathering qualitative data |
| 1998 | Gottman & others | Predicting Marital Happiness and Stability | Studied the interactional patterns in newlyweds to predict likelihood of divorce |

how the counseling profession developed and grew over time. Furthermore, as consumers of research, counselors must be capable of critical analysis of the various methodologies, statistical procedures, arguments, and conclusions of their professional literature. This analysis will not only provide you with useful knowledge but will also train you to think analytically, intentionally, and systematically about problems.

Third is the means to conduct systematic studies on topics that have professional meaning to you as a student and as a professional counselor. By understanding that research can be quite focused and can be done using a small population, practitioners who want to determine effectiveness in their work environment can proceed to engage in systematic study. Once research is understood and demystified, many practitioners recognize ways to use applied and descriptive research to help in their daily work (Heppner, Kivlighan, & Wampold, 1998; La Fountain & Bartos, 2001).

You will be expected, before becoming a professional counselor, to have a good working knowledge of basic research skills in addition to your counseling skills. At the very minimum, you must be able pose good research questions, to use clear definitions of terms, to understand sources of confusion and ambiguity and how they may be controlled, to be aware of problems associated with observation and measurement, to understand the value of documentation in the literature, and, above all, to be knowledgeable about the process of research and be motivated to learn more about it throughout your professional life.

# BECOMING AN INFORMED CONSUMER OF RESEARCH

As a student, you may be thinking, you will probably never do any research once you are out of school. Based on the experience of many practicing counselors, you are probably right, as it is relatively rare that practitioners conduct and publish studies after they have completed their training (Heppner & Anderson, 1985). Even if you never conduct your own studies, you will still be required to understand research publications in order to engage in the best and most current practices of the profession. Studying and understanding research methodology and analyses will assist you in reading and synthesizing the volumes of manuscripts published every year. You will be able to determine whether certain interventions, although statistically significant in a research article, are actually meaningful and likely to work with your specific client populations (Ogles, Lunnen, & Bonesteel, 2001).

Consider yourself fairly warned: Counseling is sometimes a very lonely profession. Much of the time is spent alone in your office, insulated from the rest of the world. You are cut off from all distractions, separated from those you care most about, and immersed totally in the world of other persons in great pain who demand your total attention. Furthermore, counseling work can become stale and predictable after a period of time. After seeing a hundred kids who won't go to class, or a hundred men who won't express feelings to their partners, or a hundred women who feel trapped in their lives, many of the issues may seem the same. One of the ways that counselors are able to remain energized in their work is by creating a larger audience for their experimental efforts. It is one thing to help a single person, or even a dozen people with a similar problem, but if you can publicize your systematic work in such a way that others may have access to your data, you will not feel so isolated; you will be part of a larger community of scholars and practitioners who pool their efforts to make sense of what is going on in their offices.

Every time you read about a new technique or model, you will use your knowledge of results to evaluate the probability of success in your work situation. Being knowledgeable about research will assist you in reading critically and evaluating the quality of the published results. You will be able to determine whether the outcomes are descriptive, important, significant, and most important, useful to you.

As a member of professional associations, you will receive many journals and other literature. You will hear presentations and attend workshops where new ideas will be presented. You will participate in discussions on the Internet. With a basic knowledge of research, you will be able to ask penetrating questions and determine whether the ideas are based on sound scientific principles.

Just as importantly, research training will prepare you to *plan* what you intend to do with your clients, *discover* what others have done under similar circumstances, *measure* the impact of your interventions, and *publicize* what occurred so that others can learn from your mistakes and successes.

# SUMMARY

Counseling is an interdisciplinary profession that has evolved from fields such as education, philosophy, medicine, and social sciences. Although all helping professionals share similarities in what they do, such as their emphasis on the therapeutic relationship, their interest in fostering client growth, and their use of interpersonal skills and research methodology, there are also several important distinctions. The counseling profession is unique in that we (1) work toward prevention rather than the remediation of problems, (2) follow a developmental rather than a psychopathological model of assessment and treatment, (3) attempt to intervene in relatively short time periods rather than establish lengthier treatments, and (4) specialize in helping people through normal life transitions and adjustments rather than only during times of major dysfunction.

Although the power and rights that we have earned through legislative acts are still not where most of us would like them to be, therapeutic counselors now enjoy an unprecedented degree of professional autonomy and respect.

# SELF-GUIDED EXPLORATIONS

1. Who are the characters and personages from history—in the arts, literature, science, religion, politics, social science, and education—who have been most inspirational to you? How have they influenced your development?

2. You find yourself in a social situation in which a number of other helping professionals (a psychiatrist, psychologist, and social worker) begin to demean what counselors can do versus what these other professionals are trained to do. Set them straight by explaining how your profession makes a unique and significant contribution.

3. Describe a piece of research that you find especially meaningful and relevant to your life. What is it about this study that you most appreciate?

4. If you were going to do an original research study that is driven by a strong personal motive of yours or related to an ongoing issue in your life, what would you choose to look at? How would you carry out the study?

5. The research and counseling processes parallel one another in that you (1) become aware that a problem exists; (2) collect relevant background information; (3) study the literature related to the problem; (4) define the variables that are involved; (5) design an intervention; (6) generate hypotheses as to what you think will happen; (7) institute the plan; (8) evaluate results; (9) discuss the larger significance of what you learned; and (10) suggest areas for further study.

Applying this same process to a real-life issue in your life, fill in as many of the steps as you can:

1. Awareness of problem
2. Relevant background
3. Related literature
4. Defined variables
5. Planned intervention
6. Hypotheses
7. Action plan
8. Predicted results
9. Significance of study
10. Areas for further study

## For Homework:

Go to the library and look through the professional journals in the field. To start out, you might consider the general ones such as: *Journal of Counseling and Development, American Psychologist, Counseling Psychologist, Psychotherapy, Canadian Journal of Counselling*, and *Psychotherapy Networker*. Next, consider those journals most relevant to the work setting or specialty areas you are considering. Because there are hundreds of such publications, you might consult with your instructor for recommendations.

Based on your brief survey, what are your initial impressions of the status research plays in counseling practice?

## SUGGESTED READINGS

Bankart, C. P. (1997). *Talking cures: A history of Western and Eastern psychotherapies*. Pacific Grove, CA: Brooks/Cole.

Beers, C. (1945). *A mind that found itself*. New York: Doubleday.

Freidman, D. K. (1992). *History of psychotherapy: A century of change*. Washington, DC: American Psychological Association.

Heppner, P. P. (Ed.). (1991). *Pioneers in counseling and development: Personal and professional perspectives*. Alexandria, VA: American Counseling Association.

Heppner, P. P., Kivlighan, D. M., & Wampold, B. E. (1998). *Research design in counseling*. Pacific Grove, CA: Wadsworth.

Hubble, M. A., Duncan, B. L., & Miller, S. D. (Eds.)(1999). *The heart and soul of change: What works in therapy*. Washington, DC: American Psychological Association.

La Fountain, R. M., & Bartos, R. B. (2001). *Research and statistics made meaningful in counseling and student affairs with Infotrac*. Pacific Grove, CA: Brooks/Cole.

McLeod, J. (2001). *Qualitative research in counseling and psychotherapy*. Thousand Oaks, CA: Sage.

Tryon, G. S. (2002). *Counseling based on process research: Applying what we know*. Boston: Allyn & Bacon.

# 3

# SETTINGS FOR COUNSELING

KEY CONCEPTS

**Professional Identity**

**Generic Skills**

**Mediation**

**Developmental Orientation**

**Remedial Orientation**

**Flexible Specialty**

**Managed Care**

# SETTINGS FOR COUNSELING

# CHAPTER 3

STUDENT: Where can I work after I get my counseling degree?

PROFESSOR: Nowhere and everywhere.

STUDENT: Huh?

PROFESSOR: You're feeling confused and frustrated because the question is more complex than you thought.

STUDENT: Actually, I'm angry because you're evading my question with that active listening stuff.

PROFESSOR: What would you like to do with your degree?

STUDENT: See what I mean? There you go again.

PROFESSOR: Okay. The reason I answered your question the way I did is that I wanted to be honest with you.

STUDENT: Yes. I appreciate that. But I'm putting all this time and work into my studies. I have a right to know what my degree will qualify me to do.

PROFESSOR: Yes, you have a right to know. You will see very few job openings in the paper under the heading "Counselor." Very few people—employers, friends, or family—will know what a counselor is qualified to do, especially when compared to a "therapist," "psychologist," and "psychiatrist."

STUDENT: This I already know. I looked in the Yellow Pages under "Counselor" and found astrologers, dieticians, palm readers, personal coaches, finance companies, and employment agencies—not to mention the usual assortment of mystics and guidance people.

PROFESSOR: That's true. However, there are also a number of fairly specific slots for counselors to fit in and a virtually unlimited market for creative professionals to develop needed services. Although your degree does not necessarily qualify you to do one particular job, there are a hundred different ways that you could put your training to work.

STUDENT: But outside of school counselors and ministers and perhaps a crisis center, college dormitory, or probation department, I've never heard of any other places where counselors can work. I mean, we're not exactly like psychiatrists—everyone knows what they do and where they are supposed to work.

PROFESSOR: That's just it. Counselors aren't as limited to working in specific settings, such as hospitals or clinics, or with specific populations, such as the personality disordered or psychotic. Counselors work with people in so many different places, from playgrounds to corporate boardrooms.

STUDENT: I know I'm supposed to get better at dealing with ambiguity and abstractions, but couldn't you be a little more specific?

PROFESSOR: Sure. But the possibilities that I name are limited by my own meager imagination. Counselors create jobs for themselves in industry, for example. It's relatively easy to convince corporate executives that profit can be increased if morale is improved among workers. We've had graduates hired to reduce absenteeism, drug abuse, and interpersonal conflicts in companies. Sometimes they also get jobs in public relations or personnel offices. In fact, what training could possibly be better for people in management at any level? Counseling teaches you to be sensitive to others' feelings, to respect their rights, and to selectively reinforce productive behavior. You learn to confront people nondefensively, to stimulate creativity, and to encourage growth at all levels. You tell me where counselors could work.

STUDENT: I just thought about all the creative roles counselors could play in a hospital, for instance. Patients don't exactly feel good about being there. Maybe a counselor-at-large could help prepare people psychologically for their operations.

PROFESSOR: Exactly. Graduates have been hired to do just that. Counselors also work as part of teams in other settings. They work with medical personnel in mental health clinics, with teachers, with attorneys, and with administrators. They work everywhere and anywhere that they can persuade people their services are helpful.

STUDENT: Now I'm really confused. How can I possibly decide which direction I should go in?

One of the major changes in the field over the last decades has been the increasing opportunities for counselors to work in a variety of settings. As the population ages, as technology and cultural changes occur more rapidly, and as people face greater stress in their lives, the need for counselors is growing in a variety of settings. Whereas once upon a time counselors only worked in schools, then moved into agency and institutional positions previously reserved for psychologists and social workers, now counselors have carved out additional territory of their own that makes it possible to offer help in diverse places.

In addition to the traditional settings in which counselors have worked (schools and community agencies), new specialties are emerging in private practice, consultation, personal coaching, the criminal justice system, and technologically-based interventions. As never before, practitioners are finding jobs in rehabilitation, substance abuse, the mental health system, student personnel, industry, and a hundred other areas. Even more innovative, counselors are finding more and more ways to use the telephone, videophone, and Internet to operate in more efficient and convenient ways (Masi & Freedman, 2001). There really are almost limitless possibilities for employment depending on the imagination, resources, and motivation of the counselor.

## WHAT COUNSELORS HAVE IN COMMON

The needs and requirements of a particular environment determine, at least in part, the adaptations and behavior of organisms in that setting. As Charles Darwin discovered in his travels, a staggering variety of species have successfully adapted to their environments—twenty thousand different butterflies, forty kinds of parrots, and three hundred species of hummingbirds. There is also potentially an endless variety of counselors, each species having successfully adapted to the demands of the work environment. Every client population, geographical area, cultural heritage, institutional policy, physical facility, and psychological climate subtly shapes a new species of counselor. It is even difficult, on the basis of the everyday practice of professionals, to recognize that they are nevertheless members of the same evolutionary family. Even so, there are probably more similarities than differences among therapeutic counselors in various settings. Before we explore the roles of counselors in the places where they work, it will be helpful to review what they all share in common.

### A Unique Identity

All counselors, irrespective of their work settings, identify themselves as part of a shared profession that is distinguished from other helping disciplines. Counseling is not the same as social work, psychology, guidance, psychiatry, or education—even though those other professionals often practice counseling in some form. Each field, however similar in its methods and goals, arises out of quite different settings. Psychiatry is a specialty of medicine. Social work came from the streets, psychology from the university, and counseling from the schools. In spite of their recent trends toward convergence, each helping profession is indelibly marked by its birthplace.

### Many Different Roles

Counselors have varied roles, regardless of the setting in which they practice. These may be grouped into several categories.

## VOICE FROM THE FIELD

I think that all counselors have to struggle with the same disturbing need to find balance in our lives. My "caretaker" role tends to get out of control sometimes. I get so overinvested in the lives of my clients that if I'm not constantly vigilant, I begin to lose focus. The boundary between myself and them becomes confused.

I find in my personal life, as well, that I restrict my self-expression and spend a lot of time trying to make sure people know that I'm human, too. I have a circle of friends who believe I'm always trying to analyze them, or in some way do my "counselor thing" with them, and the truth is that I do. This sets me apart in ways that I like and don't like.

1. *Individual assessment* comprises observation, information seeking, and interpretation of a person's behavior in areas that include performance, achievement, aptitude, personality, and interests. The results of assessment are valuable for screening, placement, diagnosis, evaluation, and planning of treatment approaches.
2. *Individual counseling* consists of those one-to-one interactions with clients in which the therapeutic process is applied to resolving personal concerns, career and educational decisions, and problems of human adjustment. More and more, counselors are called on to initiate brief interventions that very quickly and efficiently change attitudes and behavior.
3. *Family counseling* focuses on the interaction patterns that lead to dysfunctional behavior. By thinking in terms of the family system to which a client belongs, the counselor is able to intervene by understanding and changing communication patterns and coalitions of power.
4. *Group work* structures may be used to accomplish more efficiently the goals of individual counseling. Participants have the added advantages of interaction. Counselors also work in guidance groups in which they serve a more active role, designing educational exploration experiences, providing information, and stimulating personal awareness and growth.
5. *Consultation* activities involve initiating changes on an organizational level, often by working on program development. Counselors consult with the human and organizational components of systems to help the individual parts make a more unified whole. Counselors, as human relations specialists, will intervene to fix or prevent the problems that arise from interpersonal conflict. In recent times, consultation roles have been expanded to include "coaching" activities as well as traditional therapeutic relationships (Williams & Davis, 2002).
6. *Mediation* is used to help couples, business partners, or others involved in a disagreement settle their differences in an expedient and respectful way. Although this activity is often initiated at the recommendation of the court during divorce, child custody, or civil disputes, mediation can be employed as a form of structured conflict resolution and problem solving

in a variety of situations. Other forms of mediation focus primarily on helping people to understand one another and make compromises that are mutually acceptable (Winslade & Monk, 2000).

7. *Administration* plays a part in many counselors' work; it involves directing the activities of a school, agency, or organization. Public relations, quality control, fund-raising, the conducting of meetings, paperwork processing, and decision making are major components of this kind of work.

8. *Supervision* is a significant role of experienced practitioners in helping those who are less capable. The counselor may conduct in-service workshops and provide individual or group supervision sessions that may be either emotionally or behaviorally focused. Responsibility for staff training and development may also include attention to improving morale.

9. *Computer technology* is now a crucial aspect of the counselor's daily life that includes using chat rooms, distance therapy, online self-help groups, web-based programming, and Internet communications (Hsiung, 2001). Practitioners are expected to be literate enough not only to take care of word processing functions—to write reports and take care of correspondence—but also to handle other routine matters. For example, school counselors use computers to handle all record keeping and scheduling, and mental health counselors use software packages that help with diagnosis and case management. Almost all counselors are required to be fluent enough with the Internet and Web that they can access needed information and communicate with colleagues.

10. *Research* is an important part of measuring professional effectiveness. Counselors are frequently required to justify their existence and to demonstrate to funding agencies, regulatory commissions, citizens' advisory groups, and boards of trustees that they are earning their salaries. Research is also crucial in communicating the results of experimentation to other professionals so the field can continue to grow.

## A Set of Generic Skills

Regardless of their work settings, theoretical orientation, training program, and client population, counselors all use the same intervention skills. A later chapter will review in detail these universal helping skills that are employed by all human service personnel.

Counseling skills are divided into several broad categories:

1. *Diagnostic skills* involve questioning and assessment strategies to figure out what is going on with a client and formulate a plan for being helpful.

2. *Exploration skills* are used to understand the client's world and collect needed information that will be helpful in later efforts.

3. *Relationship skills* work to build a supportive alliance with clients that is conducive to openness, trust, and respect.

4. *Understanding skills* help to promote self-awareness and deep-level investigations into the nature of presenting concerns and their larger meaning.

## VOICE FROM THE FIELD

I'm working with a woman today whose 71-year-old mother is dying of uterine cancer and her 78-year-old father is binge drinking to cope with his grief. This woman is recently divorced, separated from her children, and away from her home and her friends while she tends to her parents. As if that isn't enough, she just learned that she too has cancer. She is depressed and overwhelmed.

In a situation like this, my role as a counselor is somewhat fluid. I have to pull out all the stops. I am a social worker, a psychologist, a mother, a trainer, a friend, a janitor, a nurse, a spiritual advisor, a shoulder, an ear, and a counselor. This may not be typical, but "typical" around here tends to be redefined frequently. You just have to be fluid to go with the flow.

---

5. *Action skills* help translate identified problem areas and new understanding into sequential steps toward desired goals.
6. *Group process skills* are employed in family, organizational, and consultation settings to resolve conflicts and work toward team objectives.
7. *Evaluation skills* are used to measure the effects of intervention efforts and, if necessary, make adjustments.

The use of these generic skills is by no means limited to counselors; however, we tend to depend on them as a basis for initiating the counseling process and developing an effective counseling relationship. In addition, counselors also use a wide variety of other specialized intervention skills, depending on theoretical preferences.

## A Set of Common Goals

Goals that are common to all counselors and that serve to clarify professional identity include helping clients to:

1. Work constructively toward life/career planning
2. Anticipate, plan, and react constructively to developmental issues and transitions
3. Integrate thinking, feeling, and behavior into a congruent expression of self
4. Respond productively to stress and reduce its negative impact on their lives
5. Develop effective interpersonal skills so that relationships with peers, family, and colleagues can have constructive potential
6. Assess strengths and identify weaknesses so that they may develop more personal awareness
7. Become aware of the holistic nature of life and integrate effective principles of living into psychological, physical, and social aspects of their lives
8. Develop more choices in their lives, with accompanying skills to make constructive decisions
9. Become independent of the counseling in the shortest time possible

■ | VOICE FROM THE FIELD

One of the things I love best about my job is that I get to do so many different things in any given day. Today I spent a few hours in the morning leading a group, then working on a grant that I'm writing with two other colleagues. We're trying to generate some more funds that will free us up to continue doing outreach rather than just being stuck in our offices all day.

I've had jobs before where I was seeing client after client—six, seven, eight a day. Burnout city, if you ask me. As far as I'm concerned, the more variety of things I can do, the more stimulation I feel in my work. But I was so unprepared for this stuff. In my counseling program, I mostly learned how to do one-on-one counseling with reasonably cooperative people who were motivated to get help. What I wouldn't give for such a client now! The truth is that I don't do that much individual counseling anymore—almost all groups and family work. But I guess I got a good foundation to learn the rest on my own.

## Both Developmental and Remedial Orientation

Counselors are interested in and trained for helping individuals to anticipate issues and concerns, develop adaptive life skills, respond constructively to issues and problems, and work toward psychological growth and increased personal mastery. Counselors choose and prize their role because of its orientation toward life/skill development, with an emphasis on improved problem-solving abilities and decision-making skills, as opposed to an orientation that focuses exclusively on diagnosis, evaluation, and remediation.

Although counselors can and do use their knowledge of personality theory, psychopathology, and emotional dysfunctions to work therapeutically, they often focus on prevention of problems before they become severe. Counselors tend to distinguish themselves as well-trained experts working with those who don't necessarily have severe symptoms. As I mentioned previously, many counselors operate within the mental health system doing remedial work. The principal advantage of counseling practitioners, in contrast to social workers, psychologists, and psychiatrists, is that they can help people who aren't stigmatized as dysfunctional. One need not be "sick" or "mentally ill" to seek the services of a professional counselor, whereas insurance regulations specifically mandate to the other professions that there must be evidence of a medically defensible diagnosis of mental illness or a significant disturbance of conduct before treatment can be administered.

The role of the counselor is not to instruct but to stimulate the natural growth and potential inherent in human beings (Ivey, 1991). As persons develop, they have the capability to initiate, expand, and maintain psychological growth. In fact, many (Broderick & Blewitt, 2003; Neugarten, 1968; Newman & Newman, 1999; Schlossberg, 1984; Sheehy, 1995) consider this capacity to be an essential feature of adult development. The crystallization of a client's irreconcilable conflict and the client's resulting discomfort are tools

## VOICE FROM THE FIELD

I have the same goals with almost all the kids I see. Of course, each of them comes in for a different reason and purpose. Sometimes they're having problems keeping up with class, or fighting with their parents, or maybe they're just depressed. Regardless, though, of why they come in, I still think they need a good dose of reality testing.

I try to teach each child I see the same basic messages—things like whining and complaining won't change anything, being alone sucks, causing trouble is entertaining but has certain consequences—that sort of thing. It's not that I'm unwilling to address whatever problems they bring in; it's just that I think every one of them needs to learn a few basic lessons. I think all counselors do this, whether they admit it or not.

---

often used by counselors. The client can resolve that anxiety by moving to a more mature developmental stage, which will allow for an integration of the conflict and subsequent reduction in personal discomfort.

Counselors rely heavily on the work of developmental theorists as they attempt to stimulate clients to initiate developmentally relevant growth. Developmental work focuses on client issues and may include psychosexual development (Freud, 1924), cognitive development (Piaget, 1926), psychosocial development (Erikson, 1950), career development (Super, 1957), moral development (Kohlberg, 1969), ego development (Loevinger, 1976) cultural identity development (Sue, Ivey, & Pedersen, 1996), or gender development (Basow, 1992), among many possibilities.

This core of knowledge may be described as follows:

1. Human development proceeds in a series of stages leading to increasingly complex behaviors.
2. These stages are invariant and sequential.
3. They are both genetically determined and adaptive to the culture and environment.
4. The stages alternate between periods of well-adjusted equilibrium and periods of unstable disequilibrium.
5. Growth may be encouraged by stimulating a person to restore equilibrium at a higher stage of development.
6. Wide differences in development are possible depending on the person's gender and cultural identity.
7. During adulthood, development becomes more cyclical rather than linear as people face life transitions and crises.

During counseling sessions, a practitioner employing a developmental model might be thinking something along the following lines:

This young man is 14 years old. He seems to be functioning at about age level in physical development but is considerably under expected norms in the areas of social and emotional functioning. I wonder when this lag first began to be noticeable? I must remember to check that out later.

I notice my approval seems especially important to him. Hopefully, that should give me some leverage to push him to take more responsibility for his inappropriate behavior. If I can encourage him to take some risks with me here, maybe I could get him to do the same with his parents and teachers. He seems to be perfectly capable, for instance, of controlling his anger when he has advance notice that he will be disappointed; it is surprises that throw him for a loop. I wonder how I can help him to stretch himself a bit in that area?

The work of the counselor is to help the client translate immediate issues of concern into a relevant developmental framework so the necessary growth can be identified and initiated. Pragmatically applying developmental theory, the counselor seeks to stimulate client growth toward successive stages of human maturity.

## Teamwork

A counselor rarely works alone; most counselors work in institutional or clinical settings as part of a team that is responsible for a range of activities or services, only one aspect of which is counseling. For example, many counselors work in business and industry settings, helping employees with personal, marriage, career, or substance abuse problems that can affect their work attitudes and productivity. There the counselors frequently consult their manager, as well as supervisors, union representatives, personnel department representatives, and others in the work environment. The counselor is a vital member of a team and strives to work in concert with colleagues to advance institutional goals and provide help to individual employees. Counselors also maintain an active professional liaison with community agencies, mental health clinics, and so on.

The same pattern holds true in most other settings as well. Whether counselors work in school, agency, community, or private practice settings, they function as specialists in resource identification, consultation, and individual counseling.

## A DAY IN THE LIFE

One of the goals of this text is to provide you with "voices from the field" that illustrate realistically how counselors apply their knowledge and skills in daily situations that you will face. Perhaps this can best be demonstrated if you had an idea of what a typical day was like for practitioners who operate in a variety of different settings. What follows is a realistic glimpse of counselors in each of several traditional and nontraditional roles, including a sampling of the frustrations and problems as well as their excitement and satisfaction.

These narratives are not intended to represent all practitioners who work within this specialty, or in this setting, but rather to give you a sampling of what life is like for professionals in the trenches. When you conduct your own "field studies" you can augment these stories with your own research. This will help you make some informed decisions about the aspects of the profession that you might like to investigate further.

# High School

At 7:25 A.M., when the counselor walks into his office, seven students are already waiting. Right away he knows why. There was a glitch in the computer yesterday, and third-hour English was double-loaded. The teacher about blew her fuse, but at least she has now settled down. As the counselor finishes rescheduling the last student 30 minutes later, he wonders what this activity has to do with counseling.

Scheduling classes not only is boring administrative work, but it also really eats up time, keeping him from getting to what he wants to be doing—working with kids and their problems. He makes a mental note to mention this concern in the afternoon meeting with the principal, knowing he won't even have the full support of the staff. Some of them actually prefer scheduling to counseling; they consider the work less demanding. The thought is depressing.

On the way to the attendance office to check on a student, he suddenly hears shouts and a commotion around the corner. Cringing, he moves toward the disturbance and finds two senior boys wrestling against a locker, each twice his size. Using what he hopes is his most authoritative voice, he pushes between them and manages with the help of another teacher to separate them. His heart sinks when he recognizes one of the offenders as a youngster for whom he went out on a limb two weeks ago—he was in danger of being suspended for fighting. Now this!

An hour later he feels better. The fighting business has been cleared up, and he has just finished a successful interview with a student whose parents have been pushing him toward a military career. It felt good to help him explore what he wants and to become more aware of his tendency to please his parents at all costs. The session seemed to be productive, and he felt confident that the student would make some changes.

His meeting with the principal is grim. Teachers, says she, are complaining because the counseling staff is overloading classes and allowing friends to alter their schedules so they can be together in their mischief. The counselor points out (once again) that class scheduling is administrative work and not the primary responsibility of the counseling department; further, if teachers are having discipline problems in their classes, they should consult with a counselor instead of complaining to the principal.

Lunch provides a needed break. A teacher stops by and suggests that they get together to talk about his frustrations with his job and hassles with the department chair. The talk with him seems to help. Sometimes the informal sessions over lunch seem to make more difference than all the appointments during the week.

The counselor tries to keep the afternoons open for working with kids. He has two appointments and will finish the day with a group. But he is worried

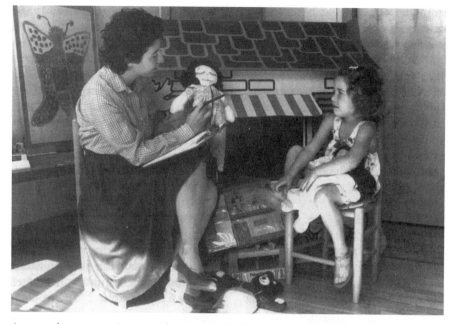

A counselor communicates with a 3-year-old child about her concerns through the use of play therapy techniques. Michael Weisbrot/Stock Boston.

about the first appointment—a 17-year-old senior who is depressed and extremely worried about smoking too much marijuana. The session is taxing, and he reflects on how difficult it is to work with kids having drug problems. The last individual appointment is a bonus. He has been working with this girl for four months now and can really see the difference. The girl has overcome her shyness, is involved in extracurricular activities, and reports a much improved relationship with her parents. She even has a boyfriend. At the finish of the session, the counselor feels great. As he is leaving for the group, the secretary motions urgently. An irate parent is on the phone demanding an explanation for her son's suspension. She's really hot. The counselor calms her down and makes an appointment to see her after school.

Now for the group: Today's topic is love. As always, he is amazed at how sensitive the kids are and how they really do confront each other as they interact. They know what honesty means.

Hurrying to meet with the irate parent, the counselor reflects on his day. It is the variety of different things he does that most stimulates him. He just can't imagine being stuck in an office all day.

## Private Practice

Through the groggy dream mist, the counselor struggled toward alertness, finally achieving enough to figure out to whom she was talking and what the situation was. She calmed the man down and firmly instructed him to take a

## VOICE FROM THE FIELD                    By Brent Bandhauer

My day starts with three phone messages taped to my door. The first call was from a parent who was worried that her ex-husband was coming to school too much. Usually he comes into my office on the pretense he's there to talk about his son, but then he tells me about all the horrible things his ex-wife does. I'm pretty sure I'm being groomed so he can count on my support in an upcoming custody hearing.

The next call was from the mom of a second grader. She was single too, but only because her husband was killed last Saturday by a drunk driver. She was wondering if she should take her children to the funeral and what she could do to make all this easier for them. I explained that in most cases children need to be part of the grieving process. They might later resent the fact that they weren't allowed to be there. I gave her some information about how children of different ages respond to death and the younger ones often won't understand the permanence. I assured her that I would include her son in my grief and loss group.

I went back to my office for some solitude. It wasn't even an hour into the day and I was feeling overwhelmed. Usually I don't feel overwhelmed until about noon. I opened a pack of mini-donuts when I was called to the emotionally disabled class. I dread such calls because it means one of the students is having a tantrum and kicking or fighting someone. I wonder why a counselor is called to calm an out-of-control student down?

I was going to eat one of my donuts, but I noticed that I was five minutes late to a class-guidance lesson and I didn't have a lesson plan ready. I grabbed my puppets since they are usually a hit with the children and I can use them to teach conflict resolution strategies to students of any age level. I got to the class and discovered a substitute. The students cheered when I walked in which was flattering, but it was much louder than if their teacher would have been there. They cheered as I walked all the way up to the front of the room and continued to cheer even as I tried to gather their attention. Finally after I gave my angriest look, which isn't very scary, they quieted down.

On my way back to my office, I decided to check my referral box. It was stuffed full. Three of them were from a student who comes in almost weekly, and two of them were from children who are already in groups, so I threw them away. The other seven were legitimate requests to come in. I added them to my list, which made nineteen individual students I wanted to see in the next two days. Overwhelmed again.

In the hallway I came across a student who had been kicked out of class. I sat down next to him and asked what he was doing out there and he told me his teacher had sent him there for no good reason. I told him I didn't know his teacher could be so mean and he smiled and said, "Yup." I worked with him to help him recognize that he could spend the rest of the day trying to get even with the teacher or he could find a way to try to get along.

After lunch, I went outside to play basketball. I try to stack the teams so the students who can't play are on my team while the other team has students who play a lot. This way I get to actually play hard in order to keep the scores even.

It was time to go to the class where the second grader lost his father. I began by asking the class what they knew. They all started to tell me about how they, too, had lost a family member. Lots of grandparents. Several dogs. A desert tortoise. And a rabbit. A couple of students seemed to feel left out and they said that their great, great grandfathers had died even before they were born.

I was getting a bit frustrated because I was trying to lead them to a point where they would suggest making the grieving boy a welcome-back card. But they just kept adding more and more people to the list of people who died. Then it occurred to me that they might be revealing hurts and that I was the one being honored with their disclosures. You see, I really strive to be available to students by hanging out on the playground, going into classrooms a lot, and being outside before and after school. Students are forever calling to me outside and in the halls, giving me great big genuine smiles when they see me, and wanting to be the one I come to their class for. I almost take it for granted that children are supposed to share personal hurts, big worries, fears, family turmoil, and love with me that I forget how important little bits of information might just be. Kids who I

*continued*

don't even remember their names come and give me a hug as if I were a favorite uncle.

I decided it didn't matter if I made it back to my office to open another pack of donuts or if I missed my afternoon class-guidance lessons. I was right where I needed to be. It took an hour before they finally stumbled on the idea of making cards. I spent the rest of the day reading cards and watching stu-

dents draw pictures of the people they cared about. The cards turned out to be heart-felt messages of concern not so much because they were worried about the boy, but because they were expressing their own feelings of loss and healing.

You can tell that I'm extremely proud to be a school counselor. I go to work happy every day because I'm loved by a whole bunch of little children.

---

hot bath, try to relax, and write his feelings down on paper. She scheduled an appointment for him the next day and then tried to go back to sleep.

The counselor has now arrived at her office, which she shares with other professionals in private practice—a few social workers, a psychologist, and a part-time psychiatrist. Her 9:00 A.M. client already sits in the waiting room, but first she returns her telephone messages. One call is from a client who wants to cancel her appointment in the middle of the day. The counselor doesn't know whether to feel disappointed because it is too late to fill that spot or relieved because now she has an unanticipated but needed break to catch up on her paperwork. Next she calls a physician whom she has been trying to reach for months, hoping to arrange a lunch meeting and discuss possible referrals. He is out of his office. Finally, she calls an insurance company that has been refusing to authorize payment for services she has already provided.

The first of six clients for the day then enters her office. The client is relatively easy to work with, is highly motivated, pays her bills on time, and will make rapid progress. The counselor struggles with herself during the session because they have just successfully completed working on the originally stated problem. The client feels great. Her marriage has stabilized. But she wants to continue the sessions. The counselor reinforces the idea that one can never have enough counseling but silently wonders if she is saying that because she means it or because she needs the money. It is such a pain for her to get new referrals.

Yet she feels so proud of her work, her competence, her ability to make a difference in people's lives. In private practice there is the constant pressure to become more skilled at helping; if not, the clients won't return or send their friends. And all over the community she can see the results of her efforts. Her reputation is slowly beginning to build.

Two more clients in the morning, then lunch; she loves the freedom of answering only to herself and decides to do some shopping and visit with a friend. She goes back to the office and an hour of paperwork—progress notes, correspondence, forms. A new referral calls, but the counselor can't persuade her to come in for an appointment because there are financial difficulties. This woman works for a company that uses a managed care system with which the counselor thus far refuses to work: "First, they will only authorize four sessions—and at bargain rates. Then, just maybe, if the client is in the throes of a nervous breakdown, they might grant another four sessions. They've got to be kidding!"

A few colleagues are free, so they have a cup of coffee together and chat about their day. One colleague in particular is feeling much stress because he has just had a draining session with a client skilled at playing games. It's back to work.

The counselor makes a few more calls, including one seeking referrals from a school system and one offering an in-service program for staff on stress management. The company agrees to let her make a presentation. She feels ecstatic: at last, a breakthrough. Then she makes a follow-up call to an ex-client who is still doing quite well and appreciates the counselor's continuing concern.

The clients file through until early evening. She feels exhausted after so many consecutive sessions. "Is the money worth all the energy it takes?" she wonders as she puts the finishing touches on her case notes. "But it is lucrative, and the freedom is wonderful, at least until the managed care system takes over completely. I like being an important part of so many people's lives, and I especially appreciate not having to answer to a boss."

## Preschool

The counselor arrives at work to find a 3-year-old hiding under a picnic table, surrounded by two teachers and his parents, all urging him to come out. Instead he screams "Never!" and continues to cry. The counselor reassures the parents, sends them off to work, and disperses the crowd of children and teachers. She then crawls under the table and sits silently for ten minutes, until the child halts his tears long enough to ask why the counselor is acting silly by sitting under a table. Without hesitation the counselor replies simply that she is a little scared today, and angry at her parents for dumping her off, and this seems like as good a place as any to hide. The 3-year-old understands immediately, nods his head, and tells the counselor that he'll pay extra attention to her today so she won't feel so lonely. He then crawls out and joins the other kids in the sandbox as if this entrance were a natural beginning to a day of school. The counselor, too, crawls out but makes her way to the morning staff meetings that she will direct in planning the day's psychological education.

After the play activities for the day have been discussed, the counselor reviews the past week's discipline problems—how they were managed and how they could have been handled differently. She reports on the outcomes of various conferences she conducted with children and their parents, then makes specific recommendations to the teachers about strategies that might be helpful in the future: "When Alice throws a temper tantrum, it is best to isolate her calmly in the 'time-out' room." "Pay special attention to Brian—give him lots of hugs today because his father beat him last night." "Don't let Jennifer test you."

As the art classes begin, the counselor works on test evaluations of the children's aptitude strengths and weaknesses, detailing plans for each child. She then spends some time with the director going over administrative chores before an appointment with parents.

The mother and father of a particularly disturbed child show up twenty minutes late and then proceed to pick at each other about whose fault it was. When the counselor tries to intervene, they turn on her and then launch into an abusive tirade against the school, the teachers, and especially the counselor for being responsible for their child's problems. They decide to pull the child out of the school, and they march up to him while he is occupied on the swings, grab him by the neck, and yell at him all the way to the car. As the child cries for his friends, the parents start arguing again about who is responsible for their having such a screwed-up kid. They spank the child for good measure, throw him into the back seat, and drive off.

Another child sees the counselor fuming, with tears in her eyes, and invites her to play on the slide. They talk about what just happened, and other children ask questions about why parents sometimes get so mad. When the kids resume their play, the counselor excuses herself to break up a fight.

The counselor is exhausted; the children are still literally running circles around her. She mobilizes her energy for the afternoon parent-education class she teaches. Eleven participants attend, almost all of them single parents who have concerns about their effectiveness. She rates the class only "fair" because she feels so tired, and a few parents are unusually rigid in their beliefs and therefore reluctant to try anything new ("Spankings were good enough for me. Why the hell shouldn't they be good enough for our kids?"). While the counselor patiently explains the negative side effects of punishment, she sees the last of the kids departing. As their cute little legs scurry off, she wonders if she is really preventing any of them from having emotional problems in the future. "I sure would like to see them about twenty years from now," she thinks. "That's an idea! I think I'll talk to the director about organizing some follow-up research."

## Mental Health Center

The community mental health center is an oasis of support in an isolated rural area. The counselor is still apprehensive about fitting into a culture that is so foreign to his experiences as a city dweller. Yet in a tight economy he felt it a necessary adjustment to go where the work is—in this case, to a large organization of social workers, psychologists, psychiatrists, health educators, and counselors who service a three-county area populated mostly by farmers and factory workers.

The day begins with a planning session for his team. Predictably, the administrator once again reminds everyone to keep up with the paperwork. The counselor groans inwardly as he remembers the stack of progress notes and treatment plans that require his attention. He is then happily distracted by a proposal to do more outreach with the aged. He quickly volunteers to head up a study group to do a needs assessment in the community and prepare materials for several grant proposals. What a coup it would be to direct his own project, especially in such an important area as counseling older adults.

Various other staff members present their reports, all jockeying for power and more resources to run their individual projects. Although the counselor deplores the politics, the personality conflicts, and the interpersonal struggles, he nevertheless jumps in with both feet so he isn't left behind. The clinical director schedules supervision conferences. The medical director reviews the medications of several clients. Finally, a half hour late, the administrator closes the meeting with tips on appropriate conduct during the upcoming accreditation audit.

Finally the real fun starts. The counselor completes two counseling sessions before lunch, the first with a family of six, two of them teenagers whose strivings for independence are hard on all of them. The second session seems calm by comparison: A depressed man discloses the emptiness in his life and his frustration in trying to find a mate.

As the counselor joins several colleagues for lunch, he rethinks how to regain more control with the family. The food is lousy, but the conversation is always lively, usually centered on bits of gossip and different perspectives on particular cases. Before he can finish dessert, he is sidetracked by the assistant director, who wants to know if she can count on his support for proposed changes in promotion policy. The counselor gives an ambiguous response until he can figure out the political consequences of taking one side or the other during the fight. He decides to be neutral—the safest plan considering his own vulnerable position.

He rushes to a group session he has scheduled with seven teenagers to help them become more vocationally marketable; they are most cooperative, possibly because they get to leave school early for the experience. The counselor absolutely loves his groups—the energy is incredible. This week the kids spend time complaining about their parents' expectations. The counselor structures a successful role-playing activity in which they act like their parents, eventually realizing that complaining can sometimes be an expression of love.

The counselor has a bit of free time before his other appointments. He meets with his supervisor about the uncooperative family, then catches up on his paperwork. All is going well until he gets the day's phone messages. One of his clients decides to discontinue treatment—no explanation, just a phone call. Now he will have to do a bunch of paperwork and follow up to close the file. One afternoon appointment talks of depressing matters so intensely that the counselor notes that even he is starting to feel depressed: "This poor woman is going to be depressed her whole life, and there's probably nothing I can do but hold her hand. That *is* depressing. I've got to put this stuff behind me. My last client is waiting. I'm so glad I thought to schedule her at the end of the day. She'll be her usual entertaining, cheerful self. It feels so fine to know that I'm partially responsible for helping her to feel so good."

## Crisis Center

The day begins with a crisis: The coffee is all gone. The crises continue—staff will be short today, so the counselor must handle more calls. The first call is from a "regular customer," a gentleman who enjoys waking himself by masturbating over the phone. The counselor giggles, then remembers her training and quickly hangs up.

The next call is a routine referral to legal aid for divorce information; next, a kid who wants information about the Xanax his mother is taking. Then—crisis strikes. A boy calls and says he thinks he just killed himself. He sounds distraught, confused. He took a bunch of pills, but he doesn't know what kind. He doesn't care anyway. He just wants to die. He just wanted to say goodbye to someone, anyone; he has no one else. The counselor tries to get his address, but to no avail; he hangs up. The counselor starts trembling, but before she can talk her feelings through, the boy calls again. This time he's laughing, screams "Sucker!" and hangs up once again. With all the lambs crying wolf, how will she ever know for sure when the games and manipulation stop? She feels abused and disgusted.

Someone is asking for her in the lobby. It's an ex-client who just dropped in to say hello and give her a progress report: He is doing fantastically, thanks to her caring work. There is no time for reveling in the glory or bemoaning the fake calls—she is late for a program at the junior high school, where she is scheduled to give a talk on drugs.

The counselor spends an hour with the kids, giving accurate information, answering questions, and discussing her observations about how children are introduced to the drug scene. Afterward one teacher solicits her advice about what he can do to help prevent further problems in the school. A few appointments are then set up to meet with any kids who wish more information. She has several valuable encounters—helping one child to work on resisting the pressure of his peers to get high and helping another to realize how dangerous it was for him to be taking pills that he couldn't identify. The counselor next meets with the school counselors to lend assistance and lead an informal workshop on strategies for fighting drug abuse.

She returns to the crisis center, spends two more hours fielding mostly routine calls, then a half hour with her colleagues discussing the frustrating morning. They mutually decide, for their own protection, that it's better to stay more detached and neutral with their clients. The counselor also vows: "I must talk to myself harder so that I don't permit the few bad experiences to overshadow the productive work that I've been doing." The thought is interrupted by the jangling phone. It is a 74-year-old woman, frightened, alone; she just wants to make human contact. The counselor spends a half hour offering reassurance and then decides to invite her over so they can talk in person.

## Street Ministry

Sam is an ordained minister, but he does not have a church. Several years ago he decided to give up his pulpit so he could more intimately and effectively help disadvantaged people in their natural habitats. Based in a soup kitchen in a poor area, Sam works with the most impoverished and neglected population in his city. Because these people would never have come to him in his church, he has decided to reach out to them.

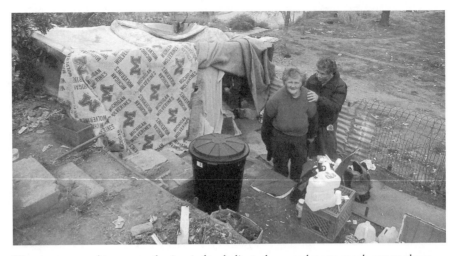

The greatest need in our profession is for dedicated counselors to reach out to those disadvantaged people who would not ordinarily seek out their services. © A. Ramey PhotoEdit, Inc.

Sam finds that most of his counseling training and religious instruction is more for his benefit than for his clients. Very little that worked in his nice, quiet office is helpful in the streets, where chaos, violence, and noise reign supreme. Yet the single most important thing of all that he remembers from his training—that without trust, compassion, and understanding, you have nothing—serves him well in his street ministry.

Because without food and shelter anything else he might do for his clients is irrelevant, Sam's first priority every morning is to help prepare and serve food to the throngs of people who are waiting for the doors of the soup kitchen to open. As he passes out bread, wipes off tables, and cleans dishes, he makes an effort to make contact with each and every person he encounters with a smile, a nod, a pat on the shoulder, a few words, or even a quick jibe. It is obvious that he is comfortable among his "congregation," and that they, in turn, have accepted him.

It is during this meal that he scans the room searching for his first client—someone in need to whom he can offer assistance. Sometimes people approach him wanting advice, a referral, or funds to feed or clothe their children, but usually he must initiate the contact. He sees a man huddled in the corner, his lip cut and cheek bruised, and escorts him to get medical attention.

On his walk back to the soup kitchen, he stops and talks to most every-one who will meet his eyes, joking, jostling, yet watching his back—the streets are a dangerous place, and he has already had more than his share of injuries while attempting to settle arguments or rescue a child from abuse. Finally he settles down on a stoop where people have learned to expect him. These are his "office hours" when he performs his most important service—referring people to places where they can get financial aid, medical attention, protective

## VOICE FROM THE FIELD

We buried one of our young people yesterday. Most likely a drug overdose. We organized the funeral and had a wake afterwards at the Center. He was a street kid who worked as a male prostitute.

I learned one major lesson yesterday. We had planned how each of the team would support a young person at the funeral and afterwards. What we didn't consider was how they would support each other and how much more significant that would be to them. So all the staff sat nearby, providing comfort when needed. I know it's an ancient image, but we looked like we were shepherds, calm and gentle shepherds, allowing the flock to move in a very large field, under the constant gaze of knowing and caring people. I realized at that moment how much support and comfort that young people can provide for one another if given the right opportunity and environment.

---

services, legal aid, or even college scholarships. Sam has developed a vast network of contacts he can draw on.

In the afternoon, with his own energy depleted by all the action, he tries to settle down with one person he can talk to—sometimes a runaway child or a pregnant teenager or a drug addict or a lonely elderly person. He has nobody standing over him telling him where he has to be; in his work, he wanders the streets doing whatever he can.

Sometimes at night, just before he falls into an exhausted slumber, he smiles to himself, feeling so good about what he is doing: counseling and helping the people nobody else cares about—the homeless and the poor who have given up hope of ever escaping their miserable existence. And yet there are other nights—sleepless ones—when he feels that he is just wasting his time—that he and a thousand others just like him couldn't put a dent in all that needs to be done.

The injured man he helped to get medical attention died two weeks later in another fight. The runaway girl he coaxed back home is now on the loose again—probably beginning her career as a prostitute. Yet Sam keeps offering soup and bread, a smile, and all the love he can give. He has nothing else to offer. And this is his calling.

## University Counseling Center

If there is one thing she enjoys most about her job in this medium-sized university, it is the diversity of her activities. Of course, there is also the excitement in being part of such a highly charged environment: young people in search of wisdom, identity, independence—and satisfying their raging hormones. But most of all she likes being part of a team in Student Services whose primary function is to facilitate the adjustment of students. And because most staff members are somewhat flexible (except for the vice president of Student Affairs, who can be a major pain), she has the opportunity to do so many things.

The bread and butter of her job description consists of the fairly routine task of helping confused students select a major (which they will probably change a few months later). Fortunately, with self-guided computer programs available, she can concentrate mostly on helping the students interpret and personalize what they have learned from the data they generated. She much prefers the group work that she does—conducting study-skills seminars; leading assertiveness training workshops; and offering seminars on HIV, drug abuse, and ethnic and cultural diversity.

Whereas her mornings are sometimes "political" (attending staff meetings, writing Student Services literature, talking to on-campus organizations), her afternoons are free to do what she enjoys. She sees several clients in fairly long-term counseling, and she especially appreciates these cases as a contrast to the relatively short-term problem solving she is often called on to participate in (with someone who is having trouble with a roommate, a parent, or a professor).

She carries a half-dozen intense counseling cases, for which she receives excellent supervision from a doctoral student who is doing an internship in the Counseling Center. This supervision (three hours per week) may be the best part of all (besides the free tuition to take any class she wants). These benefits are especially important to her, given the frustrations that are part of university life—the low salary, the power games among administrators fighting for their turf, and the repetitive nature of some of her duties.

For the seventh time this month she is on her way to conduct a human relations workshop for the resident assistants in the campus housing. Then she can hurry back for a session with one of her favorite clients. Her day will end with supervision, processing her active cases, and letting off steam about some of her frustrations.

## Counseling in Industry

Squeezed between a dozen other glass and steel structures is a building that resembles all the others. It is the corporate headquarters for a medium-sized manufacturing company that employs tens of thousands of people in the area—factory workers, skilled craftspeople, engineers, marketing and sales personnel, and administrative, financial, and support specialists.

In one suite of offices, tucked away in the back of the building and flanked by departments with signs reading "Human Resources" and "Affirmative Action," is an enigmatic label reading "Human Services." The services performed in this department are quite innovative for corporate environments.

Once it was discovered that employee morale and productivity could be increased and absenteeism could be reduced through certain support services, a number of progressive companies began hiring counselors to help their employees address personal problems that may interfere with their professional functioning. These problems may include drug and alcohol abuse, compulsive gambling, marriage and family problems, divorce adjustment, racial or sexual discrimination, developmental issues, career decision making, or conflicts in the workplace.

■ | VOICE FROM THE FIELD

My job as a rehabilitation counselor is to help people with closed head injuries—mostly accident and stroke victims—to learn to adjust psychologically to their disabilities and to work on morale to aid their recovery. I spend more time on the telephone dealing with insurance companies, medical specialists, and prospective employers than I do in face-to-face sessions with my clients.

During our planning session in the morning, we discuss cases in an interdisciplinary way so that we are clear on what role each of us will be playing in the patient's recovery process. I must say it's really fun to hear how other professionals apply their specialties—assessing areas of dysfunction, mapping out treatment programs, thinking through strategies. Although the doctors and various specialists concentrate on medical management stuff, my job is to try to bring things together—to be the liaison between the experts and the patient.

---

The Department of Human Services is staffed by three counselors, two administrative assistants, and a secretary. Their mandate is to serve employees of the company, improving their life satisfaction and helping them to resolve personal problems that may have an impact on their productivity and efficiency in the workplace. Services provided include (1) individual, group, and family counseling; (2) crisis intervention and conflict management; (3) career guidance and job placement; (4) substance abuse prevention and treatment; (5) retirement planning and counseling; (6) quality-of-work-life seminars; and (7) referral to specialized agencies in the community. The staff also coordinates its activities with those of Human Resources and Affirmative Action.

What the counselors like best about their jobs is that they have the relative freedom to implement a number of new programs that are on the cutting edge of human services. They also enjoy excellent fringe benefits and salary packages, which are the hallmark of corporate settings. And they appreciate working as part of a team of professionals who are overseeing the quality of life for thousands of employees.

On the negative side of the ledger, working for any large organization is frustrating. The work hours are fairly rigid. Most employees tend to be somewhat suspicious of what the counselors do. (Are they really there to help people, or are they spies of management who will report everything they see and hear?) Also, because what they are doing is so new, there is a certain amount of resentment and resistance associated with introducing their programs, especially among the senior employees.

On the whole, though, the counselors feel that they have a great thing going—that is, as long as upper management provides support for their programs. They also realize that, in such a small department, things work smoothly because everyone gets along quite well. As would be the case with any small group, if one member of the staff was obstructive or incompetent, things could be very unpleasant. This group does work well together, however, and its members are able to be supportive and yet confront one another when the need arises.

A number of counselors, working in many different settings, report that this last characteristic is one of the most important in any job—being part of a team in which colleagues are helpful to one another and there is a spirit of cooperation and mutual caring. Counseling is, after all, a stressful job, requiring that we have built-in components to help us function well without feeling burned out. It is for this very reason that beginning counselors look for first jobs that have very supportive environments with friendly coworkers and a benevolent supervisor who makes it feel safe to learn and grow as a professional.

# CURRENT AND FUTURE TRENDS

It is always difficult to predict future employment trends because patterns are so heavily influenced by regional funding. In some parts of the country they can't hire enough school counselors and other areas they are being laid off. The same is true with any number of other specialties. Nevertheless, it seems that the influence of forces like technology, managed care, and federally funded programs will clearly create needs in particular areas.

In rural areas throughout the world, counselors are increasingly relying on the use of distance-based modalities to reach people in need (Riemer-Reiss, 2000). This creates huge implications for future practice in which we may routinely employ the Internet and web-based modalities for consultations, instruction, or monitoring of client progress (Smith & Senior, 2001). This presents a number of advantages for clients—greater convenience, efficiency, and freedom, privacy, cost-effectiveness. There are also many disadvantages that have not yet been worked out—the potential for dishonesty and manipulation when people are not whom they say they are, difficulties in getting reimbursed for services, and specialized skills that are involved in doing this type of work (Freeny, 2001).

Although technology-based interventions will be used with increasing frequency in both rural and urban settings, there are indeed unique challenges and problems faced by clients who live in both kinds of environments. For example, families in rural areas face issues of personal and professional isolation, lack of resources and community services, and scarcity of specialists in health care. Likewise, counseling practitioners in rural areas have more complex multiple relationships and confidentiality issues, as well as fewer consultation and supervision opportunities (Weigel & Baker, 2002).

Within both rural and urban areas, there are several other problems such as the already excessive time people spend in front of their computers instead of face-to-face with people and the difficulties in helping people without access to visual cues. Someone writes to you in an email message: "I just got home from work. What a day!" If these words were spoken, you could far more easily decode the underlying meaning: Is this person exhilarated or angry or frustrated? But without such cues available, you have to ask for more

## VOICE FROM THE FIELD

When I was originally trained, we were warned repeatedly about the dangers of dual relationships and how important it is to set appropriate professional boundaries. But I live and work in a small town in which I am one of the few counselors within a hundred mile radius. There is simply no other option for people who want counseling help other than to see me. Yet I serve in parent-teacher organizations with some of these people. I see them in the grocery stores. Our children play together. I try my best to maintain a degree of distance, but sometimes it is just impossible. These ethical codes were developed for very good reasons, to protect clients' welfare, but they were also written by folks who live in New York and other big cities where they don't ever have to run into their clients on the street. But what am I to do?

---

detail and then depend so much on what people report is going on. Still, such a form of counseling is not intended to replace traditional therapeutic relationships, but rather to supplement them and to reach out to people who would never otherwise seek any help whatsoever.

One other current trend that is only going to exercise more influence on counseling specialties is managed care. Not only does managed care force practitioners to consider cost containment and efficiency when making clinical decisions, but the majority of professionals must consider ethical dilemmas reconciling the needs of their clients with those of the health organizations. Of course, whining and complaining about this situation is not going to change things; the managed care movement began as a necessary means to control spiraling medical and mental health costs. And one distinct advantage of this trend has been that we have become much more efficient in the ways we work. Yet there has also been a distinct loss of freedom and autonomy in the ways we work, and this reality must be considered when choosing a counseling specialty.

## THE VALUE OF A FLEXIBLE SPECIALTY

The days of the counseling generalist are numbered. No longer can the counselor indulge in the luxury of acting like a country doctor who knows a little bit about everything and yet nothing in depth about anything. The technology and knowledge in the field are growing so rapidly that it is impossible to stay current on subjects as diverse as Internet-based resources, genetic predeterminants of emotionally disturbed children, nutritional imbalances in geriatric senility, indirect hypnotic trance inductions, and unionism among school personnel specialists.

Most counselors, by design or by circumstances, find themselves in a flexible specialty. Because of a need in a particular community for family mediation experts, a counselor may choose to affiliate with a court system to fill the

## VOICE FROM THE FIELD

As soon as I completed the introductory course, I knew immediately the things I didn't like, even though I had no idea what I did like. The idea of sitting in an office seemed intolerable to me. I had to find something where I could move around a lot, have variety in my job, and try different things all the time. In the class on career information, I took a lot of those tests we're supposed to give to clients, but they only told me what I already knew. So I visited five different agencies and interviewed counselors in the field as part of a school project. Then I did two different internships. I tentatively settled on working with small kids because you can help them before they get into too much trouble and you get to see their changes in a matter of weeks instead of years. I also figured that if I don't like that job, I will already be prepared to work with children in any setting I choose.

---

gap. A counselor newly hired by an agency may need to adapt to handling drug-abuse cases, sex counseling, or another area in which the counselor has specialized expertise. Sometimes clientele, based on their socioeconomic or geographical background, will present similar problems of economic hardship, bored marriages, or free-floating anxiety. Again the counselor ends up reading and studying more about those particular concerns and thereby becomes an expert in dealing with future cases.

Although you probably should market yourself as a specialist in a few related areas to increase both your employability and your professional mastery, you need not become so narrow in focus that you program yourself for future difficulties. Whether you are a financier, physician, or counselor, the consequences of overspecialization can be equally undesirable, resulting in rigidity, obsolescence, and a narrow field of vision.

It may therefore be advantageous to select a particular field in which to concentrate your study while continuing efforts to survey the wide educational spectrum. Certain specialties even fit well together, depending on your interests and skills.

A survey of broad specialty areas that permit flexibility and the opportunity to develop expertise in the field is illustrated in the following list:

| Child Development | Adolescent Development |
| --- | --- |
| elementary school counseling | high school counseling |
| preschool counseling | youth probation officer |
| early childhood education | youth work in a residential facility |
| parent education | career-development specialist |
| child abuse | college placement |

| Adult Development | Interpersonal Relationships |
| --- | --- |
| adult education | marriage counseling |
| midlife transitions | family counseling |
| counseling for the aged | sex education and counseling |
| spiritual/pastoral counseling | personal coaching |
| criminal justice | divorce mediation |

| Health | Industry |
| --- | --- |
| nutritional counseling | organizational development |
| exercise and health education | corporate consulting |
| stress management | staff training and development |
| physical disabilities | employee assistance programs |
| weight loss or smoking reduction | public relations |

| University | Careers |
| --- | --- |
| student affairs | lifestyle assessment |
| residential life | career planning and placement |
| student counseling | vocational rehabilitation |
| college administration | occupational therapy |

| Addictions | Mental Health |
| --- | --- |
| substance abuse counseling | private practice |
| drug education | community mental health centers |
| crisis intervention | public and nonprofit agencies |
| primary prevention | hospitals |

## Guidelines for Selecting a Counseling Specialty

You should at least consider concentrating in one or more of the categories in the list. The task of considering them is no less overwhelming than any other career decision and needs to be based on a systematic process of solid self-evaluation and the collection of pertinent information about each subspecialty. Beginning this process early in a graduate program allows maximum opportunity for exploration and can guide your class and fieldwork so that the eventual decision on a subspecialty can emerge, rather than be forced at the last minute. The choice of some specialties will involve further training beyond your current program level, a factor that may be important for some students.

The following guidelines may be helpful in thinking about specialty areas and creating an innovative personal approach to this important task.

1. *Assess personal strengths and weaknesses.* In thinking about your personal strengths and weaknesses, strive to be extremely honest with yourself and assertively seek feedback from trusted friends, peers, colleagues, and professors. Often a disappointing specialty selection can be traced back to an inaccurate self-assessment. It is important to be scrupulous in all aspects, avoiding any tendency to be overcritical, underplay strengths, or be defensive about weaknesses. Accuracy and honesty are twin hallmarks of an effective self-assessment.

2. *Clarify values related to work.* Personal values exert a substantial impact on work satisfaction and can influence burnout, career development, and professional effectiveness. It is useful to spend some time exploring personal values and testing them within possible specialty areas. The counseling field is so large and diverse that it provides ample opportunity for individuals to seek or create work settings and specialties that are consistent with personal values. Nothing is more frustrating than choosing a career or specialty that requires considerable investment, only to discover that it doesn't feel right; for instance, that the job requires evening hours and you hate working after dark. You can avoid, or at least minimize, such disappointments and frustrations by paying careful attention to values early in the specialty-selection process.

3. *Visit as many different specialty settings as possible.* There is no replacement for reality testing in career selection. Although a specialty might sound interesting and comfortable to you, a visit to a site could provide a completely different perspective on what the job is really like. Many counseling students, for example, believe that they would like to work in a hospital setting. However, after visiting a site, they may discover that much of their work would be routine and depressing and that counselors are at the bottom of the pecking order. This awareness may cool initial enthusiasm, or it may reinforce a tentative commitment. Regardless of the outcome, decision making will be based more on reality considerations than on fantasy.

4. *Interview as many counselors in the field as possible.* Selecting a specialty depends on awareness of opportunities as well as personal preferences and goals. Interacting with professional counselors allows the student to collect a wealth of valuable information, rooted in day-to-day reality, on work situations and opportunities. A limitation of graduate education is that it is often removed from the experiences of clinicians. You can work to reduce this separation and in the process enrich the base for choosing your specialty.

5. *Maximize internship and practical experiences.* The heart of a professional training program in counseling is supervised experience. These structures provide an indispensable source of knowledge and experience for specialty selection. Seek as wide a range as possible. This is a time to

## VOICE FROM THE FIELD

It's funny, but I always thought I wanted to be in private practice. That's where the money is—supposedly. But then I talked with about a half dozen of them on the phone since most weren't willing to meet with me unless I paid for their time. I did get to interview several as well. And what I learned surprised the heck out of me.

Most of them like their work but they aren't doing that well financially. In fact, when I compared their lifestyles to that of school counselors, I realized that when you add up benefits, retirement, paid vacations, and stuff, it really isn't as good as I thought. That really opened my eyes to look at some other jobs I wouldn't have considered.

experiment and to broaden professional experiences. The field portion of your training is, in a sense, the last "free" opportunity to explore professionally. Once you have graduated, it will be much more difficult to avoid making firm commitments.

6. *Develop a future orientation.* Essayists have repeatedly observed that change is the only stable characteristic of the future. To prepare for a vital and pertinent specialty area, you will need to develop a professional orientation that looks to the future rather than the past for definition and career opportunity. For example, whereas historically school systems have been the largest employer of counselors, we can predict there will be increasing opportunities in the future for those who specialize in working with the aged. To ensure professional relevance, you will have to anticipate settings and opportunities wherein counseling skills and attitudes will be useful and in demand. Creatively forecasting the future will allow you, as a counselor-in-training, to select specialties carefully and to target emerging employment opportunities.

## SUMMARY

The selection of a specialty is, in a sense, a subgoal of counselor training. It is useful to begin the process of specialty selection early in your education but to avoid making rigid or premature commitments. Counselors need to be flexible and open to change as they develop as persons and professionals. Specialty selection is really the first step in professional development, which is an ongoing aspect of your work as a therapeutic counselor.

This chapter has provided an overview of the work of professional counselors in a variety of jobs. Each setting for therapeutic counseling is vital, dynamic, and filled with both substantial rewards and grinding frustrations. Such is the nature of the profession. Helping people, particularly within an institutional context, is not an easy task—but it does offer a unique and creative opportunity to make a difference in the world.

## VOICES FROM THE FIELD

I went all the way through my training thinking I wanted to work as a counselor in correctional facilities, if not as a probation officer. As long as I can remember, in fact, that's what I wanted to do. I studied hard, got good grades, and prepared myself as best I could for my first internship placement.

So there I was, finally, working in a prison. The first day there I sat in on a group of inmates and I was shocked. I mean shocked! They had no interest in God or religion. Every other word out of their mouths was a cussword. They had not the slightest interest in anything I had to say. All they did is stare at me as if I didn't have any clothes on.

I had no idea this is what it would be like. I mean, I saw movies and all, but still I thought I could make things different. I don't know. Maybe I still could. But I just felt so uncomfortable that I immediately switched to a different area.

---

Professional counselors work in many settings and perform a variety of tasks. Opportunities for employment in the field are extensive and require a proactive orientation. A major task for students in counselor training programs is to begin to think about their careers and to initiate careful research and planning to ensure maximum opportunity. One aspect of this planning is the tentative selection of a specialty area.

PROFESSOR: So much for our overview of the places where counselors work. Are you any more clear on what you can do with your degree?

STUDENT: You're feeling unsure of yourself and your ability to help me deal with a problem so complex.

PROFESSOR: Yes, it is frustrating. All the time I must—ah, yes, I see you have learned something. And I know how it feels to be evaded with active listening.

STUDENT: To answer your question: I learned that it is up to me to market myself for the job I really want. The counseling program provides me with a core of basic skills to apply in any setting I choose.

PROFESSOR: Yes, and it is up to me to help you in your choices by providing honest feedback about your assets and limitations concerning possible specialty areas. In addition, I need to stimulate and challenge your thinking about possibilities.

STUDENT: So I guess it's up to me to use the skills and techniques I'm learning in the program and somehow to combine them with my personal strengths and figure out what I'm going to be when I grow up.

PROFESSOR: You bet—and the process doesn't stop. In fact, right now in my own life I've been doing some thinking and evaluating. . . .

# SELF-GUIDED EXPLORATIONS

1. Imagine that it is now three years in the future and you are working in your ideal job. Describe, in detail, what a typical day in your life is like. Include not only what you are doing, but also where and how you are doing it.

2. Describe your plan for making your fantasy described on the previous page a reality.

3. Choose a counseling specialty or setting that seems intriguing to you, but not part of your current plans. Pretend that you decided to pursue that career path instead of the one described in the previous fantasy. Describe a day in your life in that setting.

## For Homework:

Write down a list of the places where, ideally, you'd like to work. Make plans to visit each one of these settings. Don't take no for an answer if you find it initially challenging to arrange these field studies. Try to make friends with someone at each site so that you will have a contact person for future internship and job placements.

Then jot down a few notes about what you learned.

# SUGGESTED READINGS

Broderick, P. C., & Blewitt, P. (2003). *The life span: Human development for helping professionals.* Upper Saddle River, NJ: Prentice-Hall.

Collison, B., & Garfield, N. J. (1996). *Careers in counseling and human services* (2nd ed.). Muncie, IN: Accelerated Development.

Gladding, S. T. (1997). *Community and agency counseling.* Columbus, OH: Merrill.

Godzki, L. (2002). *The new private practice: Therapist-coaches share stories, strategies, and advice.* New York: W. W. Norton.

Hsiung, R. C. (2001). *E-therapy: Case studies, guiding principles, and the clinical potential of the internet.* New York: Norton.

Rumrill, P. D., Bellini, J. C., & Koch, L. C. (2001). *Emerging issues in rehabilitation counseling.* Springfield, IL: C. C. Thomas.

Sandhu, D. S. (2001). *Elementary school counseling for the new millennium.* Alexandria, VA: American Counseling Association.

Schmolling, P., Youkeles, M., & Burger, W. R. (2001). *Human Services in Contemporary America* (5th ed.). Pacific Grove, CA: Brooks/Cole.

Sperry, L. (2002). *Transforming self and community: Revisioning pastoral counseling and spiritual direction.* Liturgical Press.

Thompson, R. A. (2001). *School counseling: Best practices for working in schools* (2nd ed.). New York: Brunner/Routledge.

Weikel, W. J., & Palmo, A. J. (Eds.). (1996). *Foundations of mental health counseling* (2nd ed.). Springfield, IL: Charles C. Thomas.

# 4 CHAPTER

# THE THERAPEUTIC RELATIONSHIP

## KEY CONCEPTS

Personal versus helping relationships

Power in relationships

Relationship boundaries

Holding environment

Working stage

Congruence

Working alliance

Internal narrative

Primary/advanced empathy

Initial interview

Confidentiality

Reciprocal influence

# THE THERAPEUTIC RELATIONSHIP

# CHAPTER 4

Regardless of the setting in which you practice counseling—whether in a school, agency, hospital, or private practice—the relationships you develop with your clients are crucial to any progress you might make together. For without a high degree of intimacy and trust between two people, very little can be accomplished. It is this sense of safety that is the single organizing principle of counseling, in which clients are continually checking out danger signals in the relationship with the counselor—and in all other relationships.

Make a mental list of the important relationships in your life. Include friendships. Add your parents, siblings, and other relatives. Perhaps a few teachers, coworkers, or classmates might also be considered influential in your world. Now, what do your best relationships—all those you have ever known—have in common? What are the characteristics you consider to be most crucial in your past, present, and future interactions with other people?

Important relationships in almost any context, except adversarial, have certain desirable elements—trust, for one. Mutual respect, openness, acceptance, and honesty are others. Whether we are examining personal relationships or the unique contact between counselor and client, there will be similarities. For in all kinds of relationships, helping or otherwise, we desire intimacy and intensity. And I might say that the quality we are able to create in these dimensions is directly related to the personal enrichment of our lives. I might say the same for helping relationships. I might—but I won't.

## QUALITIES OF COUNSELING RELATIONSHIPS

Counseling takes place chiefly within the context of a very special kind of relationship—one that is similar to other successful relationships but is also distinctly different. In this chapter you will explore the fundamental aspects of the therapeutic relationship, learn how these qualities are developed, and learn how several primary relationship-enhancing skills and interventions may be applied to sessions.

In a comparison between personal and helping relationships, the most outstanding distinction would be the inherent inequality of the latter. Although therapeutic relationships do resemble other kinds of intimate encounters, Josselson (1992) reminds us of some fundamental differences.

From the outset of the first encounter, the client clearly is in need of some assistance and the counselor is identified as an expert with specialized talent and skills to provide the desired help. The relationship, therefore, involves a contract in which both parties agree to abide by certain rules: the client to show up on time, and to make an effort to be as open as possible; the counselor to be trustworthy, to protect the welfare of the client, and to do everything possible to help the client reach identified goals in the most efficient period of time. The power between the client and the counselor is thus embodied in a unique structure wherein the client is primarily responsible for the content of the relationship, whereas the counselor has most of the responsibilities for directing its style and structure. Although counselors do make an effort to demonstrate complete sincerity and respect to the client, nonetheless an uneven distribution of status and power remains. After all, the relationship takes place on the counselor's home turf. There are diplomas and books on the wall. A warm professional atmosphere pervades, yet the counselor gets the more comfortable chair and, when both speak simultaneously, the counselor usually prevails.

Many practitioners, such as Rogers (1957), Boy and Pine (1990), and Egan (1998), try to minimize the power dimensions of the relationship, believing that equality is crucial to change. Feminist (Burstow, 1992; Cook, 1993; Zimmerman, 2002) and narrative (Monk, Winslade, Crocket, & Epston, 1997; White & Epston, 1990) approaches to counseling, as well, conceive of relationships that are especially sensitive to those who have been oppressed by the dominant culture. This is in marked contrast to others (Haley, 1984, 1989; Erikson, 1950; Minuchin, 1974; Strong & Claiborn, 1982), who make a strong case for the counselor deliberately and strategically cultivating a powerful position in order to be more influential. In other words, some counselors find downplaying their status to be effective in facilitating change, whereas others wish to emphasize their capability as powerful models.

Regardless of how power is conceived, almost every practitioner would agree that boundaries play a highly important role in the ways the therapeutic relationship is constructed. These limits exist not only to provide a predictable and reliable environment for clients but also to protect their safety against counselors meeting their own needs.

## VOICE FROM THE FIELD

So many of the people I see act out. They hurt themselves and others. They are always testing the limits to see what they can get away with. Even the adults act like kids in that they try to throw their weight around, but they really like it when someone tells them, "That's enough." I think that one of the most important things I do as a counselor is to create a relationship for people in which they know certain rules will be enforced every time. I don't like being so strict, but I have to for their sake.

The therapeutic relationship is also different from other interactions in that there are relatively specific objectives and stringent time limitations: The relationship exists to seek solutions, and the discussion ends once the minute hand of the clock reaches a previously agreed-on point. Thus, in addition to many of the characteristics found in other successful human relationships, the therapeutic relationship has several identifying features. Based on a review of empirical, conceptual, and clinical literature, not just in counseling but in psychology, social work, nursing, medicine, and healing in other cultures, Kottler, Sexton, and Whiston (1994) offer the following conclusions:

1. Relationships are the forum for change to take place. Regardless of the theoretical orientation that is preferred or the techniques that are employed, it is the connection between client and counselor that is the basis for all further work.
2. The relationship has an explicit goal and purpose—to end it as soon as therapeutically possible.
3. There is an understanding that one person (the counselor) has more control, responsibility, and expertise in making things go smoothly and helpfully, whereas the other person (the client) is more important.
4. The relationship is essentially one of interpersonal influence in which the counselor seeks to promote changes in the client through skills, powers, and the force of interacting personalities.
5. Therapeutic relationships exist in a cultural context. They are likely to be more helpful when they are constructed in such a way that respects the values, expectations, and needs of clients and their cultural backgrounds, including ethnicity, socioeconomic class, religion, gender, and other relevant factors.
6. The interactions are structured to make the most efficient use of time. Small talk and other meaningless prattle common to personal encounters are not in evidence during counseling, where time is viewed as a valuable commodity.
7. The helping relationship can deal with a variety of human behaviors, thoughts, attitudes, and actions—but is often focused on the expression and exploration of feelings that are rarely disclosed outside the encounter.

8. Although Rogers' (1969) "core conditions," such as realness, genuineness, freedom, acceptance, trust, prizing, and empathic understanding, are usually found within the relationship, they may not be enough to promote lasting changes.

9. For the relationship to work well, both client and counselor must come to an agreement as to the causes and etiology of the presenting complaints and what must be done to make things better. The most effective relationships are characterized by agreement on goals, consensus on methods, open communication, and a collaborative partnership.

10. The relationship is multidimensional. Most of the features described by various theorists play an important role in the process. Thus, therapeutic relationships are, in part, authentic interactions, as well as "projected" experiences in which both client and counselor distort what is happening between them based on their respective unresolved issues.

11. The relationship is dynamic and changes over time. What is most appropriate in the beginning stages of counseling (authentic engagement) is less important during the working stages when an interactional pattern has developed to accomplish therapeutic tasks. Likewise, as counseling is ending, a return to a more egalitarian relationship is more likely to be helpful than one that proved helpful at another stage.

What all these points mean is that counselors use research on best practices, combined with their own experiences, to assess for each client which sort of relationship is going to be optimal for accomplishing stated objectives. Some people in the throes of crisis need a highly supportive relationship in which they can express frightening feelings without fear of judgment and criticism. Other people need a more confrontive relationship to help them translate what they already understand into action. Likewise, relationships can be tailored for each client with an emphasis on things such as:

- Structure or flexibility
- Feelings or thoughts
- Warmth or objective detachment
- Disclosure or planning
- Consistency or novelty
- Exploration or problem solving
- Content or process

Although the therapeutic relationship is usually individualized for each client given the treatment objectives and desired outcomes, there is usually a pattern of successive stages common to almost all approaches. Greenspan and Wieder (1984) use a developmental approach to describe this predictable evolutionary process. Stability is initially established through the willingness of the client to cooperate with the structure of counseling. Attachment follows as the dimensions of trust, acceptance, and emotional interest are fostered. The final process stage includes the more traditional therapeutic work that leads to insight and change.

■  VOICE FROM THE FIELD

Long before I was a counselor, I was first a client. I will never forget what my counselor did for me, even though the ways she helped me were probably different from what she imagined. I can look back and see that she was psychoanalytic, meaning that she was pretty passive and wanted me to talk mostly about my childhood. I was willing to humor her because I just enjoyed having her mother me. Granted, she was a very withholding, coldhearted mother. But that was exactly the kind of relationship I needed at that time in my life.

My guess is that she was basically the same with all her clients. Although I now work very differently than she did with me, using the relationship with my own clients as leverage to push them, I was really grateful for my connection to her. It was probably mostly my own fantasy but it still helped me to regain control of my life. It didn't matter what we talked about in the session, I just really liked that I could count on her to be there for me.

Even more simply, there is a beginning stage to all counseling relationships in which the goals are negotiated and the patterns are established that are most likely to lead a particular client to make needed changes. For some individuals, a highly structured relationship might be best, whereas for others a more flexible pattern is optimal. During the working stage, interactions revolve around attempts to promote alternative ways of functioning, both in the session and in the client's outside world. Finally, in the ending stage, the relationship is designed principally to help the client to generalize results to other areas of life.

Evolutionary processes apply not just to how the relationship develops over time but also to the very essence of its power to promote changes. In their provocative thesis on the evolutionary basis for therapy and counseling, Glantz and Pearce (1989) noted that human beings originally functioned as part of a tribe—a close-knit unit of hunter-gatherers who depended on one another for survival. However, after several hundred thousand years of intense social existence in which people lived as part of large extended families and tribes, contemporary life has literally disbanded our intimate connections. Siblings now live in different cities from one another and from their parents. Careers require periodic relocations of family. Our cultural, ethnic, and family histories have become diluted, and our friends and family are scattered around the globe. Human beings now walk the earth more alone than ever.

It is the absence of band-like social structures that Glantz and Pearce believe has created such feelings of alienation, estrangement, loneliness, anxiety, and depression in contemporary life. Counseling in general, and the therapeutic relationship in particular, supply the nurturance, support, and caring that are now missing from daily life. It is this relationship with others, whether in individual or group treatments, that rekindles the feelings of belongingness and acceptance that were once part of tribal life.

# PERSPECTIVES ON HELPING RELATIONSHIPS

From whence has come the conception of the therapeutic relationship as we now know it? It is interesting, if not useful, to understand the origins of how therapeutic relationships evolved to their present forms.

## A Bit More of History

In modern times, helping relationships began within a religious context: Clergy members and other spiritual experts acted as go-betweens in issues between a person and God. The relationship was rigidly defined according to the values of the Middle Ages. At the onset of the Renaissance came Johann Weyer, considered by many to be the world's first psychiatrist. He condemned the archaic witch-purging practices of religious healers and instead extolled the value of a benevolent, kind, and understanding relationship between doctor and patient. A few centuries later, Sigmund Freud also gave considerable attention to the structure of patient-doctor interactions but stressed a more benign, formalized, and unobtrusive relationship. He was, of course, concerned about such things as transference—the fantasy distortions that take place—and warned practitioners of its value and danger.

Historically, the roles within the counseling relationship have not been static. Every theoretical approach you will study in the next chapters has distinct notions about how best to work with clients. Some counselors deliberately encourage dependence in their client relationships, thereby facilitating the transference struggle that Freud found to be so crucial in overcoming unresolved problems with authority. In this type of therapeutic relationship, the counselor remains aloof, dispassionate, and neutral, so as not to fall victim to an erotic involvement that could so naturally proceed from the role of omnipotent love object.

In more contemporary psychodynamic approaches that revised Freud's original prescriptions, theorists such as Gill (1982) and Kernberg (1984) speak of the relationship as a "holding environment" that provides a safe setting with clear boundaries, to help clients experience the full range of their self-destructive urges. Gill also proposed that a relationship structured around remembering the past is often not enough; it is reexperiencing and reliving prior feelings and impulses that lead to constructive work. This takes place through a relationship that helps clients access intense, unresolved feelings, express them, and discuss matters nondefensively and objectively (Kahn, 1997).

## Congruence, Positive Regard, and Empathy

In marked contrast to this rather structured sort of relationship, Carl Rogers was instrumental in defining a type of alliance with people based on nurturance, warmth, genuineness, respect, and authenticity. This relationship is a mutual involvement, a sharing of feelings in an open, accepting atmosphere;

■ │ VOICE FROM THE FIELD

I'm what you'd call a brief therapist, but I've always been uncomfortable with the rather cold and sometimes manipulative aspects of the problem-solving therapies. I'm an old-time humanist from way back when, so when I moved into a job that doesn't give me the time I once had to get to know clients awhile before I try any major interventions, I have tried to preserve my warmth and humanness in sessions even when I see someone one or two times.

I've had supervisors tell me that maybe the relationships stuff is more important to meet my needs than those of my client, and that could be true; I don't deny it. I still think, though, that people are a whole lot more willing to follow through on their homework when they feel some degree of commitment to our relationship. I just don't think you have to choose between being relationship oriented or task oriented. I really think you can do both.

the counselor accepts responsibility not only for creating these fertile conditions but also for communicating his or her own attitudes and feelings within the session. In his personal vision for creating an ideal relationship in counseling, Rogers (1961) explains: "I would like my feelings in this relationship with him to be as clear and transparent as possible, so that they are a discernible reality for him to which he can return again and again" (p. 67).

Rogers (1951) followed his early theorizing about the importance of the counseling relationship with a series of research studies during the 1950s and 1960s in which he attempted to develop some empirical evidence for his ideas. The results of these research efforts led him to conclude that there were several major characteristics of the helping relationship (Rogers, 1957):

1. *Congruence.* Rogers believed that congruence is the most important ingredient in the helping relationship and encouraged counselors to work toward developing more congruence between what they are feeling on the inside and what they are communicating on the outside.
2. *Positive regard.* This means that the counselor does not evaluate and judge clients' actions or statements; behavior is viewed neutrally, and all people are worthy of respect.
3. *Empathy.* This denotes the process of attempting to understand, from the client's frame of reference, the thoughts and feelings underlying behavior—that is, the ability to walk around in the client's shoes and know how he or she feels.

## Working Alliance

A third position is the no-nonsense instructional model of the relationship in cognitive or behavioral or other brief forms of counseling. The practitioner creates a businesslike contract with the client to meet certain specific goals, with an action plan for reaching them. In these circumstances the relationship becomes an encounter between teacher and student. The main purpose of such an affiliation is to ensure compliance to the agreed-on treatment plan. Obviously, clients will be more likely to follow through on their stated objectives when they feel some degree of commitment to the relationship.

Among a number of brief therapists (Ecker & Hulley, 1996; Quick, 1996), attempts at compromise have been undertaken in which issues related to trust and empathy are considered important—but only to the extent that they can be fostered rather quickly and efficiently. Like any other facet of helping, much depends on exactly what clients are looking for and what they need in order to feel safe enough to present themselves honestly.

Recently researchers have been exploring the counseling relationship from other perspectives. Strong and Claiborn (1982), for example, have argued that the interpersonal influence variables of perceived expertness, attractiveness, and trustworthiness all affect the counselor's ability to facilitate change in clients. The relationship is viewed as the vehicle for establishing power and influence.

In another increasingly popular paradigm, constructivists such as Anderson and Goolishian (1992); Epston, White, and Murray (1992); and Gergen and Kaye (1992) have formulated helping relationships in terms of the language and belief systems that clients bring to the encounter. All social interactions, including those that take place in counseling, are co-constructed by the participants based on their interpretations of their experiences. These internal "narratives" are altered by the dialogues that take place—conversations that are aimed at helping clients to change the ways they interpret their realities. This sort of relationship often evolves into a very active sort of collaboration in which both client and counselor try to educate one another about their respective views.

Feminist theory is also having its impact on the ways we consider gender differences as they affect therapeutic relationships. In one study of prominent women therapists, Nevels and Coche (1993) speak of the distinctly female way that relationships can be constructed. With a greater commitment to caring and connection rather than to distinctly "male" values of competition and autonomy, quite another kind of relationship develops in the counseling process, one that emphasizes greater intimacy.

Regardless of orientation, the counseling relationship is a special and necessary aspect of the therapeutic counseling encounter. Indeed, counseling effectiveness has been found to be a function of the quality of the alliance (Parloff, 1956; Truax & Carkhuff, 1967; Sexton & Whiston, 1994; Beutler, Machado, & Neufeldt, 1994). But, although the importance of the relationship is well-documented, a helping relationship in and of itself is not a sufficient condition for behavior change; it is a means to another end (Kottler, Sexton, & Whiston, 1994). As Egan (2002) has pointed out, putting too much attention on the importance of the therapeutic relationship can be as detrimental as ignoring it altogether. The purpose of all helping is to assist clients to manage their lives better. Certainly this goal is more easily achieved if the client and counselor work well together.

## VOICE FROM THE FIELD

I consider myself a relationship-oriented counselor, at least when there is enough time allocated for us to get to know one another. I feel closer to some of the people I see than some of my friends, and I'm a little embarrassed to admit that. But as much as I value the power of a helping relationship to offer support and grounding to a client, I know that sometimes it is not enough. There's a teenager I'm seeing now and we have this fabulous relationship. He confides in me, and tells me everything going on in his life. He trusts me implicitly. He likes me, and I like him as well. Unfortunately, he is still doing the same stupid, crazy things in his life that he was when he first came to me. I keep pleading with his parents to let me keep working with him, and so far they are giving me a little more time, but I know that soon they are going to yank him out of the sessions. It'll be a shame, but I have to admit that while we do relate well together, I still haven't been able to help him change his destructive patterns.

## COUNSELORS AS RELATIONSHIP SPECIALISTS

The helping relationship can be defined as a systematic and intentional attempt, using a specified cluster of interpersonal skills, to assist another person to make self-determined improvements in behavior, feelings, or thoughts. Whereas daily helping encounters such as those between parent and child, teacher and student, or supervisor and employee could also be included, it is primarily counselors who are specialists in developing these nurturing and productive encounters. May (1983) prefers the term *presence* to describe the counselor's real alliance with a client, who is less an object to be analyzed than a being to be understood. Yalom (1980), as well, states that the single most important lesson for a beginning counselor to learn is that "it is the relationship that heals" (p. 401). The therapeutic involvement with the counselor symbolically illuminates other relationships in the client's life, besides providing the opportunity for a real, caring, respectful encounter with someone who is safe. The client feels minimal danger of seduction, manipulation, or betrayal, for the stated bounds of the interaction provide for protection of privacy, confidentiality, trust, and benevolence. It is at once both refreshing and frightening to be involved with a professional who is expert at listening and nonpossessively caring.

The therapeutic relationship helps the client work through feelings of isolation, a condition that the existentialists such as Kaiser (1965) and Yalom (1980) consider the "universal symptom" of humanity. The only cure is communication with someone who is sensitive, receptive, neutral, interested, and psychologically healthy. Imagine the deep pleasure, satisfaction, freedom—the complete and total freedom—to be genuinely open with another person who is doing everything within his or her power to subjugate personal needs and

## VOICE FROM THE FIELD

I'll never forget this couple from India I once saw. They came in, sat down, and waited patiently for me to fix them. I explained what it is that I did in marriage counseling and how I did it. They nodded, then once again told me that they wanted me, as the expert, to tell them what the problem was and then to fix it. Again I explained that I didn't work that way, that my job was to help them to sort out things for themselves. Blah, blah, blah.

They were very polite and understanding but still insisted that I tell them what to do. In their country, that is how healers and helpers operate—they give advice that is expected to be followed to the letter. In exasperation, I finally said, "Okay, here's the deal," and then I proceeded to violate everything I ever learned about doing counseling. They listened carefully. The husband even took notes. Then they thanked me, promised they would do what I asked, and walked out, completely satisfied customers.

I always remember that case when I start out with a new client. It's so important to realize that people have so many different cultural expectations for what helping relationships should be like.

---

focus only on *you*. For one uninterrupted hour you have the absolute attention, full concentration, and vast resources of a specialist in building relationships. This person is caring yet honest, fully capable of perceiving things beyond your awareness and explaining things beyond your understanding. This is a relationship you can truly depend on and use as a model for the kinds of experiences you deserve.

Yalom (1980) further explains that, although the therapeutic relationship is only temporary, the experience of intimacy endures. The key to developing such a meaningful encounter, irrespective of technique, is through the full engagement with the client in the present moment:

> I listen to a woman patient. She rambles on and on. She seems unattractive in every sense of the word—physically, intellectually, emotionally. She is irritating. She has many off-putting gestures. She is not talking to me; she is talking in front of me. Yet how can she talk to me if I am not here? My thoughts wander. My head groans. What time is it? How much longer to go? I suddenly rebuke myself. I give my mind a shake.

> Whenever I think of how much time remains in the hour, I know I am failing my patient. I try then to touch her with my thoughts. I try to understand why I avoid her. What is her world like at this moment? How is she experiencing the hour? How is she experiencing me? I ask her these very questions. I tell her that I have felt distant from her for the last several minutes. Has she felt the same way? We talk about that together and try to figure out why we lost contact with one another. Suddenly we are very close. She is no longer unattractive. I have much compassion for her person, for what she is, for what she might yet be. The clock races: the hour ends too soon. (p. 415)

## VOICE FROM THE FIELD

One of the best parts of my counselor training was noticing the ways it changed all my relationships with other people. Sure, I'm more sensitive now, but I'm also more demanding for what I want in friendships. When you spend all day talking to people about their most intimate secrets, I noticed two things happened to me: One, I don't want to hear problems after I get home from work, and two, when I do talk to friends, I have a much higher standard of intimacy. I don't know if this makes sense or not because the two seem to conflict. I suppose what I'm doing is giving you fair warning that once you get used to doing counseling, you just won't be satisfied with superficial relationships any more.

In addition to sharing the attitude implicit in Yalom's moving statement, counselors are quite skilled in their ability to foster helping relationships with a wide diversity of people. Depending on the client's ethnicity, religious and spiritual convictions, gender, cultural and family background, and prior experiences, quite different sorts of relationships are indicated.

Counselors must, of course, be consistent in their ability to create constructive relationships with anyone who walks in the door. This skill and attitude take practice as well as an openness to new people. The place to start, naturally, is in your own personal life. To what extent are you able to relate to people from all walks of life?

In their study of human relationships, a number of writers (Corey, 2000; Long, 1996) found that a series of specific skills will allow you to initiate, maintain, and nurture your connections to others. Because this repertoire of behaviors is so crucial to conducting counseling successfully, they recommend that beginning students assess their degree of competence in each of several areas. For each of these categories, a few of the skills are listed that are considered most significant in creating solid counseling relationships. Read through this list and consider the degree to which you can improve your effectiveness in each of the broad categories.

As you read through your self-ratings on these items, especially those marked with a 1 or 2, you will see where you most need to improve. It is hardly expected that you would already be a master of these relationship skills; that's why we have counselor training programs to help you learn and develop them. But it should be exciting for you to consider that, by the time you have completed your education as a professional helper, you will be reasonably competent in each of these dimensions. This will, of course, not only make you a successful counselor but also help you to become more loving and intimate in all your personal relationships. A prerequisite to beginning this work is a clear understanding of the characteristics of the helping encounter.

## RELATIONSHIP SKILLS RATING SCALE

(5) All of the time; (4) Most of the time; (3) Sometimes; (2) Rarely; (1) Never

*Self-awareness*

_____ I am in touch with my inner feelings.

_____ I am comfortable with myself.

_____ I am aware of my fears, anxieties, and unresolved conflicts.

*Self-disclosure*

_____ I express my feelings honestly and clearly.

_____ I am concise and expressive in my communications.

_____ I am open in sharing what I think and feel.

*Active listening*

_____ I can focus intently on what others are saying and recall the essence of their communications.

_____ I show attention and interest when I listen.

_____ I am able to resist internal and external distractions that may impede my concentration.

*Responding*

_____ I am perceived by others as safe to talk to.

_____ I can demonstrate my understanding of what I hear.

_____ I reflect accurately other people's underlying thoughts and feelings.

*Initiating*

_____ I have the ability to put people at ease.

_____ I am able to get people to open up.

_____ I am smooth and natural in facilitating the flow of conversation.

*Attitudes*

_____ I am nonjudgmental and accepting of other people, even when they have different values and opinions than I do.

_____ I am trustworthy and respectful of other people.

_____ I am caring and compassionate.

*Managing conflict*

_____ I can confront people without them feeling defensive.

_____ I accept responsibility for my role in creating difficulties.

_____ I am able to defuse explosive situations.

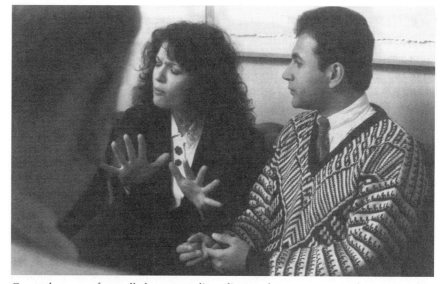

Counselors are often called on to mediate disputes between parties who are unwilling or unable to get beyond the point of blaming others for their troubles. Dick Luria/FPG/ Getty Images.

## CONFLICT RESOLUTION IN RELATIONSHIPS

As relationship specialists, counselors are often called on to mediate disputes between parents and children, husbands and wives, colleagues, friends, or extended family members. It is, therefore, critical for us not only to be experts at creating and maintaining a therapeutic relationship with clients, but also to know how to help them to resolve conflicts in their lives. So much of your time in session will be spent listening to clients complain about how poorly they are being treated by others, how unfair it is that they aren't understood or responded to the way they would prefer. Placing blame on others is thus a favorite ploy in which people avoid responsibility for their own troubles (Shaver, 1985; Tennen & Affleck, 1990; Zuk, 1984;). As long as they can blame others for not getting what they want in life, they don't have to invest the hard work and take the risks involved in changing.

Conflict also has its benefits, a phenomenon that counselors must understand before they can help to resolve relationship difficulties. Such conflicts thus have a number of positive functions as a means to release tension, promote growth, regulate distance between people, prevent stagnation, encourage dialogue, and eventually bring people closer together.

Counselors are likely to apply this knowledge to resolve conflict in basically two ways. The first involves functioning in roles as consultant, mediator, or family counselor in which they gather parties together and help them to examine the dynamics of their interactions and intervene in such a way that they respond to one another more constructively.

| **VOICE FROM THE FIELD**

I do a lot of marriage and family counseling. I invest a lot of energy in helping people really listen to one another, express their feelings honestly, own their needs, learn the art of negotiating, manage their anger productively, and honor each other's need for space and solitude. And yet when I get home, I'm ex- hausted. I feel so depleted that I don't often practice with my wife and children what I help others learn to do. Don't get me wrong: We're all pretty good to- gether. But the truth is that there is often a lot of in- congruence between my "lip" and my "life."

---

Second, counselors are likely to be called on to help individual clients come to terms with conflicted relationships in their lives, whether with bosses, spouses, friends, parents, children, neighbors, siblings, or coworkers who are disturbing them in the present, or with persons in the past who have long since moved on. In both cases, counselors generally follow a process that re- sembles quite closely a generic approach to counseling. This method of resolv- ing conflicts in relationships by moving beyond blame consists of several sequential stages (Kottler, 1994a).

1. *Identify what acts as a trigger for the relationship conflict.* This often involves instances when (a) a person's competence has been challenged, (b) a client tries unsuccessfully to win someone's approval, (c) a client fears inti- macy with someone, (d) someone won't or can't meet the client's expecta- tions, or (e) the client encounters someone who reminds him or her of other unresolved conflicts. The counselor's job at this juncture is to help clients un- derstand what sets them off in such a way that they react so ineffectively.

2. *Explore the origins of the conflict.* Difficulties in the present are often reenactments of scripts from the past. Who does this person remind the client of? Which of the client's core issues are being sparked? Counselors should look for issues related to (a) struggles for power and control, (b) the need for acceptance, and (c) problems of enmeshment.

3. *Intensify the pain.* Ironically, it is often by feeling worse that people are motivated to take constructive risks that they would ordinarily avoid. That is why counseling often involves a degree of discomfort as clients are forced to look at aspects of themselves that are unpleasant and threatening.

4. *Take responsibility without blaming.* Clients are confronted about their excuses for avoiding action. How is the client disowning the problem? What excuses is the client making? Who or what is the client's scapegoat? What are the client's fears of failure?

5. *Commit to act differently.* Clients increase their personal resolve to act by using the relationship as leverage to improve confidence, test new ideas and skills, and commit themselves to take risks.

6. *Experiment with alternatives.* The relationship becomes a safe place for clients to try out new strategies and practice new ways of thinking, feeling, and behaving.

Whether you are helping clients to move through these stages as a way to resolve their own relationship conflicts, whether you are mediating disputes between antagonists in your office, or whether you are working through impasses or impediments to progress in your own relationships with clients, there are generally several qualities that a number of research studies have found most helpful.

## PRACTICAL DIMENSIONS OF THE THERAPEUTIC RELATIONSHIP

The client usually comes to counseling with a history of impoverished relationships. With family members, friends, or colleagues, there have been some misunderstandings—even conflicts—that lead the client to seek help. The initial suspicions of a client toward new, intense relationships, even a client who feels lonely and isolated, will only be compounded within the strange, artificial boundaries of the counseling encounter.

As mentioned earlier, there is an inequality inherent in most professional relationships: The presumed expert controls most of the power. Thus the client begins the relationship at a disadvantage—unbalanced, overwhelmed, anxious, and confused. Before she or he even has the chance to adjust to the surroundings, check out the environment, and study the counselor, the session usually begins with the question, "How can I help you?" Given the difficulties present in the initial encounter, most practitioners agree—on the basis of research, theory, and experience—that the therapeutic relationship must possess certain dimensions to create a favorable climate for change.

### Commitment

As in all other meaningful contacts between people, there is an implied, if not explicit, contract in the counseling relationship to act in certain ways and follow certain agreed-on rules. The commitment to each other is both mutually and flexibly determined, but it nevertheless specifies the form and texture of the potential relationship. The counselor feels bound to this agreement with respect to promises made about what constitutes professional behavior: avoidance of self-indulgence, manipulativeness, and deceit; delivery of specified services; and total commitment, in fact, to doing everything possible to aid the client's growth.

The client is also strongly urged to feel a commitment to the relationship, although this personal contract is often difficult to enforce. By modeling honesty, the counselor encourages the client to live under agreed-on rules: to come on time, to give sufficient notice when canceling appointments, and to pay fees as negotiated. Of equal importance is the client's commitment to work with the counselor, to work on himself or herself, and to invest energy and

## ■| VOICE FROM THE FIELD

As far as I'm concerned, the objective of the first counseling session is to get the client to come back for a second one; if you can't do that, you probably can't help anyone. One of the biggest mistakes that beginners make is that they forget that one critical goal.

If you concentrate too much on asking your questions and getting forms filled out and coming up with a diagnosis, you forget that if you don't charm and persuade the client that what you have to offer is worth coming back for, then you'll have great treatment plans and nobody who sticks around to try them out on. That's why the sole relationship is so important. I know this sounds weird, but you've got to "hook" the client or all your best intentions and wonderful techniques are worthless.

---

personal risk taking in the relationship. All successful relationships a client has, whether with an attorney, a mechanic, a spouse, a friend, or a counselor, involve a commitment to be fair and just with each other.

## Trust

The development of trust in counseling relationships is crucial to productive work. The counselor's primary responsibility is to offer interpersonal conditions to the client that are likely to result in trust. But *trust* is a catchall word meaning various things and consisting of a number of factors. Several aspects of a trusting relationship are worth repeating: respect for the client's intrinsic right to be his or her own person, warm regard for the client as a unique being, and genuineness, which means being honest and real.

Although it may seem obvious to you that a counselor must be trustworthy to be helpful to a client, this trust is not as easy to maintain as it might seem. There have been serious—and unfortunately all too common—occurrences of ethical transgression in which a practitioner violates the client trust to meet his or her own needs. That is one reason why all the professions have constructed ethical codes that protect clients against exploitation.

## Empathy

Empathy refers to the ability of the counselor to truly understand the client from a unique perspective. It often involves communicating accurately the feelings and meanings of clients' statements, thereby demonstrating an active understanding of clients' concerns. Egan (2002) distinguishes between two levels of empathy: primary-level and advanced-level accurate empathy. *Primary-level empathy* refers to the interchangeability between the client's statements and the counselor's responses. At this level of empathic responding, the counselor communicates a basic understanding of the thoughts, feelings, and behavior of the client. *Advanced-level empathy* is built on the primary-level base and emphasizes the counselor's responding in a way that facilitates the deeper exploration

TABLE 4.1 | GUIDELINES FOR ESTABLISHING CULTURAL EMPATHY

1. Communicate an interest in learning more about the client's cultural identities (note plural).
2. Demonstrate an awareness and sensitivity about the client's culture, as well as a great desire to learn more.
3. Increase knowledge about the historical and political background of your clients.
4. Understand the ways that your client may have encountered oppression, discrimination, powerlessness, and prejudices.
5. Become aware of cultural differences that exist between you and your client.
6. Initiate interventions that are culturally respectful and appropriate.
7. Make use of healing practices and language that are consistent with the client's culture.

*Source:* Chung, R., & Bemak, F. (2002). The relationship of culture and empathy in cross-cultural counseling. *Journal of Counseling and Development, 80,* 154–159.

of relevant issues. Effective therapeutic counseling relationships are based on the sensitive and timely use of both levels of empathy.

While Rogers originally conceived of empathy as the means by which a counselor can understand another individual's inner experience, advances in multicultural counseling now view empathy within a cultural context as highlighted in Table 4.1 (Chung & Bemak, 2002).

## Confidentiality

An essential and unique feature of the counseling relationship (as compared with a personal or informal relationship) is the maintenance of confidentiality to ensure safety and privacy. Just as an attorney, clergy member, or physician must be able to guarantee that whatever is revealed will be considered privileged communication, trust and openness in counseling hinge on a similar promise. It is precisely the knowledge that a counselor's professional and ethical standards protect individual rights that makes it easier for the client to confide personal secrets.

When clients in counseling are often challenged as to why they spend their time (and money) to tell their problems to a stranger, they often reply with the statement that that they feel safe. They know that whatever they share will remain private. They are thus more inclined to talk about things that they may not be willing to do so otherwise.

## Benevolent Power

Interpersonal influence is that dimension of counseling that involves the application of expertise, power, and attractiveness in such a way as to foster self-awareness and constructive change. Lazarus (1981) believes that the most important function of the initial interview in counseling is to inspire hope, to

■ | VOICE FROM THE FIELD

I often play checkers with kids when they don't seem to want to talk. The thing is: You gotta make a connection any way you can. Playing a game with them to get things started sometimes loosens them up.

If they seem willing, I grab the checkerboard and we get down on the floor. We play and just kind of chat about things. With minimal coaching, they just start saying things like, "I wish my dad wouldn't yell so much," or "I hate eating lunch alone; I wish there was a friend I could be with." Then we're off and running once they've relaxed with me enough to utter just one thing that pulls up the curtain on their private world. That's what builds trust and gets the relationship going.

---

help the client believe in the process and in the expertise of the counselor as an influencer. One theorist has even created a whole therapeutic system that capitalizes principally on the placebo effects in counseling, structuring the expectations of the client to maximize favorable results. In his *Placebo Therapy,* Fish (1973) recommends using power, expertise, and the aura of omnipotence, in addition to nurturance and acceptance, to increase one's influencing capabilities in the therapeutic relationship.

Examples include evidence of expertise (for instance, diplomas on the wall), attractiveness (dress, surroundings), and power (control of the interview). Each of these social-influence parameters can be used and communicated in a manner likely to develop a constructive relationship and lead to productive change (Bandura, 1977). The use of social influence is a sensitive area because of the danger of manipulation and deceit, which do not enhance therapeutic relationships; thus, interpersonal-influence factors must be communicated openly and within a trusting, warm, and empathic context in order to minimize the potential negative effects of these elements.

## Experiencing the Therapeutic Relationship as a Client

The best way of all to get a sense of the power of therapeutic relationships, with their corresponding features just mentioned, is to experience it firsthand as a client. Some programs require you to participate in counseling as a condition of admission or graduation. The reasoning is that it is very difficult to get a sense for how counseling works if you have not sat in the client's chair.

Reading about counseling relationships is one thing. Studying the research and literature on their effects is another. Even hearing testimony from practitioners and clients about the therapeutic relationship is also educational. But none of these can replace what you could learn as a client yourself.

Apart from whatever personal issues you would have the opportunity to work on, or which interpersonal skills you identified earlier that you are in need of improving, you would be truly amazed at how wonderful it feels to be in counseling as a client. You have already experienced this before, with a spe-

**VOICE FROM THE FIELD**

For years, I felt constantly caught in a vortex about my sexual orientation. If I "come out" to people who are close but can't handle my sexuality, then I lose so much. I don't want to be a pariah. I just want what everyone else wants: happiness, partnership, fulfillment, and a chance to contribute. So I went into counseling.

What did I learn from the experience? To face myself, to sit with pain, not to run away from it. Being alone is okay now and I quite enjoy the aloneness and my own discovery. It's certainly better than fran-tically searching out the next relationship just to fill a void!

Was it useful? Counseling is a good tool for the strong at heart but not for those whose commitment to life wavers. At the end of the day, it's so bloody hard to sit and think about yourself, warts and all, with someone else in the room, with that person determined not to take responsibility for you. That's what I went for. I didn't want life the way it was for me. That's why it's hard. Feeling like an outcast who can't speak about who he loves, except in secret.

---

cial teacher or mentor, but there is something almost sacred and magical about what happens in counseling.

In order to teach your clients how to get the most from the experience you must be an expert yourself on how to be a good consumer of counseling services. If you have been in counseling yourself, then you know the games that clients play, you know the reluctance they sometimes feel, you know their struggles and inner conflicts. You know what works best and worst. Most of all, you know the power of what can happen in such a relationship.

If you have not yet seen a counselor for any length of time, I would highly recommend that you obtain this experience some time before you graduate. Among all the books I have read (and written) about counseling, all the degrees I've attained, the workshops and seminars I've attended, the demonstration videos I have watched, the conversations I've had with colleagues, and the supervision I've received from mentors, nothing was as valuable to me as the counseling relationships I've known with half a dozen clinicians during my life.

## CREATING A RELATIONSHIP IN THE INITIAL INTERVIEW

Some of the theory and research underlying the counseling relationship has been reviewed. The characteristics, components, and skills essential to these relationships can be identified. Each of these individual aspects, however, must be integrated into the person of the counselor during the interview with the client. The integration process is crucial, because the relationship variables will define the context and texture of the interaction that follows. The initial interview provides the opportunity to operationalize relationship skills and provides the first test of the effectiveness of counseling.

One of the first counseling procedures you will learn is how to conduct an initial interview to build a solid relationship with your clients and to collect relevant information that you will need in formulating a diagnosis and treatment plan. If you have not already had the opportunity to do so, it would be a very good idea for you begin practicing interview skills. This can be as simple as asking someone what he or she would like to talk about and then probing with a few questions here and there. Or, it can be a far more elaborate and systematic procedure in which you follow a detailed set of guidelines over the course of a 90-minute intake process. Regardless of the setting and clinical situation, your initial contact with a client is likely to cover several important areas.

## Establishing Rules

The relationship between client and counselor is established in the very first encounter. Even before the first words are spoken, the two size each other up, assessing the other's personal competence. The client, usually confused and nervous, will wait for the professional to begin and to define the parameters and tone for the sessions. The counselor also bides his or her time, knowing how crucial the first interchange will be to the entire therapeutic process. If ineffective or unsuccessful, the result will be unforgiving: The client will not return for more counseling. Worse yet, the client may return, but with grossly distorted perceptions of what will be involved in the future.

Perhaps the client will view the relationship as unequal, seeing the counselor, an expert, as the authority, the parent, the controller. The client may then adopt behavior appropriate to that situation, showing deference and asking questions. Transference, power, and dependence variables will exert themselves optimally as in other unequal relationships, such as those between parent and child, boss and employee, and, often, doctor and patient.

The client could also perceive the relationship as mostly equal, especially if the counselor introduces himself or herself by first name and does not respond with formal detachment. In this case the client will adapt to the situation and internally define the relationship according to his or her perceptions: "The counselor recognizes that we are equal, that what I have to say is intelligent and important, but we both really understand that I need help and I'm here because the counselor can offer it."

The initial interview, therefore, serves the function of creating and communicating rules for future interaction that are likely to be beneficial to a productive relationship. It establishes the norms for appropriate conduct and capitalizes on the trust, respect, acceptance, and warmth that are so much a part of the therapeutic encounter.

Remember, the client doesn't know how to be a "good" partner in this process; it is your job to teach the person about how to get the most from the experience. This starts with establishing appropriate norms for behavior.

## Planting Hope

The client is often motivated to make an appointment out of a sense of helplessness. People rarely pay money, risk embarrassment, or inconvenience themselves to visit a professional if there is another way to resolve their con-

## VOICE FROM THE FIELD

I never have an adolescent show up at the door seeking help. It just hasn't happened to me. So if they're there, it's because somebody else is making them come—a parent or teacher or somebody. So now I have to be up front with them in the very first session, and I've got about 15 minutes to grab their attention.

"I know there must be some problem," I tell them, "or you wouldn't be here. It's not my job to change you. I don't even think you need to be fixed.

You can make that choice for yourself. At this point, I just want to find out who you are. After we get to know each other, then we can look at some aspects of your life that you might want to change. That's up to you." Saying something like that usually works for me. They appreciate me being honest. They can tell I'm not playing games. That makes whatever else we do together a lot easier.

cerns. Counseling is usually the last resort, the final step before self-destructive acts are likely to occur.

Clients show up at the first session ambivalent about their behavior and unable to trust their feelings. They want help; they want to change. Yet they have also invested themselves in preserving the status quo and will therefore often resist, on some level, the interventions of the counselor. They want reassurance, easy solutions to their problems, and simple answers to their complicated questions. But most of all they want to believe that they can learn to trust themselves. Clients want to hope that working for the future is worthwhile. They want to believe in their capacity to make needed changes in their lives. They want to hope that, eventually, their pain will diminish and will someday be replaced by something better. Clients have hope that we, as professionals, know what we're doing, that we actually can make a difference. Therefore, favorable expectations for treatment, consistent with what can be delivered, must be quickly established in the initial interview.

This could sound something like the following introduction:

I am so glad that you came to see me at this time. Although I can see how much you are suffering, and what a difficult struggle you are going through right now, I want to assure you that this pain does not have to last much longer. In fact, I am willing to venture that you are already feeling better since you showed up here. It feels good to tell somebody else about what is going on and to know that you have been heard and understood.

Although I can't give you any guarantees about how long it will take to resolve your problems, since much of that depends on you, I can tell you that I have helped a lot of other people who have presented similar issues. I would expect that you will notice some improvement within a very short period of time.

Of course, you don't want to make promises you can't keep, or exaggerate what you can deliver. But it is important to let the client know that relief is on the way.

## Assuring Confidentiality

Confidentiality is the verbal contract between two people in which the counselor promises to keep private the communications heard in counseling and the client agrees to believe the promise. Unless such an understanding and basic level of trust can be reached, it is unlikely that the relationship can proceed any further.

For this reason the issue of confidentiality is always discussed early in the initial interview, both to allay fears about how private the sessions will be and to convince the client that the relationship will be safe and sacred, impervious to the questions of a curious parent, spouse, employer, or judge. The therapeutic relationship thus begins with a mutual commitment—that of the counselor to work ethically and competently in the best interest of the client while safeguarding privacy, and that of the client to be as open, truthful, and self-revealing as possible. These commitments will form the temporary bond of the relationship until real respect and intimacy evolve as a function of working together.

## Assessing Expectations

Often in conjunction with delivering a statement about confidentiality, the counselor further defines the therapeutic relationship to ensure that both parties enter into the verbal contract in ways that will be compatible and satisfying.

Clients can come to the first session with fairly outlandish notions about what is possible, probable, or likely to occur. These unrealistic expectations may include any of the following:

- "I talk. You listen. Then you talk. I listen. We take turns until one of us gets too bored."
- "I tell you my problems. Then you tell me yours. Afterward, I can figure out what I should do by what you have done."
- "I tell you my dreams and then you tell me what they mean."
- "You're like a lie detector. Whenever I don't tell the truth or exaggerate a little bit, or go through my standard lines, you interrupt me and tell me I'm full of crap."
- "You give me a tissue and hold my hand and tell me everything will be okay. That's what a helpful person should do."
- "I tell you my problems. You tell me what to do so I can change situations that keep me from getting what I want."
- "You agree with me that it's mostly other people's fault that I don't get what I want."

Images of a friend, father/confessor, nurturing mother, lover, coach, consultant, teacher, and coach all emerge in the client's mind as models for what the therapeutic relationship will be like. Many of the misconceptions and distorted expectations can be cleared up after they are discussed in the interview. As the counselor explains what counseling is and how and why it works, the client's images can be modified to reflect a more accurate portrayal. In this process, client and counselor discuss who will do what, in what order, and what is likely to happen as a result of the fulfillment of these expectations. By the time this component of the initial interview is over, both client and counselor should have negotiated a mutually agreeable set of goals for what will take place.

## Collecting Information

Before the counselor can really go to work, some form of data collection usually needs to take place in the first interview. The extent and depth of this activity will depend on the theory to which the practitioner subscribes; a psychoanalytic counselor might spend several entire sessions creating a history, whereas a strategic counselor would devote much less time, limiting the focus to specific information about the presenting problem.

Other models for collecting relevant background information about a client's environment are available, most including some preliminary explorations into the client's development, the evolution of the problem, and a description of self-defeating behaviors. In addition, the counselor should find out which solutions have already been tried and why the client is seeking help at this particular time. Finally, a history is usually collected of relevant medical information, family background, and developmental issues that may be related to the presenting complaints.

Most clinicians have a list of favorite questions to elicit useful information about how the client characteristically functions. Insightful queries can also create greater intimacy, openness, self-disclosure, and trust in the relationship. The following questions often facilitate the self-examination process and produce valuable data for the counselor. Simultaneously, the client begins to experience the excitement and discomfort of looking inward. Answer these questions for yourself as you review them:

- Who are the most important people in your world, and how do you spend time winning their approval?
- Who else knows that you are having this difficulty, and what will you tell them?
- What is your favorite part of each day?
- When you feel a lot of pressure, what kinds of things do you usually do to calm yourself?
- When are the specific times in your daily life in which you feel most uncomfortable and out of control?

Regardless of the questions or data-collecting model selected, the intention in the initial interview is to complete a preliminary inventory of the client's complaints, symptoms, and concerns.

## Identifying Problems

The identification of a client's complaints eventually leads to a working diagnosis. Because counselors aren't restricted to a medical model that limits labels to categories of psychopathology, they are able to concentrate on functional diagnoses that describe specific behavior patterns for each client. Counselors do not need to think exclusively in terms of "neurotic," "schizophrenic," or "dependent personality." Instead, efforts are made for the counselor and client to label problems and issues in specific, operational, and useful ways during the initial interview.

Regardless of which diagnostic model is employed (see Chapter 8) the intention is to take inventory of all the areas in which the client may need work and to prioritize which ones will be the focus first.

## Beginning Intervention

In addition to the traditional uses of the initial interview to begin the therapeutic relationship and collect useful information, Kovacs (1982) feels that other goals take even greater precedence. The counselor must intervene in the very first session on some level "to make at least a small dent in the stasis into which the patient has been locked for some time now" (p. 148). Counseling starts immediately in the first session. It is not enough merely to initiate the relationship, fill out forms, set goals, or create structure. These steps are but the means of bringing a sense of commitment to the counseling relationship.

Especially in today's climate of brief therapy and pressure from managed care organizations, it is crucial that some sort of intervention or actual counseling take place in the first session. This can be as simple as a mild confrontation or exploration of the client's thoughts and feelings, or can involve a more elaborate strategy to initiate the treatment plan. Much depends on how much time you have allocated with a client. If you think this may be a relatively long-term case (more than eight sessions) then you have the luxury of using the first session to gather information and then plan interventions in later sessions. If, however, this will be a brief relationships (less than three or four sessions) then you must begin the therapeutic strategy right away. Regardless of the length of treatment, keep in mind that a client will not return for a second appointment if the first one perceived as less than satisfactory.

## First-Session Agenda Review

I'll never forget my very first counseling session in practicum. I saw my client sitting in the waiting room looking nonchalant as she turned through a magazine. Yet I was so terrified I couldn't make myself go out there to get her. I was desperately afraid I would freeze completely once we got behind the one-way mirror. I just knew I would forget everything I ever learned and sit there open-mouthed and dazed.

As an act of desperation, I hurriedly wrote out a "cheat sheet," including a list of all the things I should remember to do in the first session. Naively, I believed that if only we got through all these steps, then it would be a perfect first interview.

As it turned out, the client caught me staring at the paper on my lap. I had no choice but to bring it out in the open and explain that this was the outline for our session. To my surprise, she was impressed that I was so well organized and she insisted that we check off each item one at a time. To this day, I still have my yellowed and frayed cheat sheet, which looks something like this:

## VOICE FROM THE FIELD

Good counselors are nosy. We ask lots of questions, sometimes directly, but most often we just probe to get things going. One of the best ways I learned how to ask effective questions was by trying things out in my personal life. I get bored at parties anyway and I'm impatient with small talk, so at social gatherings I try to get things going by challenging others to ask me any question they want and, within reason, I'll answer it honestly. There are a few exceptions, of course, but I've learned with practice that there is hardly anything that I wouldn't talk about. Then we each take turns trying to come up with better and better questions designed to get people to be revealing. My favorite one of all is: "What is the one question you're most afraid I'll ask?" Then I ask them to answer it.

*Opening.* Begin the interview dynamically and enthusiastically, sensitizing the client to the excitement of change.

*Route.* Find out through which avenue the client decided to seek help, how the decision was made, and why this particular choice was made.

*Reason.* Find out why the client is deciding to get help now.

*Experience in counseling.* Ascertain whether the client has had any previous experience with counseling. If so, ask who she or he has seen and what it was like.

*Expectations.* Explore what the client's expectations are for treatment. Do they relate to previous counseling experience? What does the client believe will happen?

*Definition.* Correct any misconceptions and unrealistic expectations by providing a definition of counseling, detailing how the process works.

*Confidentiality.* Discuss confidentiality in an effort to establish trust.

*Search for content.* Identify areas appropriate for counseling content, including presenting problems, self-destructive behavior, and unresolved conflicts.

*Important people.* Explore the people most important in the client's world, especially those who have a vested interest in the treatment outcome.

*Functional levels.* Assess the functional level of the client across a broad spectrum of behaviors—intelligence, resilience, confidence, exercise, sleeping and eating routines, dexterity, perceptual and cognitive capacities, life skills, and values.

*Structure.* Determine a structure for the particular client and counseling situation that will make significant progress likely to occur.

*Commitment.* Secure a commitment from the client to change and to work toward counseling goals.

*Goals.* Specifically work with the client to define realistic goals for the counseling that can be reduced to subgoals for and between future sessions.

*Summary.* Have the client evaluate what his or her perceptions and feelings are about the first session.

*Closing.* End the first session, solidify the relationship, and set future appointments.

This list may seem comprehensive, and it does include quite a number of elements, but this still doesn't cover all the territory. You would hardly be expected to cover all these features in one session, but they do form a rough structure for how you would proceed. By way of summary, your principal job as a counselor is to create an alliance with your clients in which you establish a degree of trust and intimacy. This must be done efficiently and effectively or your clients will develop unrealistic expectations—or they won't come back.

The steps of an initial interview translate into several core therapeutic tasks: (1) establishing a bond between you and your client, (2) providing preliminary information regarding what counseling is and how it works, (3) assessing client issues and expectations, (4) instilling a sense of hope, and (5) obtaining a commitment to be patient and to work hard in the sessions. From these humble beginnings, the success of all future counseling efforts is firmly established.

## RECIPROCAL INFLUENCE IN HELPING RELATIONSHIPS

In a theological perspective on what he calls a "soulful relationship," Moore (1994) describes the poetics of intimacy that operate between people who are understanding one another. Although he is speaking primarily of the attachments in friendship, Moore offers a more mystical view of what happens in counseling as well: "The idea of a soulful relationship is not a sentimental one, nor is it easy to put into practice. The courage required to open one's soul to express itself or to receive another is infinitely more demanding than the effort we put into avoidance of intimacy. The stretching of the soul is like the painful opening of the body in birth" (p. 30).

The most frightening and challenging aspects of being in a relationship with a client involve this mutual revealing of selves. Although we are careful to avoid self-indulgence, inappropriate self-disclosure, or putting the focus on ourselves in sessions, we nevertheless reveal ourselves in infinite ways. Our very presence in the room, meeting the client in an open, frank, and focused manner, invites mutual scrutiny. Just as we are systematically assessing what is going on with our clients, so too are they checking us out. They attend to every nuance in our voice and manner. They ask themselves, continually, what it means that we said or did something a particular way. Indeed, they come to know us almost as intimately as we know them, and that occurs without us having to tell a single story about our own lives.

The relationship between client and counselor is thus among the most intimate connections that can exist between human beings. Clients will tell you things that he or she would not tell a best friend, whisper to a lover, or even write in a journal. With the structured safety, rules of confidentiality, insulation from distractions, and permission to be as authentic as possible, this relationship can be as close to perfect as exists in this world.

The influence that takes place in therapeutic relationships moves in both directions simultaneously. Just as we do and say all within our power to change the client in directions we see as most profitable, so too is the client working hard to have an impact on us. This is the best part of the job—the growth and learning that comes from our relationships with our clients. It is the worst part as well—it is from such interactions that we retain the legacy of other people's pain.

## SUMMARY

Considering the energy, motivation, courage, and desperation required for a client to initiate the first appointment, anxiety during the first encounter is usually quite high. This initial interaction in the counseling relationship is marked by fear—fear of what might or might not happen; fear that there is no cure; fear that there is a cure but that it will involve a lot of work; fear that the counselor might tell someone else about the session; fear about what friends, family, even the receptionist might think about the fact that the client needs help; fear of revealing deeply guarded secrets; and perhaps most of all, fear of entering into an intense human relationship.

That the counselor is able, often within the first few minutes, to relieve a client's apprehensions is a testimony to the consummate skill of the professional who is experienced at relationship building. Everything in the easy manner and the calm self-confidence of the counselor indicates that this is a person who is comfortable with intimacy. The soft smile, soothing voice, relaxed posture, and interested eyes all communicate an authenticity that helps the client trust, open up, and feel prized. Rapport is developed not by accident, nor by magic, but by the deliberate efforts of the well-trained counselor who understands the core conditions of nurturance in human relationships and can create them at will.

## SELF-GUIDED EXPLORATIONS

1. Describe one of the most influential helping relationships you have ever experienced. What was it about this relationship that was so powerful and influential?
2. One important skill involved in building therapeutic relationships is asking open-ended, exploratory questions. If you could ask a stranger only three questions and had to give a lengthy talk on the essence of what this person is like based on the answers given, what questions would you ask?
3. Answer the questions you just created.
4. Describe the relationship that is most conflicted in your life right now. Then follow the steps of resolving conflicted relationships that are described in the text to work through your difficulty:
   a. What most often acts as a trigger for the conflict to begin or escalate?
   b. How is this present conflict familiar to you in terms of other difficulties you have experienced in the past?
   c. What are the hidden benefits for you in this conflict?

    d. In what ways are you disowning responsibility for your share of the problem?

    e. What do you vow to do to change the ways you react to the situation?

    f. What are some of the creative strategies you might try to break through the impasse?

## For Homework:

The "Hot Seat" is an exercise in which participants agree to answer any question asked of them as honestly as they can. It is used to build intimacy in groups, but also to train counselors to ask good probing questions that collect valuable information and promote insight. Take the questions you generated in this chapter as a starting point and practice deepening your primary relationships. Take turns with friends or family members asking questions and then answering them.

Write down a few of the favorite questions that you want to remember to use in the future.

## SUGGESTED READINGS

Brammer, L. M., & MacDonald, G. (1999). *The helping relationship*. Boston: Allyn & Bacon.

Derlega, V. J., Hendrick, S. S., Winstead, B. A., & Berg, J. H. (1991). *Psychotherapy as a personal relationship*. New York: Guilford Press.

Egan, G. (1998). *The skilled helper: A systematic approach to effective helping* (6th ed.). Pacific Grove, CA: Brooks/Cole.

Feltham, C. (1999). *Understanding the counseling relationship*. Thousand Oaks, CA: Sage.

Gelso, C. J., & Hayes, J. A. (1998). *The psychotherapy relationship: Theory, research, and practice*. New York: Wiley.

Kahn, M. (1997). *Between therapist and client: The new relationship* (rev. ed.). New York: W. H. Freeman.

Kottler, J. A. (1994). Beyond blame: A new way of resolving conflicts in relationships. San Francisco: Jossey-Bass.

Rogers, C. R. (1980). *A way of being*. Boston: Houghton Mifflin.

Rosenthal, H. (1998). *Before you see your first client*. Holmes Beach, FL: Learning.

Stark, M. (2000). *Modes of therapeutic action: Enhancement of knowledge, provision of experience, and engagement in relationship*. Northvale, NJ: Jason Aronson.

Welch, I. D. (1998). *The path of psychotherapy*. Pacific Grove, CA: Brooks/Cole.

Zimmerman, T. S. (2002). *Balancing family and work: Special considerations in feminist therapy*. New York: Haworth Press.

# COUNSELING
# APPROACHES

PART 2

# 5 CHAPTER INSIGHT-ORIENTED APPROACHES

KEY CONCEPTS

Good theories

Constructivist approach

Feminist approach

Multicultural context

Client-centered

A way of being

Active listening

Existentialism

Presence

Psychodynamic

Defense mechanisms

Transference

Here and now

Unfinished business

Narratives

# INSIGHT-ORIENTED APPROACHES

## INTRODUCTION TO THEORY CONSTRUCTION

Theory has been both a plague and a challenge for students since pre-Socratic times when philosophers would aggressively query their disciples about the meaning of life. Certainly the contemporary student finds little solace in historical precedent for his or her own struggles to understand the differences among the various theoretical systems that are part of the counseling profession. "What good is theory?" students often ask. "I want to be a counselor, not a philosopher."

Yet confusion abounds within the realm of counseling itself, as the differences of opinion on the structure of the therapeutic relationship have shown. Whereas some of the more insight-oriented counseling approaches focus on creating an authentic human encounter for its intrinsic healing properties, the action-oriented approaches use the relationship as a means to another end. And even within a particular orientation there is much disagreement as to style, form, and content. Carl Rogers, for example, proposed that it is the realness of the encounter that is important, and so he described an insight theory that encourages naturalness, genuineness, and humanness in the relationship. On the other hand, Sigmund Freud's insight theory postulated that the relationship should be as anonymous and formalized as possible so that the client can work through resistance and transference issues.

A theory, therefore, is a blueprint for action. The counselor's choices of interventions, reactions, analysis, and understanding all flow logically from a theoretical model of what people are like, what is good for them, and what conditions are likely to influence them in a self-determined, desirable direction (Geis, 1973). Some students may be surprised to learn that counselors actually have quite complex and well-developed theories of metaphysics (how the world works), ethics (how people should act), logic (cause–effect relationships), ontology (meaning of human existence), and epistemology (how people know) (Kottler, 1994b). It is precisely these theories that guide what a counselor does with a particular client at a particular moment.

Theories are valuable because they organize knowledge and information in an easily retrievable fashion. They are no more or less than models for consistency in action; they permit all practitioners, whether of architecture, medicine, or counseling, to repeat those strategies that have worked previously in similar circumstances (Argyris, 1974). Theories, of course, have other useful functions, such as attempting to simplify the world and developing rules to explain, predict, or guide behavior.

Although they are valuable constructs for aiding action, theories are not indelibly inscribed in stone as truth. In fact, Cottone (1992) has made the case that because counseling and related professions are not cast in the same scientific ideals as those embodied in, say, a theory of relativity, we would be better off looking at paradigms that represent a bigger picture of what we do. For example, instead of looking at the individual theories as presented in this chapter and the next one, he prefers instead to organize our conceptual knowledge into four broad categories that encompass a number of subgroups that have elements in common. Whether we are talking about theories or paradigms, we are dealing with the conceptual knowledge that guides our behavior.

When you study the various counseling approaches, remember that each is a single attempt to explain the therapeutic process, albeit with emphasis, values, and strengths in some areas and limitations in others. In deciding which ideas have the most personal relevance for you, bear in mind the attributes of good theories set forth by Burks and Steffire (1979) long ago: Good theories are clearly and precisely described, as simply expressed as possible, comprehensive in scope, useful in the real world, and valuable in generating new knowledge and research.

In theory construction, we are indirectly trying to establish a basis for predicting (1) a client prognosis, (2) likely consequences of certain interventions, (3) connections among experiences (and non-experiences) in a client's life, and (4) the impact of our therapeutic efforts. But because no prediction can ever be 100 percent certain, we also use theory to approximate some degree of consistency. Theories are working hypotheses, subject to change and revision as new information about the world, our clients, and ourselves becomes available. We cannot accurately and precisely describe what we see; instead, we filter our experiences through slightly focused images and inadequate language that approximates what we think we perceive. Theory is, in a sense, our beliefs about how we explain reality (Burks & Steffire, 1979). Furthermore, this reality is hardly an absolute thing but rather subject to the unique and subjective ways that each of us creates meaning based on our assumptions, language, culture, and social norms (Gergen, 1994; Schneider, 1998).

Bateson (1979) described a few of the problems of theory construction in science by listing many of the inherent logical weaknesses in the ways we organize our knowledge:

1. Science can never prove anything, not only because prediction is imperfect and our methods of collecting data are flawed but also because proof occurs only in the realm of abstraction.

2. In human perception, all experience is subjective and hence colored by individual perceptions, as well as by unconscious motives. We can be certain that the reports of our senses will be slightly distorted, viewed through individual prisms that have been shaped by unique genetic structures and cultural experiences.

3. Explanations are the results of descriptions, and these descriptions can be organized in more than one way. Convenience determines how things are classified, and, no matter which model is used, some information will be lost or downplayed.

4. For a theory (and hence its predictive power) to be perfect, it would have to deal with factors that are 100 percent controllable. Far from the whimsical, impulsive nature of the human world, even physical laws are minutely capricious.

5. Theories are constructed from information. Information is subject not only to inadequate description and arbitrary classification but also to flawed methods of measurement. Researchers in counseling, for instance, have been debating for decades about whether it can even be reliably demonstrated that therapeutic interventions cure people because we can't agree on definitions of cure, much less figure out a way to measure the degree to which it occurs.

## Approximation of Truth and Reality

As a beginning counseling student, it would be advisable to view each of the theoretical systems represented in these chapters within the aforementioned human context. Each theory is an approximation of truth, one person's or group's attempt at explaining phenomena that are difficult to understand and virtually impossible to describe fully. These theories, as with all other human structures, are imperfect working hypotheses subject to distortions, biases, and limitations.

It is suggested in this initial exposure to the major theories of the field that you don't worry so much about learning all the minute details but instead concentrate on the bigger picture. These two chapters are intended primarily to introduce you to some of the basic terms and language of theory in the counseling profession. This will give you a head start for later courses, in which you will be expected to actually apply the concepts to your work with clients.

One other thing to keep in mind is that, historically, most of the popular theories in counseling were invented by white, upper-middle-class older men and so reflect the biases and perceptions of this group. Yet it is a remarkable fact that their innumerable contributions to the field were made in spite of

## VOICE FROM THE FIELD

There is no more confusing and frustrating thing for me than struggling with all the theories I've been bombarded with over the years. At first, I was a client-centered counselor 'cause that's what almost everyone was where I was trained. I could reflect those feelings with the best of them. Then I was assigned to a new supervisor at work who was real keen on Gestalt therapy; he even grew a beard to make himself look like Fritz Perls. I'm pretty easygoing, so I learned that stuff too—and learned it well.

To make this short, I've been through a half-dozen others and I loved 'em all—Adlerian, Reality, Ericksonian, others I can't even remember. Now I'm at a point where the various theory fads don't faze me any more. I've been able to take the best parts of each theory I learned and merge it into my own ideas about what is going on with clients. The bottom line for me, and any other counselor worth a damn, is that I have a clear plan for how to proceed with my clients.

their race, upward mobility, age, and lack of multicultural experience. Several conceptual forces are having a tremendous impact on expanding the applicability of counseling theory to a much more diverse population.

In a constructivist approach to counseling, any theory is adapted in such a way as to reflect the individual values, culture, gender, language, and perceptions of each client (Anderson, 1990; Efran, Lukens, & Lukens, 1990; Gergen, 1991; Neimeyer & Mahoney, 1999). Rather than approaching clients with our preconceptions about what their experiences might mean, we work instead to help them create their own meanings based on their cultural and perceptual background. Although we look at constructivist thinking later as a particular approach to counseling, almost all theories are now being looked at through this lens that: (1) recognizes multiple versions of "reality," (2) looks at "truth" as relative to a person's underlying assumptions, (3) considers cultural roots and traditions, and (4) examines how language and social norms shape perceptions of ourselves, others, and the world (D'Andrea, 2000).

The main task of the counselor taking a constructivist or social constructionist approach (the latter places more emphasis on the ways that language, culture, and social context shape views of reality) is to help people to examine the meaning of their life experiences and recreate alternative narratives that are more empowering. One could also say that, regardless of theoretical allegiances and what one calls oneself, this is what most practitioners do these days.

In a similar vein, feminist approaches to counseling theory, such as those described by Burstow (1992), Enns (1993), Cook (1993), and Worell and Papendrick-Remer (2001), urge practitioners to adapt their theories in such a way that greater balance is placed on values other than those emphasized by the dominant male culture. This means that any of the theories that will be reviewed must take into consideration differences in gender roles, as well as diversity and complexity in human experiences. This is especially the case with regard to individuals who are not members of the dominant cultures that have influenced principally the development of the most popular theories.

### ◼ | VOICE FROM THE FIELD

I have read dozens of books about constructivism and at first I got lost in the language and terms they favor. Stuff like "postmodernism," "deconstruction," and "analogical listening." It felt like I had to learn a foreign language first before I could ever hope to understand what the heck they were talking about. Then I'm suspicious anyway about supposedly new theories on the scene that are just old ideas repackaged a bit differently.

After considerable study, and a lot of conversations with colleagues, I now understand how useful constructivist thinking can be to promote greater humility, flexibility, and sensitivity. It forces me not only to challenge my client's assumptions, but my own beliefs about the way things are. I also really enjoy the collaborative role I play with clients in which we become "coauthors" of new stories in their lives, rather than merely accepting what they think happened as "truth."

Finally, theories are increasingly examined within a multicultural context in which practitioners are encouraged to adapt their methods to fit the needs of diverse clientele (Sue, Ivey, & Pedersen, 1996). As we will explore in a later chapter, a client's culture does not just include ethnicity and race but all the different ways that people define their primary identity including sexual orientation, profession, geographical region, religion, and other factors. Furthermore, it is important to examine critically the inherent biases of each theory, especially as it reflects the personal values and cultural assumptions of its inventors (Hayes, 1996).

You will wish to read the following sections openly and critically. Assume that each theory has some merit and value, some practical use and interesting ideas that can help you better understand the process of counseling. It would be helpful to assume, as well, that each of these theoretical orientations has its limitations with some clients, with some practitioners, and in some settings and situations.

The distinction between insight theories (this chapter) and action theories (Chapter 6), although a convenient demarcation of counseling approaches, is hardly a clear-cut one. No longer can we say that any theory is now applied in the "pure" form in which it was invented. Insight practitioners who identify strongly with psychoanalytic or existential frameworks nevertheless make use of behavioral structures to help their clients translate insights into action in their lives. And even the most staunch cognitive and behavioral practitioners will sometimes help their clients understand the source of their suffering. During a research project (Kottler & Carlson, 2002) in which we interviewed twenty of the most prominent theorists about their experiences with failure, we discovered that they routinely refer to one another's work and collaborate. This means that it is no longer possible to tell where one theory begins and another ends.

The theories grouped together in this chapter have one principle in common: It is through the process of self-awareness, self-understanding, and self-revelation that true growth occurs. Whether in a gradual clarification of feelings or in a brief spurt of insight, whether facilitated through open sharing or in-depth interpretations, whether focused on the present, past, or future, the theories treated in this chapter work through the process of self-discovery. Their unifying dimension is the belief that insight into one's problems, along with a grasp of implications, connections, consequences, and perspectives, is a necessary prerequisite before any real and lasting change can occur.

# CLIENT-CENTERED COUNSELING

## Aliases: Nondirective, Person-Centered, Humanistic, Rogerian, Self Theory

Before Carl Rogers entered the scene, therapeutic counseling was largely a directive, prescriptive enterprise consisting of advice, diagnoses, interpretations, and authority. With the publication of his books (Rogers, 1942, 1951), the field was irreversibly pushed in the direction of giving clients more autonomy and responsibility for their treatment. Client-centered counseling caught on quickly because of its optimistic philosophy, which emphasized the wonderful potential of humans to learn, grow, and heal themselves when given the opportunity within a nurturing therapeutic relationship. Further, nondirective counseling became attractive to North Americans as their first native-born approach, one that stressed positive concepts and relatively simple interventions.

Rogers also strongly influenced two other theorists who were later to refine and adapt his ideas, thus reaching a larger audience. Robert Carkhuff and his colleagues ingeniously combined techniques of behavioral analysis into a helping model that presented simplified counselor skills as the essence of constructive intervention. Carkhuff also helped to convert Rogerian philosophy into a system of action. Thomas Gordon is another adapter of client-centered counseling; he created a popular educational system for training parents (Gordon, 1970) and teachers (Gordon, 1974) by applying the skills of "active listening" to clarify a person's feelings.

In more recent times the client-centered approach has been championed by such writers as Boy and Pine (1990), Wertz (1998), and Bugental, Pierson, and Schneider (2001), who have sought to bring Rogers' concepts of humanism into the mainstream of all counseling practice. Since all counseling is essentially a relationship and human activity, Kelly (1997) has proposed that even the most technically oriented practitioners still make use of humanistic concepts in their work.

## Basic Assumptions

Most client-centered counselors are in basic agreement on the following points:

1. Human beings are growth oriented and tend toward self-actualization. This natural process of development toward higher stages of moral, emotional, and behavioral evolution can be facilitated by professional helpers

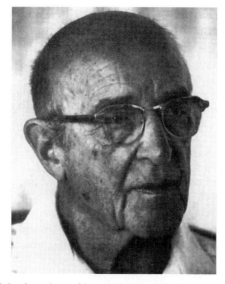

Carl Rogers, one of the founders of humanistic psychology and client-centered counseling, was known for his emphasis on creating relationships with students and clients that were caring and compassionate. © Center for the Study of the Person, courtesy of Carl Rogers Memorial Library.

who are able to stimulate the inherent capacity for progress in clients who are temporarily stymied or faltering.

2. "Every individual exists in a continually changing world of experience of which he is the center" (Rogers, 1951, p. 483). This proposition emphasizes the central importance of the individual and the subjective nature of personal experience. No matter how empathic you try to be, you can still never really know the full experiences and perceptions of another person.

3. An important vehicle for change to occur is the therapeutic relationship that exudes qualities of trust, openness, acceptance, permissiveness, and warmth. The degree to which the counselor is able to create this nurturing atmosphere will influence the client's possibilities for growth.

4. The legitimate focus of counseling content is on affect and through exploration of feelings. Both interpersonal relationships and the self-concept may be improved by becoming aware of feelings about oneself and others and by learning to express these emotions in sensitive and self-enhancing ways.

5. The universal goals of counseling are to help people to be more free, intentional, ethical, contemplative, and human. This means that time is spent in sessions helping clients to examine their values and personal characteristics so that they may become more humane and caring in their relationship with self and others.

6. The client/student has primary responsibility for the course of treatment/study—what constitutes appropriate content and whether, ultimately, it succeeds. Thus a goal is shared by client and counselor and a mutual understanding of the client's world.

7. Human beings are intrinsically good and trustworthy. They will instinctively move, in a deliberate way, toward goals that are satisfying and socially responsible. Irresponsible or socially undesirable behavior emerges from a defensiveness that alienates human beings from their own nature. As defensiveness declines and persons become more open to their own experiences, they will strive for meaningful and constructive relationships.

In a way, talking about techniques violates the very philosophy of a client-centered approach because this is more a "way of being" with a client than it is a "way of doing." Nevertheless, beginning students are anxious to translate this elusive but powerful orientation to helping into something concrete that can be seen, touched, or applied. More recent developments of the person-centered approach, such as emotionally focused therapy (Greenberg, 2002; Greenberg & Safran, 1987), have included theories that are far more structured and that respond to the current demands by managed care for increased accountability and specific treatment goals.

## Favorite Techniques

Client-centered counseling is hardly technique oriented, preferring instead to explore curative variables and focus on developing solid relationships with clients. Nevertheless, there are a few standard intervention strategies. The bread-and-butter technique of the client-centered counselor (as well as of many others) is reflection of feelings, also referred to as active listening. This skill is now so universal and generic that is used by virtually all practitioners of every theoretical persuasion.

Communicating from a posture of empathic understanding, the counselor intently attends to a client's verbal and nonverbal messages, interprets the surface and underlying meanings, and then formulates a response that demonstrates a deep-level understanding of the client's experience. This technique has several advantages:

1. Although it is the most difficult counseling skill to master, it is relatively simple to learn and fosters an open and honest helping relationship. At its most basic level, the beginner listens carefully to the underlying feeling that is expressed and then communicates back what is heard:

   CLIENT: I don't know what's going on with this situation. The more I think about it, the more . . . I just don't know.

   COUNSELOR: You sound really confused.

2. Even if the reflection of feeling is inaccurate and ignores the client's actual messages, it still encourages further self-exploration.

   COUNSELOR: You sound so angry at your brother for not writing you to join him.

   CLIENT: No. Not really. I'm not so much angry at him as I am frustrated at myself for not telling him it was important that I go.

## VOICE FROM THE FIELD

I'm what you'd call a humanistic counselor in today's climate. That doesn't mean I sit around like Rogers did, nodding my head like a friendly grandfather and concentrating only on reflecting the feelings of my clients. I don't mean to demean the limits of that sort of approach, but I think if Rogers was still alive he would have continued to evolve his thinking to make it more responsive to the demands of what we have to do.

I use a lot of different techniques in my work, actually. I've gone to workshops on just about every-thing I can. What makes me humanistic, though, isn't so much what I do in my sessions but what I'm after in my work and how I think and feel inside. I truly believe that it is through my relationships with clients that most work is accomplished. I think it's ridiculous even in brief therapy to solve client's problems without helping them to understand the source of their feelings and to express them in more constructive ways.

---

3. It helps the client to feel reassured that he or she is deeply understood and accepted.

   STUDENT: I really think it's stupid to give us an exam in a class like this that emphasizes skills instead of stuff to memorize.

   PROFESSOR: You feel as though I don't treat you with enough respect, and you also have some real concerns about how well you are doing in this class.

4. It clarifies a client's feelings so that the situation may be viewed more objectively.

   CLIENT: My father always butts into my life when he can't take care of his own.

   COUNSELOR: You are really afraid that, although you love your father very much, you may follow in his footsteps as a disaster in love relationships.

5. It provides an opportunity for emotional catharsis, bringing relief of pent-up tensions and pressure.

   CLIENT: I don't know how I feel about it.

   COUNSELOR: You're afraid to let yourself feel.

   CLIENT: You're damn right I am! I gave that bastard the best years of my life. I don't know whether to cry, scream, fight, or give up. I'm so confused.

6. It encourages the client to move from superficial concerns to deeper, more significant problems.

   CLIENT: I don't know. I've just never had good study habits. You have any tricks for doing better on true-false exams?

   COUNSELOR: You have some real reservations about your ability to discipline yourself. You sometimes feel as though you aren't smart enough to hack college and are afraid that, even if you do study, you'll flunk out anyway.

Like any of the techniques presented in this book or in your counselor training, in order to make them part of you and your natural style of interacting with others, you must practice them in your daily life. Active listening skills can be learned rather quickly even though it takes a lifetime to master them. You can get a head start by finding as many opportunities as you can—with your friends, family, classmates, coworkers—to really listen and respond actively to what they say. This does not mean that you should be counseling family and friends in your personal life, just that you can choose to listen and respond more attentively to the people you love the most.

Remember that when you are applying this approach to helping clients, your job is not to solve problems or offer advice, but rather to reflect back to others the essence of what you heard. It is their job to take this feedback and integrate it in such a way that it makes sense to them, that it facilitates deeper level understanding, and that it motivates them to make needed changes.

## Criticisms of Client-Centered Counseling

Although a valuable and—at the time of its inception—radical departure from usual procedures, client-centered counseling can be criticized on several grounds:

1. It may give too much responsibility to the client and reduce the role of the counselor as the trained expert. Clients don't often know what they are feeling.
2. It may be somewhat naïve in its view of clients as naturally evolving and lofty in goals that may not be possible. Counselors, for example, may be unable to create "unconditional positive regard," because everything is ultimately conditional.
3. It does not respond to the difficulties encountered in translating feelings into action.
4. It is narrow in its focus on feelings and tends to ignore thoughts and behavior.
5. It may overemphasize the importance of relationship factors, which may be a necessary but insufficient condition for therapeutic change.
6. It is not useful for clients who are in crisis and require directive intervention.
7. It tends to be more useful for highly verbal clients and less appropriate for those who have difficulty expressing themselves.
8. It may overfocus on issues of freedom, autonomy, and independence—distinctly North American values—and underestimate the importance of socio-cultural influences that are prevalent in other cultures and countries.

Whereas the client-centered approach has been legitimately criticized for placing too much emphasis on individual issues, while neglecting systemic and cultural forces, more contemporary practice has used Rogers' ideas to identify one's own values and biases and the importance of treating each person as unique. This no longer means looking solely at the client's self, but also looking at the cultural context for self-development (MacDougall, 2002).

## ▐ VOICE FROM THE FIELD

I remember when I first learned active listening in my counseling program what a difference it meant in so many of my relationships. At first I was so awkward at it that every time I slipped it into a conversation I thought I'd get caught, that a friend or one of my kids would accuse me of acting like a counselor with them. But what I discovered is that adopting this stance helped deepen all my relationships. It taught me to listen more deeply and respond more compassionately. The fact is that in most conversations, people don't listen to one another very well; they are never giving all their attention. Ever since I first learned these skills I made a commitment to myself that I would give the people I love the same kind of quality attention that I give my clients.

## Personal Applications

Principles of client-centered counseling can help you to:

1. Create greater self-awareness, especially with regard to your feelings, and thereby expand growth and congruence. It helps you to create a growth orientation and encourages an active attitude toward life and personal growth.
2. Gain appreciation for the importance of genuineness, unconditional regard, acceptance, and empathy in dealing with other persons. This may help you to stifle or mute the critical voice inside your head.
3. Take more responsibility for your own education and life experiences. The person-centered approach emphasizes self-empowerment.
4. Recognize the importance of exploring your feelings, risking, and sharing them with others. You can therefore practice in your own life what you want for your clients.

## EXISTENTIAL COUNSELING

### Aliases: Humanistic, Phenomenological, Experiential

Existentialism is a particularly rich and difficult theory because it intersects so many different fields. It had a long and distinguished career as a philosophy long before it was recruited to the more practical dimensions of reality in therapeutic counseling. Beginning with Socrates and continuing onward into the twentieth century, such well-known philosophers as Kierkegaard, Neitzsche, Heidegger, Husserl, Tillich, and Marcel have led an international search for the ultimate meaning of human existence. These complex philosophies were later absorbed into the world of art (Cezanne, Picasso, Van Gogh, Chagall) and literature (Kafka, Camus, Sartre, Dostoyevsky). Existentialism has now been translated into a style of living, a way of being that encourages a person to use and accept anxiety constructively (May, 1983). Fortunately, it is not necessary to fully comprehend existentialist philosophy in order to make use of its concepts in therapeutic counseling. For our purposes, we will concentrate our discussion on its practical applications.

Among the several theorists who were responsible for translating existential philosophy to practical reality, Viktor Frankl (1962) adopted this mode of meaning-making thinking as a survival strategy in Nazi concentration camps during World War II. The main determinant, according to Frankl, of an inmate's likelihood of living or giving up and dying was the ability to create a personal meaning to the experience: "If there is a meaning in life at all, then there must be a meaning in suffering. Suffering is an ineradicable part of life, even as fate and death. Without suffering and death human life cannot be complete" (p. 106).

Whether a rationalization or justification of the unjustifiable, Frankl observed the importance of the basic existential hallmarks in the everyday life of anyone who suffers humiliation and pain—in a hospital, death camp, or counselor's office. Freedom, choice, being, responsibility, and meaning are the ideas that helped him to survive and those that help clients to flourish:

> We who lived in concentration camps can remember the men who walked through the huts comforting others, giving away their last piece of bread. They may have been few in number, but they offer sufficient proof that everything can be taken from a man but one thing: the last of the human freedoms—to choose one's attitude in any given set of circumstances, to choose one's own way. (Frankl, 1962, p. 104)

The implications of this brief statement are profound, not only for the counselor who is helping others to find their way, but also for ourselves. So often people come to us feeling trapped in their lives, without hope, without choices, as if they are in a prison with no escape. Yet the bars are of their own creation because of a refusal, or inability, to accept responsibility for the choices in their lives. Feeling trapped is the result of not recognizing freedom. That is one of our jobs as counselors: to help people find the meaning in their suffering, to help them to make choices that lead to greater freedom.

Rollo May (1958) introduced these compelling ideas, previously restricted to the European continent, to North American psychotherapists and counselors. The focus of therapeutic intervention is to help clients become responsible for their choices, to manage their freedom and thereby transcend the meaninglessness of their lives, moving into a more authentic existence. May contributed a series of books on love, power, creativity, anxiety, freedom, and various other issues of existential relevance. His goal was to assist the client to develop insight regarding the life forces that can be mobilized to overcome the existential crises of powerlessness and freedom:

> After many a therapeutic hour which I would call successful, the client leaves with more anxiety than he had when he came in; only now the anxiety is conscious rather than unconscious, constructive rather than destructive. The definition of mental health needs to be changed to living without paralyzing anxiety, but living with normal anxiety is a stimulant to a vital existence, as a source of energy, and as life enhancing. (May, 1981, p. 191)

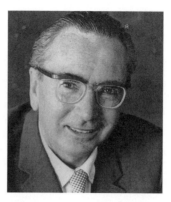

Victor Frankl, one of the founders of existential therapy, developed his approach while trying make sense of the pain and suffering he witnessed in the Nazi concentration camps. His book, *Man's Search for Meaning,* is cited by librarians as among the most important works of the last century. Courtesy of the Harvard University Archives.

If anxiety has its usefulness, so too does the concept of death to the existentialist. Yalom (1980, 2001) writes about the idea of death as the primary savior of humankind because it motivates an intense appreciation of life's value. By confronting our own vulnerability, the ultimate threat to our existence, we are made aware of people and things that are truly important. Death and the companion existential issues of isolation, meaninglessness, and freedom are seen as the legitimate focus of counseling. Yalom was able to translate much of the confusion, complex language, and abstract ideas of existentialism into a system of helping and an attitude for the helper, complete with methodologies for analyzing and solving human problems.

Existential counseling is richly endowed in its affiliations with Rogers' client-oriented approach, Maslow and Shostrom's self-actualization psychology, and Freud's theory of psychoanalysis. Far from postulating a rigid set of therapeutic procedures, the existentialist offers a way of thinking about clients and their concerns, about humans and their dilemmas, and about life and its puzzles (May & Yalom, 1995). In its more recent forms of evolution (Mahrer, 1996; Strasser & Strasser, 1997; Watson & Bohart, 2001) existential approaches have been more highly structured and responsive to the demands of managed care.

## Premises of Existential Counseling

The existential approach has been minimally concerned with the techniques and specific interventions of counseling, concentrating instead on philosophical principles that aid the understanding of the client. As an insight-oriented theory, its main goal is to help people find personal meaning in their actions, their lives, and their suffering. A counselor working from an existential posture would assist people primarily to develop the range of their choices, and hence their freedom to develop in new ways.

VOICE FROM THE FIELD

I'm an existentialist. I think. But then I've never been sure what that means. If it means being fascinated with what we are all doing here on this planet, then count me in. If it means helping clients to sort out what their meaning and purpose in life is all about, then that's what I do. No extra charge either. I just kinda throw it in with whatever else they have in mind they'd like to accomplish. I just think that human beings are drawn, maybe even driven, to figure out meanings behind things, including their own behavior. And I see that as my job to help them.

---

Clients who present the symptoms of existential anxiety (lack of meaning, fear of death, isolation, avoidance of responsibility) can be helped to become more capable of determining the outcome of their daily life. They become aware of their fears. They understand the significance and personal meaning of their refusal to enjoy freedom. They confront the naked fact that each person, from the moment of birth, stands alone. Yet, far from necessarily condemning the self to loneliness, we may choose to take responsibility for our aloneness, our freedom, our choices, and the consequences of what we choose. "The one who realizes in anguish his condition as being thrown into a responsibility which extends to his very abandonment has no longer either remorse or regret or excuse, he is no longer anything but a freedom which perfectly reveals itself and whose being resides in this very revelation" (Sartre, 1957, p. 59).

Similar to the client-centered counselor (which is often included in this same family), the existential practitioner seeks to enter into the client's world and, remaining in the present, to use the therapeutic alliance—the relationship—as a fulcrum by which to lever more involvement and commitment to living, to being. This process of counseling and change is more than a little ambiguous. The existential approach is a philosophy, an attitude, a way of thinking, analyzing, and experiencing; it is, therefore, difficult to describe specifically how the counselor acts, even though a few techniques reluctantly emerge from the theory.

The basic distinguishing features of an existential approach include the following:

- A focus on issues of freedom
- A confrontation with fears of death, alienation, and aloneness
- An emphasis on taking responsibility for one's life
- A compatibility with other, more action-oriented, theories
- A challenge to discover the meanings behind one's choices and actions
- A search for a personal philosophy to guide daily life

Existentialism is basically an attitude toward living and, as such, emphasizes the role of understanding and insight into the human condition. The counselor works toward knowing the client rather than knowing *about* him or her. The process of knowing includes the three separate modes of human existence: the client's natural, biological world; the interpersonal world; and the uncharted territory of the solitary individual in relationship to him or herself. It is the counselor's presence with the client rather than any specific technique that encourages growth to greater autonomy. Presence involves more than being physically together with the client; it means being with the person in body, in spirit, and in every possible way so that you can be perfectly open and accessible to whatever is presented (Bugental, 1991).

## Criticisms of Existential Counseling

Existentialism is often misunderstood by philosophers and can be obtuse to those who are untrained in this discipline. It has been described as a particularly abstract, ambiguous, mystical theory that is difficult to apply to the circumstances of everyday living. Also, because the philosophy is so intellectually complex, it is not often appropriate for clients who are of low to average intelligence, or for people with severe emotional and cognitive disturbances. Needless to say, other individuals who are in the midst of a crisis or who are barely surviving in their basic economic needs are going to be relatively unconcerned with their "existential angst" or "phenomenological nonbeing" as compared to other, more pressing problems.

The existential approach is also hard to study because it is nonempirical and doesn't lend itself to scientific scrutiny. Further, although practitioners of this theory are extremely versatile and flexible in their willingness to use a variety of techniques, relatively few specific interventions are available.

## Personal Applications

Stop reading for a moment. Put your hand on your heart. (I'm not kidding. Do it. Now!)

Feel your heart beating. Feel it pumping through your chest. Duh-dum. Duh-dum. Duh-dum. About once every second, 60 times every minute, 360 times every hour, it beats without your awareness. Feel it beating right now, pumping away as if you don't have a care in the world.

Your heart is a muscle, squeezing blood in and out, circulating it throughout your body and brain. It is also a muscle that is wearing out. This very second, as it continues to beat, it is slowing, inevitably, wearing out. Each of us is allocated only a certain number of heartbeats before the heart just stops beating altogether.

Now think about all the heartbeats that you waste every minute, every hour, every day. Think about all the heartbeats you give away when you're bored and wile away time as if you have all the heartbeats in the world. But you don't. Maybe a hundred left. Or a thousand. Or even a million. But the number left is finite.

So the question remains: What do you intend to do with the precious few heartbeats you have left?

If you actually followed this process, if you really paid attention to its implications, your heart is probably beating a little quicker right now. Thinking about death and our eventual demise is terrifying. Yet according to the existentialist, it is actually death that saves us, that motivates us to live life more intensely and passionately. If every heartbeat is a gift, if at any moment your heart could stop beating, or an artery could explode in your brain, or a piano could fall on your head, what choices are you making to become more intensely involved in living and to accept responsibility for your decisions?

If that doesn't get your attention, you weren't listening.

# PSYCHOANALYTIC COUNSELING

## Aliases: Psychoanalysis, Analysis, Freudian Psychotherapy, Psychodynamic Therapy

The profession of therapeutic counseling can be traced to Sigmund Freud and his early experimentations with hypnosis and the "talking cure," in which he allowed hysterical patients to reveal their innermost unconscious desires. From the late nineteenth century until his death in exile from his native Austria at the outbreak of World War II, Freud not only revolutionized our conceptions of human psychology but also single-handedly recruited an army of psychoanalytic thinkers to continue his work. Carl Jung, Otto Rank, Alfred Adler, Wilhelm Reich, Karen Horney, Theodore Reik, Franz Alexander, Harry Stack Sullivan, Erik Erikson, Erich Fromm, Heinz Kohut, and Anna Freud form an impressive list of theorists, brilliant in their own right, who were able to expand, revise, and adapt the psychoanalytic approach to their respective settings, situations, and personalities. As a footnote, even the creators of completely new schools of counseling, such as Fritz Perls, Albert Ellis, Eric Berne, and Rollo May, were once practicing psychoanalysts who grew beyond the confines of traditional psychoanalysis.

An additional point of clarification: There is a difference between *psychoanalysis*—the orthodox application of Freudian theory—and *psychoanalytically oriented* therapy, which makes use of some Freudian concepts but is more flexible in their application, according to the preferences of the practitioner. Some theorists have successfully abbreviated psychoanalytic methods into a short-term psychodynamic approach that can be more efficient, economical, and appropriate for counseling settings (Book, 1998; Davanloo, 1978; Levenson, 1995; Mander, 2000; Schwartz, 1997; Strupp & Binder, 1984). Our discussion will focus on some of the more universal and practical ideas of psychoanalytic theory—those that are most relevant to the practice of counseling.

## Basic Psychoanalytic Concepts

Traditional psychoanalysis is quite complex and time consuming. Its practice requires five years of intensive postdoctoral training, which includes undergoing personal treatment as well as seminars in order to have a working knowledge of the theory. Most of its practitioners have doctoral or medical degrees, although private practitioners in social work and other disciplines also have favored this theory historically.

Many terms of psychoanalysis have crept into our everyday language—for example, *ego, catharsis, unconscious, defense mechanisms,* and *rationalization*—making a basic understanding of some important ideas necessary for any practicing counselor. Even for those who have no intention of ever using this particular style of helping, the conceptual vocabulary of psychoanalysis has become crucial as a mode of communication with other professionals, as an orientation toward analyzing the etiology and development of human problems, and as a foundational base for constructing new counseling strategies. The following sections discuss some of the most basic psychoanalytic concepts.

**Layers of Awareness**   Freud introduced the concept of different levels of awareness that motivate behavior. He postulated that there are several regions of the mind: the conscious mind, which contains those thoughts and feelings that are always accessible; the preconscious mind, which holds elements on the edge of awareness that, with minimal effort, can be made immediately accessible; and the *unconscious mind,* which harbors the secrets of the soul.

Each layer of awareness can be peeled away, providing deeper access into the human psyche, only by permitting unconscious thoughts to surface. This task may be accomplished through analysis of dreams, free association of thoughts, catharsis of feelings, and interpretations that provide a level of insight sufficient to release unconscious, inhibiting desires and facilitate their continued awareness.

**Stages of Personal Development**   As a medically trained physician, Freud had a particular interest in neurology and the instinctual basis of behavior. He thus viewed the development of human personality as following a series of biologically determined stages, each an expression of the pleasure principle—the child's insatiable urge to reduce tension and maintain psychic equilibrium by self-indulgence in oral, anal, or genital preoccupations. Freud's original conception of psychosexual development is often paired with a more recent adaptation by Erik Erikson (1950), which has more contemporary relevance for counselors seeking to understand the orderly progression of human development. Freud was concerned mostly with early childhood development and its impact on later life; Erikson's stages more accurately reflect growth throughout the life cycle, with a particular emphasis on social influences.

**Structure of the Psyche**   The healthy personality, according to Freud, consists of three separate systems, which function harmoniously and cooperatively to satisfy a person's basic needs and desires. Each of these aspects of personality is less discrete than the structure suggests and should more accurately be considered as an approximate description of processes that influence who you are and how you react to the world around you.

The *id* is the source of all energy and instinctual drives. Its sole psychological function is to reduce tension, discomfort, and pain at all costs. The id is impulsive, demanding, and infantile in its wishes, acting without thought or consideration of consequences.

The *ego* is the contact between the id's uncontrolled energy and the world of reality. The ego rationally, intelligently, and logically attempts to harness and moderate blind action. The ego is an integrator, pacifier, negotiator, and compromiser that seeks in socially acceptable and appropriate ways to fulfill a person's needs.

The *superego* is concerned primarily with moral issues. It is the ideal part of yourself, as contrasted with reality or pleasure. Operating as your conscience, it strives for perfection and virtuousness. In its battle waged against the hedonistic id, the superego often takes home the spoils of "pride" or "guilt," depending on the ego's chosen resolution of the conflict.

**Defense Mechanisms**    The defense mechanisms are a major contribution of psychoanalysis to practicing counselors. According to their descriptions, the defenses used by the ego to guard against perceived attack are analogous to the workings of our body's immunological system to maintain a constant equilibrium of fluid temperature, pressure, and content. Change is the enemy. Just as we are unaware of the antibodies in our bloodstream when they are activated to fight foreign protein molecules, our psychological defense mechanisms operate without our conscious awareness in an attempt to reduce anxiety and lower tension. They are ingenious strategies, impressive in their variety and flexibility; but these unconscious mind-directed defenses make the job of counseling and facilitating changes much more difficult. Better we should recognize the opponents that will be resisting our best treatment efforts:

Repression: The selective exclusion of painful experiences of the past from conscious awareness; a form of censorship used to block traumatic episodes.

Projection: The art of putting onto another person those characteristics that are unacceptable to yourself, such as accusing someone of being angry when we are actually feeling the anger.

Denial: The distortion of reality by pretending that undesirable or unacceptable events are not really happening. In contrast to repression, denial occurs on a preconscious rather than unconscious level.

Sublimation: The disguised conversion of forbidden impulses into socially acceptable behaviors. For instance, athletes may unconsciously choose their profession as a way to release aggression. Creative enterprises such as da Vinci's paintings or Shakespeare's sonnets were seen by Freud as sublimated sexual desires.

Reaction formation: Used to counter perceived threats, the substitution of an opposite reaction for the one that is disturbing. Guilt can be replaced by indignation, hatred by devotion, or resentment by overprotection.

Rationalization: The intellectual misuse of logic to overexplain or justify conflicting messages. For example, "It doesn't matter if I type the paper or not; I'll probably flunk the class anyway."

CHAPTER 5 INSIGHT-ORIENTED APPROACHES 131

## VOICE FROM THE FIELD

Any counselor, regardless of where she works, had better know the language of psychoanalysis down cold. Everybody in the field uses the jargon. Besides, with all the jokes about Freud and psychoanalysis, you won't know when to laugh unless you know the theory. Just kidding.

The theory does give you a foundation for other stuff you'll learn. I don't know too many people, ex-cept a few in private practice, who even use the the-ory that much any more. Well, lots of people use it but don't necessarily apply it the way Freud intended. Still, it is absolutely a brilliant framework for helping clients understand their past, and especially how that affects their present behavior. When I do family coun-seling, for example, there are some psychoanalytic ideas I use to look at family-of-origin stuff.

Displacement: The rechanneling of energy from one object to another, as when an infant sucks a finger or another object in place of the desired breast.

Identification: The incorporation, in exaggerated form, of the values, atti-tudes, standards, and characteristics of persons who are anxiety provok-ing, as when a child punishes herself or himself for being bad.

Regression: The retreat to an earlier stage of development because of fear. Any flight from controlled and realistic thinking may constitute a regression.

Fixation: The tendency to remain at one level, interrupting the normal plan of psychological development. It is generally a defense against anxiety and results from the fear of taking the next step in psychological development.

In general, defense mechanisms are methods used by the ego to deal with anxiety. They tend to distort, hide, or deny reality and hinder psychological development. They are essential to the infantile ego because of the lack of ego strength; however, they will persist when the ego has not matured sufficiently. One goal of therapeutic counseling, from the perspective of psychoanalytic theory, is to foster the healthy development of the ego.

## Criticisms of Psychoanalytic Counseling

Traditional psychoanalytic counseling has been criticized on a number of grounds, many of which relate to its deterministic philosophy and inflexible closed-system approach:

1. The expense and time involved in psychoanalytic treatment are consider-able, requiring lengthy training for the counselor and treatment for the client that could run into years.
2. It is not useful as an approach for treating large numbers of people who require counseling services.
3. There is an overemphasis on the role of insight and very little emphasis on making life changes.

4. The approach is based on experiences with neurotic rather than normal populations and may be skewed in the direction of sickness instead of health.
5. The concepts of psychoanalytic theory are difficult to research and support empirically.
6. Traditional Freudian psychoanalysis places excessive emphasis on basic instinctual desires and forces, ignoring the effects of social and cultural factors. Perhaps more than usual for theories developed by white males, it is gender and culturally biased.
7. It is not useful for persons in crisis who require immediate relief of symptoms.
8. The theory has traditionally been criticized as strongly culturally and gender biased, but that is what you would expect from an approach developed more than a century ago. Just as in every other theory currently practiced, efforts have been made to make the theory more responsive to issues of client diversity.

Criticizing Freud's ideas, especially the rigidity with which some psychoanalysts function, has become so fashionable that many valuable therapeutic concepts have been discarded in the backlash. In part to answer their critics and in part to make the treatment more realistic, the core of psychoanalytic thinking has been preserved by some theorists in a new short-term form of therapeutic counseling. More focus is placed on specific problem areas. The treatment is more individually designed, and the counselor confronts resistance more directly. Efforts are made to establish time limits for both length of treatment and specific goals. The clinician plays a more active role in interpreting transference issues and in linking them to previous relationships. Efforts have also been undertaken to make psychoanalytic treatments more responsive to the needs of managed care systems (Mander, 2000; Schwartz, 1997).

## Personal Applications

One of the distinguishing features of psychoanalytic theory is the strong emphasis placed on applying the concepts and techniques to one's own life. In a revealing letter to a friend, Freud remarked on his own painful struggles with self-analysis, which eventually led to further refinements of his ideas:

15.10.97.

IX. Bergasse 19

My dear Wilhelm,

My self-analysis is the most important thing I have in hand, and promises to be of the greatest value to me, when it is finished. When I was in the very midst of it, I suddenly broke down for three days, and I had the feeling of inner binding about which my patients complain so much, and I was inconsolable. . . .

It is no easy matter. Being entirely honest with oneself is a good exercise. Only one idea of general value has occurred to me. I have found love of the mother and jealousy of the father in my own case too, and now believe it to be a general phenomenon of early childhood. (Freud, 1954, pp. 221, 223)

The theory and techniques of psychoanalysis naturally lend themselves to personal experimentation; it was that exact method that Freud employed in their invention. Interpreting dreams is an especially fruitful method of understanding our unconscious desires and avoiding resistance, because even our defense mechanisms sleep at night. Other techniques designed to unlock the secrets of the soul include hypnosis and free association. In applying any of these strategies to ourselves, it is crucial to follow Freud's imperative that we be entirely honest about our desires, wishes, and motives.

# GESTALT COUNSELING

## Originators and Basic Concepts

Gestalt counseling has distinguished roots that go back to the very beginning of psychology as a discipline. Scientists interested in the process of learning and perception noted that problem solving is less a gradual phenomenon as it is a critical moment of insight. Kurt Koffka (1935) and Wolfgang Kohler (1929) spent considerable time between the world wars creating certain laws of behavior that could be used to explain the process of learning. For example, they noted that we tend to perceive things grouped together as clusters, according to their proximity to one another, and that we learn to focus our attention selectively on those events, situations, or stimuli that provide internal psychological equilibrium, even though we may thereby distort reality.

The basic goal of Gestalt theory is to describe human existence in terms of awareness. Gestalt counseling has been influenced philosophically by existentialism and psychologically by humanism. Each of these influences has reinforced experience as the central concept on which awareness is built. Gestalt therapy focuses on the *what* and *how* of behavior and on the central role of *unfinished business* from the past that interferes with effective functioning in the present. By helping individuals more fully to experience the present—the "here and now"—Gestalt counselors facilitate greater self-awareness and understanding.

Gestalt counseling is most closely associated with Fritz Perls (1969a), who organized the contemporary Gestalt movement in California and was its central figure until his death in 1970. Gestalt counseling is essentially experiential rather than theoretical and to a large extent is strongly influenced by the character and person of the practitioner. This was certainly true in the case of Perls, who was a charismatic personality.

Gestalt counseling stresses the role of personal responsibility in the development of awareness and experiencing of feelings. Unfinished business from the past is brought into the present, and the impasse it represents is dealt with therapeutically. The term *stuck* is used to describe the inability to resolve issues and thereby avoid dealing with the "now." *Polarization* is another key Gestalt concept; it refers to the various parts of the self that are in conflict. In his autobiography, Perls interrupts the flow of his narrative to conduct an internal dialogue between his polarized, conflicted selves:

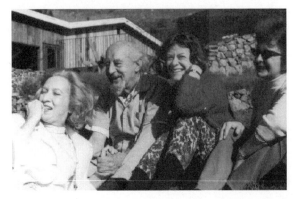

Fritz Perls was the charismatic leader of the Gestalt therapy movement, an approach to counseling that emphasizes direct experience and staying in the present moment.
Courtesy of Esalen Institute.

TOPDOG: Stop, Fritz, what are you doing?

UNDERDOG: What do you mean?

TOPDOG: You know very well what I mean. You're drifting from one thing to another.

UNDERDOG: I still don't see your objection.

TOPDOG: You don't see my objection? Man, who the hell can get a clear picture of your therapy?

UNDERDOG: You mean I should take a blackboard and make tables and categorize every term, every opposite neatly?

TOPDOG: That's not a bad idea. You could do that. . . .

UNDERDOG: So what do you want me to do? Stop letting the river flow? Stop playing my garbage bin game?

TOPDOG: Well, that wouldn't be a bad idea, if you would sit down and discipline yourself. . . .

UNDERDOG: Go to hell. You know me better. If I try to do something deliberate and under pressure, I get spiteful and go on strike. All my life I have been a drifter. (Perls, 1969b, pp. 117–118)

## Techniques of Gestalt Counseling

Gestalt counseling could be seen as the more pragmatic sibling of existential theory. Whereas the latter is heavy on philosophy and light on practical strategies, the latter is absolutely loaded with hundreds of techniques that are used by practitioners of all orientations.

## VOICE FROM THE FIELD

I've always been intrigued by Gestalt stuff but never really got a handle on it. I think I probably do a lot of Gestalt-type work, but I'm never sure what that means. I remember one time I saw a book in which Perls was interviewed and the cover said something like, "Fritz finally reveals the secrets of what his theory is all about," or something like that. I bought the book, got home, and dipped into it right away. The first question was, "So Fritz, tell us what your theory is all about." Not only did Perls not answer the question but within minutes he had the interviewer pretending he was an airplane.

I love this goofy stuff—even if I don't know what it means. Maybe Perls would consider that progress because he was so anti-intellectual. Anyway, sometime soon I intend to experience this theory more since you can't really learn it by studying it from the outside.

**Hot Seat**   This technique requires an individual to be the focus of attention and answer all questions with complete honesty and sincerity. The participant is challenged to be the "here-and-now" self at all times, a task that is quite difficult, considering the intensity of questions that could be posed: "What is your most common fantasy?" "What in your life are you most ashamed of?" "Which person in the group are you most attracted to and why?" This is an exercise that I find particularly interesting to use in classes when demonstrating how to ask good open-ended questions, the kind that generate a lot of reflection and exploration. You will also find that this works equally well in social situations to foster greater intimacy.

**Resentment Expression**   Perls believed that it was essential to express resentments, which, if unexpressed, are converted to guilt. To take an example: Make a list of all the things about which you consciously feel guilty. Now change the word *guilt* to *resentment*: "I feel guilty because I do not spend enough time with my children" becomes "I resent having to spend time with my children." Exploring and expressing the resentment can help a person become unstuck and work through unfinished business.

**Double Chairing**   This technique is designed to help persons to experience the opposite poles of the self. The counselor explores a problem with a client and identifies the opposing feelings. Two chairs are then set up, and the client is instructed to take one and talk to the empty chair from one (specified) pole of the issue. On instruction from the counselor, the client moves to the second chair and talks from the opposite perspective. For example: "I can't stand the way my wife puts me down for everything, and I won't take it. I won't spend another minute in that house. I'm going to ask for a divorce and stick with it. Being alone is better than this misery." From the opposite pole: "Even though I feel very dissatisfied and maybe even angry with my wife, I really need to try harder to make this marriage work. We have a lot of years invested, our kids deserve an intact home, and I really don't like the idea of being alone and starting over. Besides, I'm not the easiest guy to live with." The purpose of this technique is to increase the awareness of feelings, resentments, fears, and issues from each pole of the individual's experience.

**Owning the Projection**    In this exercise the client is encouraged to apply his or her projections to himself or herself to demonstrate how we sometimes avoid our negatively perceived qualities and traits by putting them onto others. For example, a client says to a group member, "I think you are manipulative" and then says, "I am manipulative." Or, "I don't think you are trustworthy" and then, "I don't think I am trustworthy."

## Criticisms of Gestalt Counseling

As is immediately evident from this brief presentation, Gestalt counseling is considerably different from the other insight theories in that little attempt has been made by its creators to explain concepts and more emphasis has been placed on experiential aspects. Consequently, the Gestalt approach is rich in strategies to help the client and counselor stay in the "here and now" and work toward greater integration of the self's polarities.

But Gestalt counseling has been soundly criticized for its lack of a clearly articulated theory and its limited empirical base. Among other criticisms are these:

1. There is a tendency for counselors to be overly manipulative and controlling.
2. Gestalt counseling is sometimes viewed as anti-intellectual because cognitive thinking factors are greatly de-emphasized.
3. Gestalt counseling is sometimes viewed as gimmicky and having a high potential for abuse.
4. It sometimes encourages a "do your own thing" attitude, which can create a sense of irresponsibility.
5. There is very little emphasis on acquiring behaviorally useful life skills.

## HONORABLE MENTIONS

You have probably heard that are literally hundreds of counseling theories currently in practice and at least two dozen that may be considered relatively common. I don't mean to slight any particular approach by not including it in this chapter or the next one. Because of space limitations I can only give you a sampling of a few representative approaches. In latter courses you will have the chance to study these theories, and many others, in greater depth. Other books devoted exclusively to counseling theory can provide you with greater detail (see Capuzzi & Gross, 2001; Corey, 2000; Kottler, 2002; Wedding & Corsini, 2001 as examples). And, of course, you will want to read many of the theorists' original works when you have chance.

I would, however, like to mention a few other insight-focused therapies that have been influential in the field. The decision not to give them as much space as the ideas discussed previously is based solely on my belief that they *currently* exert less influence on the field than those previously mentioned. These theories are potentially as valuable or useful as the ones that have been presented; a theory's inclusion is a matter of personal opinion about what is most appropriate for beginning students to learn first. I am sure your instructor will point out other theories that I've neglected or underemphasized and will encourage you to examine them in greater depth. Your instructor may also take issue with the way I've classified these theories as "insight" or "action" oriented when, in fact, this simple dichotomy does not do justice to the complexity and flexibility of these approaches.

## Adlerian Counseling

Alfred Adler, one of Freud's disciples who went his own way, developed a remarkably integrative theory for his time—one that combined some of the premises of psychoanalysis with a more pragmatic approach that emphasized such ideas as: (1) the social context for human behavior, (2) the interpersonal nature of client problems, (3) the cognitive organization of a client's style of thinking, and (4) the importance of choice and responsibility in making decisions.

Adlerian counselors, although subscribing to the tenets above, are quite flexible in their style of practice. After all, they hold much in common with some of the existential practitioners (the emphasis on personal responsibility), the cognitive therapists (the focus on the subjective perception of reality), the psychoanalysts (attention to dreams and the unconscious), and even the behaviorists (the focus on specific tasks to be completed).

A resurgence of interest in Adlerian approaches has been evident in recent years, due in part to the systematic organization and explication of Adler's ideas by authors such as Lundin (1989), Sweeney (1998), Watts and Carlson (1999), and Dinkmeyer and Sperry (2000). Prior to these contemporary spokespeople, it was primarily Rudolf Dreikurs who popularized Adler's work. Dreikurs (1950) formulated five basic norms of Adlerian theory:

1. *Socially embedded:* All problems are basically social problems and emerge from the need to belong and find a place in the group. A well-adjusted person is oriented to and behaves in line with the needs of the social situation. A maladjusted person has faulty concepts, feelings of inferiority, and mistaken goals and is overly concerned with what others think of him or her or with what is in it for him or her.

2. *Self-determining and creative:* Adler believed that life is movement and that individuals have the power to change interactions by what they do. The belief that individuals can change and are active participants in their lives is the basis for such optimism.

3. *Goal directed:* Behavior, according to Adler, is directed toward goals that are inferred from the consequences of behavior. Looking for causes of behavior is unproductive because they are unknowable and, even if known, cannot be changed. Goals, once recognized, can be modified and represent a behavioral choice.

4. *Subjective:* Reality is as we perceive it and is not absolute. Adler further believed that it is not what happens to us that matters, but how we feel about it. As a result, Adler emphasized interactions and movement in all relationships as the units of analysis.
5. *Holistic:* Human beings are integrated, whole, and incapable of being reduced to discrete units. One must deal with the entire person.

In Adlerian theory, feelings of inferiority are the basis of anxiety and are destructive to clients. Inferiority feelings are not feelings in the usual sense but are a belief system or a reasoning process about how one should be. One's response to inferiority feelings is the basis for character formation.

Adler (1958) believed that the purpose of counseling is to restore faith in the self to overcome these feelings of inferiority. The process of counseling contains four steps for the individual:

1. Become aware of prejudices. Recognize that as children we learned that we were not good enough as we were; thus, we were urged to do better.
2. Stop being afraid of making a mistake. Overconcern with error encourages more, not fewer, mistakes. Further, it is human to make mistakes; do we expect ourselves to be superhuman? Mistakes reflect an opportunity to learn if they are accepted and if we avoid discouragement.
3. Cultivate the courage to be imperfect. Working to resist self-evaluation and to do our best to respond to the needs of a situation is preferable to feeling inadequate because we could improve performance. We don't have to be any better than we are.
4. Enjoy the pleasure in an activity. It is important not to reduce pleasure in life by being overly concerned with success, failure, or prestige. Learning to do one's best and accepting the outcome increase the pleasure in life.

The Adlerian approach is concerned with helping individuals develop a lifestyle that is socially responsible and personally fulfilling, one that allows for growth and a holistic integration. A person who is psychopathological is discouraged and has lost faith in the ability to change.

## Narrative Therapy

Based on constructivist principles described earlier in the chapter—as well as contributions by White and Epston (1990), two innovative clinicians working in Australia and New Zealand—this approach has been described as the "third wave" (after Freud and the problem-solving therapies described in the next chapter) of conceptual evolution. Whereas the first wave concentrated on the individual's troubled personality and the second wave focused on family systems, the third narrative wave "draws attention to far larger systems, such as the daunting cultural sea we swim in—the messages from television advertisements, schools, newspaper experts, bosses, grandmothers, and friends—that tell us how to think and who to be" (O'Hanlon, 1994, p. 23).

Narrative approaches seek to help people to "re-story" their lives—to change the narratives about what took place. As such, it is part of the constructivist movement described earlier that emphasizes the cultural/linguistic influences on how our assumptions about reality are formed. In one sense, it is similar to rational-emotive and cognitive therapies described in the next chapter in that its focus is on altering perceptions of events. Unlike these theories that concentrate mostly on internal dialogue, however, the narrative approach more broadly examines how reality is interpreted within a cultural context.

Through a series of "circular questions," the counselor demonstrates respectful curiosity about the client's experience: "I'd like to know about you. Help me to understand your story." Rather than labeling or analyzing the client's experience using interpretations and reflections, the counselor instead draws out the client's own narrative:

- What happened when you were younger that helped prepare you to deal with this?
- What do you realize now?
- What will your next step be?
- Who will be most appreciative?

Further, the process follows a series of stages that begins with "externalizing the problem," a method quite at odds with other approaches that emphasize accepting responsibility for your troubles. The focus instead is on helping clients to deal with the problem as an enemy to be defeated. Next, the client is helped to explore all the ways this problem has been disruptive, to himself or herself and to others. Exceptions are identified in which the client was able to keep the problem at bay, as well as an alternative narrative constructed in which the client is portrayed in a more fully functioning light (Monk, Winslade, Crocket, & Epston, 1997).

Although this theory could easily have been included in the next chapter on action-oriented approaches because of its use of several unique interventions, it is presented here as one example of constructivist insights that seeks as its aim to change the ways people view their realities. In that sense, it is similar to both existential approaches that help clients to find meaning in their lives and cognitive approaches that are more directive in confronting the ways that clients interpret their experiences.

## Feminist Therapies

There is no single feminist therapy but rather a school of thought that also is rather "constructivist" in orientation. Similar to narrative therapy just mentioned, a person's experience of a problem or issue is shaped by forces within our culture, the influence of language, and especially the way that power is exercised.

No doubt you have noticed that most of the theoreticians who have shaped the fields of counseling and therapy were "old, white guys." It has only been in the last few decades that influences from marginalized groups have been integrated into mainstream thinking.

Most Feminist approaches to counseling all share certain beliefs that guide clinical practice (Enns, 1997; Worrell & Papendrick-Remer, 2001):

1. Males and females develop in unique and sometimes different ways. These differences related to language, worldview, values, and perceptions should be honored and respected in counseling.
2. Women and various minority groups have been marginalized historically. Thus dealing with issues of power is an integral part of therapeutic work for those who feel powerless.
3. Political/social/cultural influences are often at the core of many presenting complaints. Individual concerns are examined within this broader context.
4. Alternative diagnostic systems are needed that are not so biased against traditional female behavior. Thus what has been described as "hysterical" (overemotional) or "dependent" (socially considerate) have often been treated as a form of psychopathology.
5. Women's unique "voices" have been underappreciated and disrespected.

Of course, with all this emphasis on gender differences we can sometimes neglect shared experiences. There has been considerable misunderstanding about feminist therapies, associating it exclusively with women's issues. In fact, this theory is equally liberating for men as women as it defines gender roles with more flexibility. Just as women have been trapped in certain norms and roles, so too have men. Feminist therapies seek to help all clients gain insight into the choices they have made and how they have been shaped by the gender expectations of their cultures.

## SUMMARY

In this chapter we have looked at some of the more prominent insight-oriented theories that influence therapeutic counseling. There are, of course, many we have neglected, such as the other psychodynamic approaches of Jung, Alexander, Bordin, Sullivan, Reich, and Fromm; some of the "expressive" therapies (transpersonal, bioenergetics, drama, or dance therapy); approaches from the Far East (Morita or Buddhist approaches); or some more recent innovations that are both insight and action oriented (Eye Movement Desensitization Reprocessing). Part of the task of developing into a mature professional counselor is coming to terms, on a personal and intellectual level, with the many options available. At some point in your training you will be expected to make some hard choices about which approaches are most suitable to your personality, interpersonal style, work setting, and client needs.

Each of the insight approaches presented offers the counselor a framework for understanding the client's world and a methodology for promoting greater self-awareness and self-understanding. It is assumed that such exploration and knowledge will lead a client toward making desired life changes. It is also believed that the presence of the counselor and the relationship between counselor and client provide nonspecific curative effects that are helpful in the process of being and becoming.

## SELF-GUIDED EXPLORATIONS

1. Many approaches to counseling are based on helping clients understand how and why they have developed particular behavioral, emotional, or cognitive patterns. As a result of studying several of the insight-oriented theories (psychoanalytic, existential, Adlerian, Gestalt, client-centered, etc.), describe some of the insights you have become aware of about your own characteristic personality style.

2. Describe a time in which some dramatic insight or realization provided a major change in your life. What was it that helped you translate that awareness into constructive action?

3. Helping clients to identify and explore their feelings constitutes a significant part of insight-oriented counseling work. What are some of your feelings that you struggle with on an ongoing basis (for example, anger, envy, jealousy, frustration, anxiety, shame, depression, sadness, cynicism, fear of failure)?

4. A number of coping mechanisms are used by people to deal with threatening material that might arise in counseling sessions or in life. Which of these do you recognize as part of the characteristic style with which you protect yourself from perceived attacks? Describe specific examples.

| | |
|---|---|
| Repression | Rationalization |
| Projection | Displacement |
| Denial | Identification |
| Sublimation | Regression |

5. Existential theory is concerned with living more in the present by accepting how precious is each breath we take. Consider how fleeting your own time is on this planet. On one end of this continuum is your birth; the other end represents your death. Place a mark on the line to represent where you are now in your life span. Write down any reactions, thoughts, and feelings that come up for you as you reflect on how much of your life is over and how much time you have left.

Birth _____ Death

6. In small groups, talk to classmates about the ways you have been limited by your gender role. How have you felt your choices restricted and options minimized because you are a man or woman?

7. Think about a loss you have experienced in your life. This could have been the death of a loved one, the ending of a love relationship, or perhaps a loss of a part of yourself. Take a constructivist approach to exploring this issue in greater depth by asking yourself (or writing in a journal)(Neimeyer, 2002):

   • What sense of this loss did you make at the time it first took place?
   • How have your perceptions and views of this experience changed over time?

- If you were to revisit this loss right now (close your eyes for a moment and let yourself access some of the residual feelings), what still remains present for you?
- How has this loss affected and influenced your life since then, including your decisions, priorities, and choices?
- What lessons did you learn as a result of this experience that have both strengthened and limited you?
- How might you "re-story" this loss in such a way that its meaning and significance are honored yet you might draw increased strength and resilience from the experience?

As one example of how loss and trauma can be reconstructed in more self-enhancing ways, champion bicyclist Lance Armstrong recovered from (potentially) terminal cancer to win the Tour de France more times than any other North American. In talking about his loss and life-threatening illness, Armstrong (2002, p. 73) says: "It was the best thing that ever happened to me. Now I have a template for how to overcome something, how to prepare for something. I looked at the illness as an athletic event. The cancer was the competitor. I wanted to win.. . . . When I recovered, I applied that focus and ethic to cycling. It taught me a totally new level of commitment."

## For Homework:

Talk to classmates or interview others about those times in their lives in which some insight or self-understanding became an impetus for significant, enduring changes. Find out what it was about their experiences that made the most difference. Write down which themes seemed most prominent.

## SUGGESTED READINGS

Armstrong, L. (2002). *It's not about the bike*. New York: Berkley.

Bateson, G. (1979). *Mind and nature*. New York: Bantam.

Book, H. E. (1998). *How to practice brief, psychodynamic psychotherapy*. Washington, DC: American Psychological Association.

Corey, G. (2000). *Theory and practice of counseling and psychotherapy* (6th ed.). Pacific Grove, CA: Brooks/Cole.

D'Andrea, M. (2000). Postmodernism, social constructionism, and multiculturalism: Three forces that are shaping and expanding our thoughts about counseling. *Journal of Mental Health Counseling, 22*, 1–16.

Dinkmeyer, D., & Sperry, L. (2000). *Counseling and psychotherapy: An integrated, individual psychology approach*. Upper Saddle River, NJ: Merrill.

Kottler, J. A. (2002). *Theories in counseling and therapy: An experiential approach*. Boston: Allyn and Bacon.

Mander, G. (2000). *Psychodynamic approach to brief therapy*. Thousand Oaks, CA: Sage.

May, R. (1983). *The discovery of being*. New York: W. W. Norton.

Monk, G., Winslade, J., Crocket, K., & Epston, D. (Eds.). (1997). *Narrative therapy in practice: The archaeology of hope.* San Francisco: Jossey-Bass.

Neimeyer, R. A., & Mahoney, M. J. (Eds.) (1999). *Constructivism in psychotherapy.* Washington, DC: American Psychological Association.

Perls, F. (1969). *In and out of the garbage pail.* Lafayette, CA: Real People Press.

Rogers, C. (1980). *A way of being.* Boston: Houghton Mifflin.

Schneider, K. J., Bugental, J. F. T., & Pierson, J. F. (Eds.)(2001). *The handbook of humanistic psychology: Leading edges in theory, research, and practice.* Thousand Oaks, CA: Sage.

St. Clair, M. (1996). *Object relations and self psychology: An introduction.* Pacific Grove, CA: Brooks/Cole.

Sweeney, T. J. (1998). *Adlerian counseling: A practitioner's guide* (4th ed.). New York: Brunner/Routledge.

Wedding, D., & Corsini, R. J. (2001). *Case studies in psychotherapy* (3rd ed.). Itasca, IL: F. E. Peacock.

Worrell, J., & Papendrick-Remer, P. (2001). *Feminist perspectives in therapy.* New York: Wiley.

Yalom, I. (2001). *Momma and the meaning of life: Tales of psychotherapy.* New York: HarperCollins.

# 6 CHAPTER

# ACTION-ORIENTED APPROACHES

KEY CONCEPTS

Brief counseling

Behavioral counseling

Operant conditioning

Reinforcement strategies

Systematic desensitization

Flooding

Rational emotive behavior therapy

ABC theory of emotions

Irrational beliefs

Strategic counseling

Reality therapy

Multimodal therapy

Expressive therapies

# ACTION-ORIENTED APPROACHES

# CHAPTER 6

The theoretical perspectives presented in the previous chapter emphasized the importance of self-awareness and understanding in the counseling process. The primary medium used in insight-based approaches is verbal intervention designed to promote the client's exploration and understanding of presenting complaints. In this chapter, we will examine theories that stress, not insight, but interventions that lead more directly to relief of symptoms. These approaches blend an emphasis on action with verbal processing to accomplish specific therapeutic goals. Furthermore, they are designed as brief treatment models.

I would like to mention once again that although, for the purposes of this textbook, I have divided theories into those that primarily focus on understanding versus those that more directly promote action, most practitioners help their clients do both. Of course, the particular treatment plan and approach employed would depend on several factors, such as how much time is available and what the client needs.

Action-oriented approaches to counseling are generally characterized by their reliance on behaviorally specific interventions and outcome measures. The counselor in these approaches works actively to structure sessions so that concrete, observable, and measurable goals can be established and accomplished. The role of the counselor tends to be active and directive, working with the client to structure the sessions. Action-oriented counseling gives less attention than insight theories to the therapeutic relationship and to process, interpretation, and insight. Instead, its proponents

## VOICE FROM THE FIELD

I think the thing that most surprised me when I got out of my training program was how different my job was from what I was led to believe in my classes. Although I'm a school counselor, I've heard the same thing from friends who work in other places as well. You see, we did so much reading and got so much practice working with clients who supposedly would come for a prescribed period of time—six months, or even ten sessions.

Then I got this job where I'm really lucky if I get to see a kid more than twice. I'm just so busy doing other things that I run around putting out fires. During the rare instance when I get to sit down with someone and actually do counseling, I've got maybe twenty minutes before an interruption. Out of necessity, I've had to learn to adapt everything I learned to work in very brief periods of time.

For a while, I thought about starting a small private practice on the side, just so I could keep my regular counseling skills sharp. But I've learned from friends that with all this managed care stuff going on, they're lucky to see anyone more than a half-dozen times. Still, even that would be a luxury for me.

---

emphasize a more objective and scientific approach to counseling that makes use of a variety of techniques and structures.

The field is currently undergoing dramatic reshaping of its primary mission, not just in the traditional domain of school counseling but in all of the other specialties, including community counseling, mental health counseling, rehabilitation counseling, marriage and family counseling, and pastoral counseling. Increasingly we are being called on to make a difference in clients' lives in briefer periods of times, to prove that our efforts have had an impact, and to be accountable to third parties for our relative successes and failures.

The climate in the community, the popular media, and insurance companies tends to be more and more skeptical that we are indeed being helpful. Consequently, most counselors feel pressure to plan some sort of therapeutic tasks with clients that can be implemented quickly and can be measured as to their effects. Action-oriented theories are becoming increasingly popular as a framework for preparing some sort of intervention, specifying how long the treatment will last, and determining what outcomes can be expected when the counseling is over.

Quite a number of new volumes are being published each year to help all counselors, even those who are insight oriented, to respond to the demands of the marketplace and the realities of everyday practice. Whether we like it or not, we are being forced by managed care organizations to make adjustments in the ways that we help people, greater emphasis being placed on swift, efficient, and measurable methods (Littrel, 1998; Presbury, Echterling, & McKee, 2002) Even school counselors are jumping on the bandwagon of brief counseling models because they have always been required to help children in just a few sessions (Murphy, 1997; Sklare, 1997).

Regardless of the setting and circumstances in which you intend to practice or the clientele you intend to reach, it is highly probable that proficiency will be required in at least one brief counseling approach, no matter how much you prefer to work with more in-depth, long-term cases.

# BEHAVIORAL COUNSELING

## Aliases: Behaviorism, Behavior Modification, Behavior Therapy

The influence of behaviorism on counseling has come a long way since B. F. Skinner and his rigid prescriptions for human control and manipulation (Skinner, 1938, 1953). Once viewed as a radical counterpoint to the humanism of Carl Rogers and Abraham Maslow, behavioral principles have been assimilated into the mainstream of therapeutic counseling to the extent that even insight-oriented counselors regularly use many of the behavioral techniques, such as thought stopping, goal setting, assertiveness training, relaxation training, systematic desensitization, self-management, and other methods of skill acquisition. Ironically, the reverse is true as well: Relationship variables emphasized by client-centered counselors are also part of the ways behavioral counselors operate; if for no other reason, clients are more inclined to follow through on prescriptions if they feel some degree of commitment to the counselor and accountability to the relationship (Cormier & Cormier, 1998).

So many different kinds of behavioral treatments are currently in practice that it is difficult to lump them all together into a common camp. Some emphasize cognitive features; others stress reinforcement, modeling, self-control, or behavioral analyses. Nevertheless, most behavioral approaches have the following elements in common (Spiegler & Guevremont, 1998):

1. An emphasis on the present rather than on the past.
2. Attention to changing specific dysfunctional behaviors.
3. Reliance on research as an integral partner for developing and testing interventions.
4. A preference for carefully measuring treatment outcomes.
5. Matching specific treatments to particular presenting problems.

These factors common to behavioral approaches are now being integrated more and more into many other counseling styles.

## Early Background

The term *behavioral counseling* was first introduced by John Krumboltz. He suggested that counselors should remind themselves that the purpose of their activity is to foster behavioral changes in clients; thus all counseling is ultimately behavioral (Krumboltz, 1965). From a behavioristic perspective, counseling can be viewed as the systematic use of procedures to reach mutually established therapeutic goals that will resolve client concerns and conflicts

(Thoresen, 1969). The behavioral approach therefore views counseling less as a philosophy of life and more as a set of principles to be used in a targeted and situationally specific manner.

Although the behavioral approach to counseling has many variations, most proponents agree that clients' problems are the result of maladaptive learning patterns; treatment thus takes the form of learning new life skills. Concepts central to the work of a behavioral counselor include: (1) behavioral assessment and identification of target symptoms; (2) reinforcement (both operant and classical); (3) social modeling of skills and desirable behaviors; (4) skills training (that is, assertiveness or stress inoculation); (5) environmental changes that will encourage identified goals; and (6) objective measurement of changes over time. In many ways, behavioral counseling is viewed as an educational process that borrows heavily from learning theory and emphasizes the acquisition of more adaptive ways to act.

The work of Ivan Pavlov, with his salivating dogs and their responses to the ringing of dinner bells, John Watson's discovery that neurosis can be induced by scaring infants, and B. F. Skinner's fascination with teaching pigeons to play table tennis are important milestones in the development of behaviorism. Those early research efforts were translated into action techniques for promoting systematic client change (Garfield & Bergin, 1994; Kanfer & Goldstein, 1991).

John Dollard and Neil Miller (1950) attempted to combine psychoanalytic insights and practical learning principles into a science of human behavior. Joseph Wolpe (1958, 1969) worked to apply Pavlov's classical conditioning to systematic desensitization. Julian Rotter and Albert Bandura worked independently on a behavioral approach that stressed the impact of social learning and modeling concepts, in which context behavior is shaped by the interactions of an individual personality with significant others. Kanfer and Phillips (1970) used Skinner's operant model as a basis for developing the methods we now know as "behavior modification." Within the counseling literature, significant contributors such as John Krumboltz (1966), Carl Thoresen (1969), and Ray Hosford (1969) have been active in translating learning-theory principles into therapeutic practice.

The theory of behavioral counseling is deceptively simple. We are born into the world basically empty headed, with a few reflexes. All our values, attitudes, preferences, emotional responses, thinking patterns, personality styles, and problems are the result of learned behavior. We are shaped by our environment, reinforced and molded by the world around us. A systematic and scientific approach is used to (1) identify specific behaviors in need of elimination or acquisition, (2) set objectives that are reasonable and desirable, (3) collect data on the client's functioning levels, (4) design and engineer initial change efforts, (5) isolate and diminish client resistance, (6) modify distracting variables, (7) monitor and assess the impact of planned interventions, and (8) make alterations as needed in the treatment plan (Gottman & Leiblum, 1974; Spiegler & Guevremont, 1998).

# Behavioral Technology

One valuable tool of the researcher in general—and of behaviorists in particular—is the use of time-series charts for graphic portrayal of client change. This method helps the counselor to study a single case intensively, plotting baseline data and the results of therapeutic interventions. It aids in quantitatively and specifically describing the behaviors targeted for changes, as well as in noting the effects of any action. In Figure 6.1, the counselor has available at a glance a summary of the client's presenting problems and the results of several attempts to change the behavior.

A strength of the behavioral approach is not only its assessment procedures but also its wide variety of treatment strategies. Its technology of helping is consistently and reliably applied to produce observable client changes, which the behaviorist is skilled at identifying, measuring, and changing. Many behavioral methodologies are now part of the repertoire of every therapeutic counselor; some are discussed here.

*Operant-conditioning procedures,* including those based on the work of B. F. Skinner (1953) and other researchers, are methods in which the frequency of behavior may be increased or decreased according to the type and timing of stimuli presented. In *positive reinforcement* strategies the counselor hopes to increase behavior by rewarding the client. Implicitly, the most subtle head nods, "uh-huhs," smiles, and twinkling eyes positively reinforce the client's talking, trusting, and opening up. Operationally, this methodology is used in *token economies* with a variety of normal and maladjusted client populations, often in classroom settings, to spell out and encourage acceptable behavior as it spontaneously or deliberately occurs. Participants receive rewards in the form of points or privileges in exchange for their cooperation and lose points for obstructing progress.

The counselor's task is to (1) identify the specific target behaviors in need of upgrading; (2) discover situation-specific, individually designed rewards that motivate a given client; (3) administer the reinforcement soon after the target behavior is displayed; and (4) slowly wean the client from any dependence on the external motivation in favor of internalized, self-administered reinforcers. These same principles would hold true for any other operant procedure.

*Negative reinforcement* also produces an increase in desired target behaviors such as assertiveness, but it does so by removing a stimulus that the client perceives as aversive. Resistant clients, for example, can rid themselves of the inconvenience and discomfort of their counseling sessions only by being more cooperative and working faster to change.

*Punishment* strategies are used to reduce the frequency of a client's behavior by presenting an aversive stimulus. Unfortunately, many parents and teachers rely too heavily on this strategy because of its seeming convenience, even though it usually produces negative side effects in the child such as withdrawal, aggression, and generalized fears. Another problem with punishment

FIGURE 6.1 | EFFECTS OF INTERVENTIONS ON CLIENT'S RELATIONSHIP
WITH SPOUSE

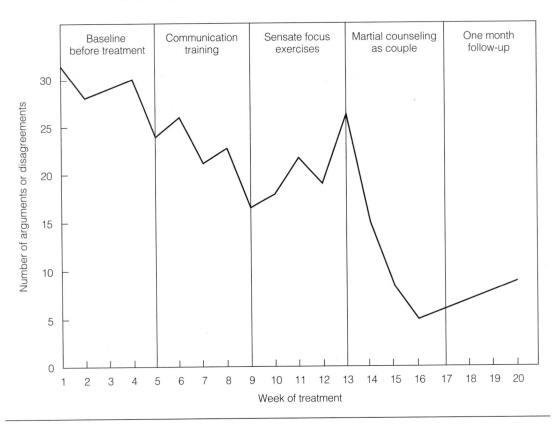

is that its effects are brief and the behavior that is stopped often reappears at a higher level of frequency. Punishment may be used in conjunction with other operant procedures, such as in a weight-loss program in which the client writes a self-contract such as the one shown in Table 6.1.

The behavioral counselor has a variety of other standard techniques that have developed from laboratory research on conditioning processes.

*Extinction* involves the removal of the reinforcement for a given behavior, such as ignoring a child's temper tantrum. Two factors should be kept in mind when using extinction: (1) During the initial phase, after the reinforcer has been removed, the target behavior increases dramatically; during the second phase, the behavior decreases; and (2) extinction, once implemented, must be applied systematically and consistently.

*Covert reinforcement* uses mental images that function as reinforcers and can be generated by the client. The client is asked to imagine a situation in which he or she might refrain from an undesirable behavior. The counselor then instructs the client to visualize the reinforcing image.

TABLE 6.1 | SAMPLE CONTRACT

| | |
|---|---|
| **Goals:** | To lose 15 pounds in sixty days. To change my eating habits to include more fruits and vegetables and less chocolate. To exercise three times per week for no less than 20 minutes. |
| **Procedures:** | I will limit myself to 1,500 calories per day and restrict all eating activities to the dinner table. Snacks and in-between meals are strictly forbidden. |
| **Consequences:** | Daily reward: For each day I am able to stay within my calorie limit, I am permitted to play my tuba for two uninterrupted hours. |
| **Daily punishment:** | For each day I violate my calorie limit, I will set my alarm for 3 A.M., wake up, and vacuum and clean the house from top to bottom. |
| **Contract reward:** | If I am successful in losing 15 pounds within two months, I will treat myself to a four-day skiing weekend and buy myself a new outfit in a smaller size. |
| **Contract punishment:** | If I am unsuccessful, I will agree to do all housekeeping chores for a month. |

Signed _____ Date _____

Witness _____

---

*Contingency contracting* is the use of a behavioral contract that defines the necessary contingencies on which a reinforcer will be presented (see Table 6.1). Clients decide how often and at which levels they desire the reinforcer, thus shaping their own behavior.

*Shaping* is a process in which complex terminal behaviors are reinforced in approximate successive stages. The client receives consistent reinforcement in small steps as movement is made toward the ultimate goal.

In *classical* or *Pavlovian conditioning,* a presented stimulus elicits automatic responses. *Systematic desensitization,* an example of classical conditioning developed by Joseph Wolpe (1958,1982), is the most common of these methodologies; clients are taught to substitute relaxation responses for anxiety when confronted by previously frightening situations such as tests or social events.

This method initially involves teaching the client how to relax. Next, a hierarchy of perceived threat is developed in which the client lists minimally stressful scenes (for example, watching a film of someone receiving an injection) and works toward progressively fearful images (receiving a flu shot in the arm).

The counselor will usually use a hypnotically calm, relaxing voice, even pacing the words . . . to . . . the . . . rise . . . and . . . fall . . . of . . . the . . . client's . . . breathing. The client is instructed to relax each muscle in the body, to imagine all tension draining away, to visualize a floating, drifting scene on the beach, perhaps feeling the warm sun and cool sand, hearing the waves crash against the surf, seeing birds sailing high above. After the client reaches a state of total relaxation, she or he is asked to work through the fear hierarchy, systematically reducing any tension with learned relaxation responses. After a few practice sessions, almost anyone can learn to inhibit his or her anxiety.

In *flooding*, an opposite strategy is employed to erode the stimulus/response sequence. A phobia, fear, or bad habit can be extinguished by bombarding the person with the stimulus until fatigue sets in or until (in the case of a habit) the stimulus loses its pleasurable value. While lecturing on this subject, I was confronted by a disbelieving student who aggressively asked, "If this stuff works, how could I use it to stop smoking?" I flippantly replied, "Lock yourself in the closet with a pack of Camels, and don't come out until you're done smoking them all," never once considering that the student might actually follow the advice. A week later the student showed up in class again to report his story:

> I wasn't sure if you were kidding or not but I decided to try this behavior stuff anyway. I bought a pack of unfiltered cigarettes, went home, told my mother I was doing an experiment for school, and proceeded to lock myself in the bathroom. Since I usually smoke filtered menthols, I was, at first, a little surprised that I actually enjoyed the first two cigarettes. I even thought to myself, "Not only is this not going to work, but now I'm going to be addicted worse!" By the fifth cigarette I noticed I was feeling a little dizzy, and by the seventh the smoke was starting to burn my eyes. I finally started to get really sick by the tenth. I guess I must have passed out because the next morning I woke up in a pool of vomit with a cigarette burn on my leg. Not only will I never smoke again, but I can't even stand being in the same room with someone else who is.

This student's experience illustrates not only the effectiveness of behavioral strategies but also the importance of carefully monitoring their application so that abuse and harm can be avoided. Because the counselor has a more forceful role in behavioral counseling, the client's rights and freedom of choice are jeopardized unless great caution is taken to ensure that the ends justify the means and that the client is fully informed about the implications, dangers, and limitations of a given procedure.

## Criticisms of the Behavioral Approach

Behaviorism has been criticized most often because of its narrow focus on observable human behavior and its lack of attention to feelings and thoughts, which also make up a significant part of a person's functioning. In addition, the behavioral approach works only with the presenting complaint, which could be a symptom of underlying intrapsychic conflicts. Many insight-oriented theorists therefore believe that symptoms thus cured will inevitably be replaced by others, because the internal condition of the client has not been altered.

As an action-oriented approach, behavioral counseling has also been criticized as mechanistic, manipulative, and impersonal because it downplays the role of the therapeutic relationship and all but ignores the value of self-understanding in the change process. Because it also works toward empiricism (that is, specificity or quantification), prediction, and control, it often sacrifices the values of intuition and artistry in change endeavors.

# RATIONAL EMOTIVE BEHAVIOR COUNSELING

## Aliases: Rational Emotive Therapy, REBT, Cognitive Behavior Therapy, Rational Behavior Therapy, Cognitive Restructuring

Feeling confined and bored by the rigid structures of traditional psychoanalysis, Albert Ellis (1962) developed a system of counseling based on principles of logic and rational analysis. Ellis has written hundreds of books and articles—even songs and coloring books—to further refine and popularize his theory of rational emotive behavior therapy (REBT). He has remained remarkably (perhaps even rigidly) consistent through the years, attempting to live his life as a model of rational functioning. In the past few decades he has devoted himself to collaborating with researchers (Ellis & Whiteley, 1979; Ellis & Grieger, 1986) to establish a more solid empirical base for the theory. More recently, he has been working to integrate his model with other fashionable ideas of constructivist thinking and brief therapy (Ellis, 1995, 2001), even calling it a kind of humanistic counseling because of its emphasis on unconditional self-acceptance (Ellis, 1996). While this is quite a stretch, REBT and other cognitive therapies have been integrated into the mainstream of what almost every counselor employs at times.

Many REBT offshoots put more emphasis on the rational-educational process (Maultsby, 1984) or the cognitive-behavior components (Beck, 1976; Cormier & Cormier, 1998; Mahoney, 1974, 1995; Meichenbaum, 1977). Other theorists such as Arnold Lazarus (1981, 1993, 1995) have expanded a basically cognitive-oriented model to a more integrative approach he calls multimodal therapy because it addresses not only cognitions but also all the other facets of human experience (see "Honorable Mentions" at the end of the chapter). Each of these adaptations has more similarities than differences (Weinrach, 1996).

There are definitely differences in therapeutic style. Whereas Ellis prefers a more confrontational, "in-your-face" approach, others such as Aaron Beck, Michael Mahoney, Donald Meichenbaum, and Arnold Lazarus structure a more collaborative type of interaction. In other words, those who object to the more abrasive aspects of Ellis' interpersonal style have been able to adapt the cognitive approach to fit a gentler and kinder context.

All the proponents of cognitive approaches are in basic agreement that the legitimate focus of counseling ought to be modification of the way people think.

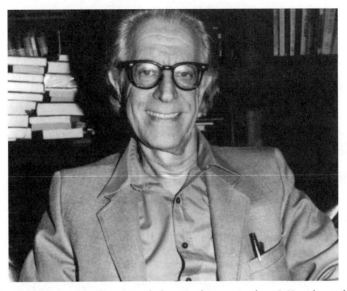

Albert Ellis developed rational emotive behavior therapy in the 1960s, about the same time that Carl Rogers was working on his humanistic approach. Ellis was instrumental not only in bringing attention to the role of thinking in change processes but also devising one of the first truly brief therapy approaches. Courtesy of The Albert Ellis Institute.

## Basic Points of REBT

A thunderstorm, missed appointment, critical comment, failing grade, and flat tire are all examples of daily occurrences that can make us feel upset, right? Not so, according to Ellis and company.

> My approach to psychotherapy is to zero in, as quickly as possible, on the client's basic philosophy of life; to get him to see exactly what this is and how it is inevitably self-defeating; and to persuade him to work his ass off, cognitively, emotively, and behaviorally, to profoundly change it. My basic assumption is that virtually all "emotionally disturbed" individuals actually think crookedly, magically, dogmatically, and unrealistically. (Ellis, 1988, p. 581)

Nobody or nothing outside of ourselves can cause us to feel anything. There is no "bad-temper button" on our foreheads that anyone else can push to make us angry on demand. Granted, many things that people do or events that occur are highly conducive to letting us upset ourselves. Nevertheless, it is our choice, due to years of lazy negligence and wallowing in our irrational beliefs, to interpret the world negatively and consequently to feel depressed, anxious, guilty, or frustrated.

The primary goal of cognitive therapies is to help clients identify their patterns of irrational thinking, those habitual beliefs that lead one to misperceive reality, and subsequently learn alternative tools of thinking that are, in real-world terms, more logical, consistent, rational, and scientific. According to the ABC theory of emotions (see Table 6.2), it is evaluative thoughts (B) rather than the

## VOICE FROM THE FIELD

Of all the theories I've used—and believe me, I've used a bunch—RET is the one I found most useful in my own life. I don't even practice it that much anymore with my clients, but I still use it every day inside my own head. So often, I get down on myself because I feel like I'm failing my clients or not doing as good a job as I should. Then I hear Ellis' voice in my head, confronting me about my "shoulds" and absolute judgments. It really does work miracles.

Why don't I use it anymore with my clients? I don't know. I guess I just got bored with it after awhile. It's not that it stopped working; really, it's powerful stuff. It's just that I got tired disputing the same old irrational beliefs over and over. I moved on to something new and more dynamic. But I still use it sometimes with clients who really seem like good candidates for a more confrontive, thinking approach.

---

traumatic situation itself (A) that will primarily determine the emotional reaction (C). This response will be an extremely negative emotion unless the person vigorously challenges the validity of assumptions, thereby disputing irrational beliefs (D) and making a new, more desirable emotional response (E) more likely.

Thoughts or behaviors are viewed as irrational if they create significant emotional conflicts with others, block constructive goals, do not adhere to objective reality, or needlessly threaten life. Originally Ellis proposed eleven separate irrational beliefs (Ellis & Harper, 1975), which he later simplified to four basic ideas. He believed that the original beliefs were dysfunctional inferences based on the following core, dogmatic ideas (Ellis, 1991).

**Awfulizing** "Awfulizing" is the habitual exaggeration of reality by "disasterizing" about the future, focusing on the worst possible outcome:

- "OK, I'll study to take the dumb test again, but I'll probably never pass it."
- "It's just *terrible* that we have to live through this divorce."
- "I can't believe this *catastrophe*—can you just imagine my shame when I found out he was already married?"
- "Yeah, sure, my speech went well, but what a *total flop* when those people in the back left early."

Because it can never be proved that anything is totally bad and because things can always turn out worse than they actually did, "awfulizing" makes a major emotional tailspin out of a minor disappointment. By keeping expectations to a minimum and countering exaggerations with more appropriate, realistic interpretations of life's unexpected events, such irrational beliefs can be neutralized.

**"I can't stand it"** As a corollary and companion to the irrational belief represented by "awfulizing," this belief also distorts the relative significance of things when they don't go our own way. For those people with a low tolerance for frustration, life's normal setbacks take on gargantuan proportions of pain.

TABLE 6.2 | ABC THEORY OF EMOTIONS

**A**

**Activating Emotional Experience**

Reading chapters on counseling approaches that present a dozen complex theories

**B**

**Belief or Interpretation of Experience**

"I feel so stupid that I can't understand all of this stuff."

"This is terrible. I'll never be a good counselor since I already feel lost."

"I should be able to pick this stuff up faster."

**C**

**Consequences**

Anxiety

Fear

Confusion

Frustration

Anger

**D**

**Disputing Irrational Beliefs**

"Of course I feel overwhelmed—that is what an introductory student is supposed to feel when presented with an overview of the field in just a few weeks."

"Just because I don't understand everything about these theories doesn't make me a stupid person—just a person who will have to work a little harder and have more patience."

"This isn't a terrible situation—it's only difficult and slightly uncomfortable."

**E**

**Emotional Effect**

Relief

Mild tension

Mild annoyance

Excitement

---

In reality, we can stand everything but death—up to and including having to go to the bathroom desperately with no facility around. Indeed we grit our teeth, cross our legs (unless walking quickly), and bear the pain until we can find release. This metaphor is typical of those a counselor might use to illustrate humorously the childish foot stomping we resort to when confronted with disappointment.

**Musterbating**   The use of "musts," "shoulds," and "oughts" is, Ellis believes, the cornerstone of all emotional disturbance. The use of these words, and the underlying thoughts they represent, implies that a person expects special treatment and that the forces of the universe have to cooperate to provide what is demanded.

- "I *must* do well in *all* situations and circumstances, and, when I don't, it's awful."
- "I *must* be loved and approved of by *everyone* to feel worthwhile."
- "They *ought* to have given me the job. I deserved it. It just isn't fair."

There is nothing inherently fair and equitable about the world we live in. In spite of our expectations and demands that we get what we want and feel we deserve, rarely does the world cooperate. To expect it to do so is irrational.

As with any of these irrational beliefs that are both language and culturally based, it is critical that necessary care be employed to adopt the concepts to fit the client's background. In a study of how REBT is used in Spanish-speaking countries like El Salvador, Spain, Costa Rica, and Columbia, Lega and Ellis (2001) found that whereas "musts" are still present in client's irrational thinking but there are differences in degree, form, and style, just as one would expect in another language. Basically, what "musterbating" represents is evidence of rigid, absolutistic thinking, and this is what is challenged.

**Self-judgments**   Evaluating oneself or others in absolute terms of good, bad, right, or wrong, and therefore condemning less-than-desirable performance, represents the fourth kind of irrational belief.

- "I completely blew the whole interview; I'm a horrible counselor."
- "I'm just not comfortable at parties because I make such a fool of myself."
- "You're not a very good mother to let your kids have so much freedom."
- "He's a real idiot and can't do anything right. If I were in his place . . ."

It is irrational to expect perfection of oneself or others, on any level, because such a goal is impossible. Treatment of this irrational belief involves teaching clients to rate their behavior rather than their personhood and not to permit themselves to dislike other people but only to disapprove of things they might do (or not do).

According to the tenets of cognitive-based counseling, all human beings have each of the irrational beliefs in varying quantities, although their effects, intensity, and destructive potential will depend on the individual. Essentially, the counseling strategy involves defining, discriminating, debating, and disputing the client's irrational thinking patterns while substituting alternative thoughts that are more appropriate and logical. So the reasoning goes: If we can change how we think, we can change how we feel and therefore how we behave.

## Criticisms of Cognitive-Based Therapies

1. Human beings are multifaceted, with feelings as well as thoughts. Critics suggest that REBT puts undue emphasis on thought processes to the

exclusion of many legitimate feelings, thereby contributing to repression and denial of feelings.

2. REBT is probably less effective with some kinds of clients—those who already have problems with overintellectualizing or who don't have the capacity to reason logically (young children, schizophrenics, some clients with character disorders, or clients with minimal intelligence).

3. Many cognitive-behavioral counselors complain of boredom and burnout from continuously repeating the same arguments and processes with all clients.

4. REBT is difficult for some professionals to practice if they are not outgoing and combative and don't enjoy vigorous debate and confrontation.

5. Because the counselor's role is so verbal, active, and directive, the client may feel overpowered, dominated, and not responsible for the outcome.

## Personal Applications

Among counseling approaches, REBT lends itself particularly well to personal adoption by the professional. Ellis has said repeatedly that, by talking our clients out of their crazy beliefs, we cannot help changing our own in the process. Other REBT practitioners report that they have noticed themselves becoming more psychologically healthy as they become more experienced clinicians. Ellis and Wilde (2002) describe how this approach can be applied to a series of cases, demonstrating the kind of parallel process that can occur in which practitioners confront their own issues with perfectionism and low frustration tolerance as they challenge these beliefs in their clients.

Personally useful ideas from REBT include the following:

1. The idea that, because we create our own emotional misery through distorted thinking, we can potentially change these negative feelings by changing the way we think about our situations. A highway accident, critical comment, and missed appointment can all be viewed as inconveniences or disasters, depending on our point of view.

2. The technique of carefully monitoring our language for words such as *should, must,* and *ought,* which may imply irrational beliefs. As we become more aware of illogical language, we start to hear faulty phrases in others and ourselves: "She makes me so angry" (how can anyone make you feel anything without your consent?); "This weather is so depressing" (rain is just rain—it's your interpretation that makes it seem depressing); "It just frustrates me so much" (don't you mean, "I frustrate myself over what I perceive is happening"?).

3. The structure of mentally rehearsing difficult tasks for the future or painful events of the past to relieve anxiety and work through unsolved irrational beliefs. These imagery techniques are helpful, for instance, in allaying fears for an upcoming interview in which penetrating questions can be asked: "What's the worst that could happen? Even if I mess up the interview and perform less than perfectly, does that mean I'm not a good counselor and will never be competent? And even if that were so, what does that have to do with my 'goodness' as a human being?"

# STRATEGIC COUNSELING

## Aliases: Strategic Family Therapy, Problem-Solving Therapy, Brief Therapy, Tactical Therapy, Ordeal Therapy

Perhaps the most exciting change in the direction of therapeutic counseling to occur in many years, strategic counseling combines the methods and theory from a number of disciplines into a dramatic action-oriented helping model that often requires but a few sessions to rid clients permanently of their presenting complaints. Milton Erickson—psychiatrist, hypnotist, wizard—grew up physically handicapped. He discovered ways of getting other people to do things for themselves or for him without having to ask. As a professional adult, Erickson developed new ways of helping people through the uses of metaphor, paradoxical instructions, hypnotic suggestions, and other elaborate and sophisticated communication devices (Haley, 1973).

Richard Bandler and John Grinder (1975) systematized what Erickson did intuitively by creating a communication model of counseling that diagnoses a client's personal style and then matches the helper's mode to ensure greater rapport and influence. The efforts of a Gestalt therapist and a linguistics professor were thus merged to create *neurolinguistic programming,* a system of eye watching and language patterning that allows counselors to persuade clients to change on conscious and unconscious levels.

Jay Haley (1976) and Cloe Madanes (1983) were also strongly influenced by Erickson but moved in another direction, one that emphasized symptoms in the context of family systems. In collaboration with the "Palo Alto Group," Haley, his mentor Gregory Bateson, and a host of skilled researchers, theoreticians, and clinicians in sociology, education, medicine, anthropology, and psychology, combined forces to revolutionize strategic counseling with families.

Haley and his associates sought to examine individual problems as metaphors for patterns that exist in the family. A child who develops problems in school has found a way to distract the parents from their own troubles. As long as they focus on the child's delinquent activities, they function as a cohesive team. Once the child recovers, the parents begin their bickering anew. Haley sought to break the destructive chain by analyzing and changing the patterns of communication among family members. He was later to refine his theory into a form of "ordeal therapy" in which the goal is to present a therapeutic problem more difficult than the client's presenting concerns (Haley, 1984).

While Haley and other family therapists such as Virginia Satir and Salvador Minuchin were laboring on the East Coast, the Palo Alto Group continued to flourish, culminating in the publication of two works that describe the art and science of doing counseling briefly and strategically. In *Change: Principles of Problem Formation and Problem Resolution,* Watzlawick, Weakland, and Fisch (1974) described a new way of looking at problems: as a vicious-cycle process in which the client's attempted solutions only maintain the problem. The child acts out, for example, because his parents nag; his parents nag because he acts out. The authors argue that the only efficient way for a therapist to intervene in such a system is to assume a "maneuverable" position having maximum flexibilities while limiting the client's avenues of escape. Therapists provide specific descriptions of various tactics that effectively change the ways a client can respond, thereby forcing the client to choose other, more self-enhancing responses.

Strategic, problem-solving, or brief approaches to counseling, whether in an individual, family, or group context, are among the hottest movements in the field today. Innovations by de Shazer (1991), O'Hanlon (1994), White and Epston (1990), Quick (1996), Zeig (Haley & Zeig, 2001) and others have encouraged practitioners of any number of theoretical persuasions to be more creative and pragmatic in the ways they promote client changes. Even counselors who see themselves as primarily relationship oriented in their work with clients have been willing to experiment with these methodologies that encourage shaking things up a bit.

I recall feeling so frustrated with a client who had not been responding to anything I, or anyone else I consulted about the case, could think of. We had built what I thought was a solid relationship. We were following a path that I had been down many times before, a direction that I was quite familiar and comfortable with; I knew what I was doing wasn't working but I was at a loss as to where to go next. I had reached a point where I hoped this client would just go away.

My partner in private practice at the time sat me down, I think mostly because he was tired of listening to me complain about how stuck I felt with this case. Applying the principles of a problem-solving approach, he had me take inventory of all the things I had done previously that hadn't worked, even though they were methods that I liked very much and had served me well many times before. His gentle guidance was essentially getting me to promise that I wouldn't do those things any more but would agree to do something else, anything other than what I had already been doing. When I begged for his advice about where I should start next, he showed that same enigmatic smile that I favor when clients ask me what to do. With a shrug, he asked me if it really mattered as long as I didn't continue with what I had already been doing.

It took several weeks before the client and I found the right combination of things that made our relationship work and made the counseling helpful to him in terms of resolving his initial difficulties. What made all the difference to us, even in a style of treatment that was more insight rather than action oriented, was a problem-solving approach in which the focus remained on what we were doing that was working and what was not proving to be helpful.

The simple methodology implicit in this case study is now so much a part of the way most counselors think and function that strategic approaches have become as much generic practice as have the contributions from client-centered, cognitive, or behavioral theories. Many practitioners, from all walks of life and work settings, function as brief, strategic counselors when they ask a series of questions designed to move clients toward resolution of their problems (Quick, 1996; Sklare, 1997):

- What's the trouble?
- Why are you here and what do you expect?

- How is that a problem for you?
- When, where, and with whom does the problem occur?
- What are some exceptions when you don't experience this as a problem?
- If you woke up tomorrow without the problem, what would be different?
- If your problem was solved by a miracle, what form might that take?
- What have you already tried to solve the problem that doesn't work?
- What have you tried that *does* work sometimes?
- When is the problem not a problem?
- When is the problem the worst?
- How did you manage to overcome your problem in previous exceptions you described?

## Strategic Interventions

The strategic practitioner follows an orderly sequence of steps: understanding the dynamics of the client's relationships, identifying the sources of conflict, and planning a strategy for change. The principal strength of this approach, however, lies not with its innovations in theory but rather with its creative, often radical prescriptions for change.

The great majority of the contributors to brief, strategic counseling would agree on the basic assumptions that (1) the counselor's role is highly active and directive; (2) counseling need not take a lot of time to be effective; (3) analyzing family and individual communication patterns is crucial to understanding the client problems; (4) intervention efforts are action oriented, with insight downplayed; (5) strategies are all individually designed to match the client's personal style and situation; and (6) if one strategy doesn't work, try something else.

Strategic methods are often provocative. They tell us to do things that just a few years ago we learned not to do: Be active, directive, controlling, and mysterious. The counselor, as an expert, accepts responsibility for designing treatment methods that are effective. The task of getting clients to respond differently to their life situations requires artistry and skill in persuasion, motivation, and influence, as well as a sense of humor and of the absurd (Haley, 1984; Madanes, 1990). Here is a sampling of some flexible, unusual, and ingenious strategies.

*Pretending* is a strategy that Madanes (1984) prefers when working with children who have disruptive symptoms irritating to their parents. After the child has been deliberately directed to engage in the symptoms, they lose their controlling power. Other forms of directive intervention involve shifting the power in a family, changing the family members' style of interaction, and posing paradoxical tasks: The client is given instructions that the counselor hopes she or he will disobey. With clients who wished to lose weight, for example, Milton Erickson was fond of ordering them to gain 5 pounds before the next session. If they complied, they demonstrated the potential control they had over their weight—the ability to increase (and, by implication, decrease) it at will. More likely, however, they would think Erickson crazy, deliberately disobey the order, and lose weight, thereby following the road to recovery.

Many other brief, strategic interventions, such as *metaphorical directives, power shifts,* and *reframing,* will be described in the chapter on marital and family counseling. The action orientation of the strategic approach is already evident: Counselors seek to influence behavior dramatically by disrupting existing life patterns. Because much of strategic counseling is intuitive and creative, it requires a solid base of clinical experience and supervision before it can be safely and effectively used. This approach to helping tends to work best with complex family systems and with individuals who have strong commitments to maladaptive behavior.

It is certainly significant that the managed care movement is exercising such influence in the field that counselors of all persuasions and theoretical orientations are finding creative, innovative ways to shorten their treatments. Many of the insight-oriented theories presented in the previous chapter have been shortened, including even those that are based in psychoanalytic and other longer term methods (Davanloo, 1978; Mann, 1973; Sifeneo, 1992). Some theorists, responding to the demands of the marketplace, have even created treatments designed to be conducted in a single session (Bloom, 1997; Talmon, 1990). Others have tried to preserve the sanctity of depth-oriented, relationship-based counseling within a more pragmatic, briefer application (Ecker & Hulley, 1996).

## Criticisms of Strategic Counseling

Although brief, strategic interventions can be quite dramatic and effective in helping clients, especially those who are resistant or who feel stuck, there are also a number of problems associated with their use:

1. The client is not given primary responsibility for the content or focus of the session; it is clear that the counselor is the authority in charge.
2. The process is often deliberately mysterious, so the client doesn't understand what has happened or why.
3. Insight is unnecessarily downgraded or totally ignored as a distracting variable, even though self-understanding is an important goal of many clients.
4. Ethical problems are potentially associated with such explicit influence and control. There is some danger if directives are misinterpreted or used irresponsibly.
5. Because the focus of this approach is on solving problems, it could rely largely on a male-oriented, control-based methodology that is inconsistent with the values of some cultures.
6. Many of the strategies are intuitively constructed and are therefore difficult to learn and apply reliably. Many of the successful cases presented in the literature and in training workshops were constructed by teams of experts working from behind one-way mirrors, an option not available to most practitioners in the field.
7. There is a limited empirical base for these approaches, and by their nature they prove difficult to research.

## Personal Applications

Strategic counseling emphasizes a flexible, pragmatic approach to solving problems. Thus it helps the practitioner to be quite creative, inventive, and even playful in his or her outlook. Many of the therapeutic principles applied to client issues are equally helpful in working through conflicts of your own, especially when following a few rules:

1. When you try something and it doesn't work, don't do the same thing; try anything else other than what you are doing. For example, if you repeatedly push on a door to get out of a room, and nothing happens, pushing harder is not likely to work either. Operating strategically would have you do the opposite: Try pulling. Although there is no guarantee that this will be any more successful, at least it gets you out of a situation in which you are stuck repeating the same thing over and over.

2. When you are facing a problem that feels insurmountable, reframe it in a way that makes it more manageable. Imagine, for example, that you are feeling discouraged because you keep "failing" at something that is important to you. Morale can be substantially improved by casting the term *failure* in a different light: Not succeeding at something is simply a means of gaining greater experience and practice.

3. Typical of the innovative ways that strategic counselors tackle difficult problems, O'Hanlon and Weiner-Davis (1989) describe a dramatic method of change called "time travel." Assume that you are a client who feels stuck. First, you are asked to practice traveling into the past and future through the use of fantasy. Once you can easily move forward or backward at will, you are asked to travel into the future to a time when your problem is resolved. Are you there yet? Okay, then—what did you do to fix your problem? You can then retrospectively "look back" from your perch in the future and tell yourself what you need to do.

Strategic and problem-solving approaches to counseling are not strictly classified as theories because they emphasize pragmatic utility over conceptual purity. They are representative of a more technical approach to helping people in which each collaboration with a client presents an opportunity to invent a new solution to a problem.

# HONORABLE MENTIONS

I mentioned in the previous chapter, limited space requires that you are exposed to only a few theories representative of those that are action oriented. Your instructors, coworkers, and other authors could easily suggest that models other than those described be included. The good news is that you will most likely have at least one other course devoted exclusively to studying theories in greater depth. Nevertheless, here are a few others that deserve honorable mention.

## Multimodal Counseling

Among several other action-oriented practitioners, Arnold Lazarus has sought to combine features from several theories into a flexible system for analyzing and treating clients' problems. Originally a behaviorist, Lazarus was influenced by the behavioral therapy of Joseph Wolpe and, later, by the cognitive therapy of Albert Ellis. He has endeavored to create an approach to counseling that is behavioral in its systematic analysis, comprehensive in its scope of exploring the total person, and pragmatic in its selection of techniques (Lazarus, 1981, 1993, 1995).

This theory is called *multimodal* because it seeks to understand and intervene at the levels of all seven modalities of the human personality. People are capable of experiencing sensations, feelings, thoughts, images, observable behavior, interpersonal responses, and biochemical and neurophysiological reactions. These human components are conveniently organized into the acronym BASIC ID, in which each letter represents a different modality that can be used to explore and change behavior. Multimodal assessment thus permits the practitioner to understand at a glance (1) how the client characteristically functions; (2) how, where, and why the presenting problem manifests itself; and (3) how specifically to use the profile as a blueprint for promoting change.

One distinct contribution of this approach is that it avoids the use of formal diagnostic labels and psychological jargon in favor of more down-to-earth terms. It also encourages the counselor to design individualized treatment strategies for each client.

## Reality Therapy

William Glasser (1965, 1990, 1998) is credited as the founder of reality therapy, which reflected his dissatisfaction with contemporary psychoanalytic theory. It is an essentially didactic approach that stresses problem solving, personal responsibility, and the need to cope with the demands of a person's "reality." Reality theory is based on the assumption that all individuals need to develop an identity, which can be either a "success identity" or a "failure identity."

Reality therapy has been enjoying a resurgence of interest in the past few years due in part to renewed focus on the role of personal responsibility in life problems and to several recent publications (Glasser, 1990, 1998; Wubbolding, 1990, 2000; Glasser & Breggin, 2001) that have adapted his original ideas to contemporary problems in schools and society.

The counselor's job is to become highly involved with the client and to encourage motivation toward a plan of responsible action that will lead to constructive behavior change and a "success identity." The reality-therapy approach is active, directive, and cognitive, with a strong behavioral emphasis that makes use of contingency contracting. The counselor assumes simultaneous supportive and confrontive roles with clients.

Reality therapy is a short-term treatment that has been widely used in schools, institutions, and correctional settings. It is a fairly simple therapeutic approach, at least to learn the basics, and can be mastered without lengthy training and supervision. The disadvantages of reality therapy include its tendency to reward conforming behavior, the danger of the therapist's imposing

▊ | VOICE FROM THE FIELD

I've always found reality therapy to be my preferred theory because it kind of gives you a road map. You have an idea of where you are with a client—and where you need to go next—at any moment. I really like that structure.

I don't think I'll hurt anyone with it either. Basically, what I'm doing is helping people to evaluate for themselves the consequences of their behavior. I don't have to be the expert.

---

personal values of reality, and its tendency to treat symptoms rather than possible underlying causes.

## Expressive Therapies

Expressive therapies include a variety of therapeutic approaches that, although loosely integrated, all rest on the assumption that primarily nonverbal media are effective in the release and resolution of clients' problems. Whereas most of the other theories presented in this chapter rely primarily on cognitive and behavioral factors, expressive therapies tend not to rely on language and thus are able to bypass much resistance and to intensively explore underlying conflicts and dysfunctional issues.

Frequently the use of expressive therapy is not theoretically isolated but occurs as an adjunct to other theoretical modalities. I offer several examples of these alternative approaches to balance the more traditional modalities that we have previously explored.

**Art Therapy**   Art therapy has long been a form of treatment for children, helping them to express feelings actively as well as to talk through images represented in their drawings. The *Journal of Art Therapy* contains suggestions for using materials to promote better cooperation in children, for gathering data for diagnoses, and especially for helping people become more creative and emotionally expressive. Practitioners resort to such alternative therapeutic media as musical instruments, games, sculpture, photography, drawing, cartooning, poetry, journal writing, puppetry, and drama when verbal strategies are ineffective (Gladding, 1998). Resistances and emotional blocks can therefore be bypassed through these treatment strategies and through others such as drama, music, and dance therapies that are primarily nonverbal.

**Music and Dance Therapy**   Movement is a popular form of expressive therapy, used with music or without. There is even the American Dance Therapy Association that seeks to guide practitioners who employ such methods in their work. As with most of the other nonverbally mediated treatments, this strategy has the advantage of bypassing intellectualization and verbal defenses with the intent of helping people to become more self-expressive, more in touch with their bodies and minds, and more inclined to explore their potential in creative ways.

**Biofeedback**    Another action method that can be used to improve client control, biofeedback gives clients accurate information about their psychophysiological responses. Readings can be taken of bodily functions such as brain activity, heart rate, muscle movement, blood pressure, and skin responses to improve muscular and neurological control. Katkin and Goldband (1980) suggest that biofeedback may be applied to teach relaxation skills and thereby to reduce general tension, to control migraine headaches, to modify vascular disorders such as hypertension, to better tolerate chronic pain, to relieve sexual dysfunctions, to control seizure disorders, or to prevent stress-related problems.

**Play Therapy**    Most counseling with children employs some kind of play, whether it involves drawing, playing cards or games, building structures, dressing up in costumes, or playing catch with a ball. Beginning from about age two until the teen years, but especially during the early childhood and elementary school years, play is the primary form of expression for children. The counselor seeks to establish trust with the child, as well as to facilitate communication and even solve problems, through the interactive nature of play. The whole spectrum of different counseling theories have their own approach to play therapy, but each of them emphasizes action rather than merely talking about issues (James, 1997; Straus, 1999).

**Hypnotherapy**    Another area that requires additional training and certification for counselors is hypnotherapy. Hypnosis has been applied widely in therapeutic situations since Freud's day—by behavioral counselors who wish to intensify systematic desensitization techniques, by psychoanalysts to access the unconscious, and by many other clinicians who use imagery, rehearsal, and fantasy techniques. Whereas hypnosis has most commonly been integrated into weight loss and smoking-cessation programs, its methods of inducing relaxation and hypersuggestibility are also used in working through many forms of client resistance.

**Exercise**    Other more natural forms of handling stress have evolved through the popularity of structured exercise programs. Many people have discovered the therapeutic benefits of activities such as running, walking, bicycling, rowing, aerobic dance, swimming, weightlifting, and the martial arts.

It is only recently that mental health and medical experts have begun to recognize the potential benefits of exercises such as running to improve creativity, confidence, self-control, and well-being, as well as to reduce negative addictions, boredom, anxiety, and depression (Sachs & Buflone, 1984). Running and similar activities have thus become integrated into many therapeutic programs as adjuncts to treatment, as transitional support systems after counseling has ended, or even as a sole means of psychological and spiritual rejuvenation. Some therapists, such as Glasser (1976), recognized a while ago that positive addictions such as running can combat self-destructive patterns and be a form of self-medication for stress.

## Bibliotherapy

Perhaps it is fitting that we end this chapter on action approaches by talking about the importance of supplementary reading assignments, not unlike the suggested readings at the end of each chapter. Routinely, quite a number of therapists who come from different theoretical orientations recommend to their clients that they read certain books that complement or reinforce the ideas that come up in sessions. There is a long and honored tradition for clinicians to suggest self-help or psychology books, or even novels that deal with relevant themes (Joshua & DeMenna, 2000; Stanley, 1999). Some bibliotherapy approaches look toward particular populations such as therapeutic books for children (Pardeck & Pardeck, 1993) or for women (Chrisler & Ulsh, 2001). For example, Pardeck and Pardeck (1993) did a survey of feminist therapists to determine which were their most frequently recommend books to female clients (you might want to write these down). Although the list is now somewhat dated, the most commonly cited book was *The Courage to Heal* (Bass, 1988).

As you develop experience, and broaden your own reading interests, you will collect your own favorite sources to recommend to people. Most of those books that I recommend the most include fiction like Michael Dorris' *The Yellow Raft in Blue Water* about a story of abuse told from the perspective of a child, mother, and grandmother, each of whom believes the others are at fault, or Barbara Kingsolver's *Poisonwood Bible* about a family's struggle to understand one another in the midst of their immersion in a foreign culture. There are also dozens of excellent self-help books on the market that you might use to supplement the work you do with people. In fact, whenever I encounter an area in my work in which I find very little written, that motivates me to do my own research in that area in order to supply needed resources. A couple of examples include my interest in helping people understand why they struggle with their solitude (*Private Moments, Secret Selves*, 1990), why they tend to blame others for their conflicts (*Beyond Blame*, 1994), the meaning of their crying (*The Language of Tears*, 1996), and how to reinforce the work that is done in therapy (*Making Changes Last*, 2001).

Lest you think that adjunct structures must be limited to books, quite a number of counselors also make use of films to supplement their sessions (Solomon, 2001). Clients with obsessive-compulsive disorder might be asked to watch *As Good As It Gets*, or who have enmeshed attachments might watch *What About Bob?*, or who have alcohol problems might watch *Leaving Las Vegas*. The main point I'd like to make is that it is never too early in your career to start collecting good books, films, and other media that might supplement and strengthen the work that you intend to do. Remember the key to action-oriented methods is that talk is not enough; people have to go out in the world in order to *do* things in order to make the changes last.

# SUMMARY

The previous chapters on counseling theory have reviewed some of the most popular therapeutic systems currently in use. Action-oriented approaches mentioned in this chapter place more emphasis on the technique and technology of change.

At this juncture, your state of confusion is probably unavoidable, if not desirable. It is overwhelming to study so many different explanations of how best to do counseling, especially when each system appears to have attractive components.

On an unconscious if not deliberate level, your mind is already sifting through the vast array of new ideas and making decisions about what to reserve for further study and what to throw out because of apparent clashes with your values, personality, skills, and interests. In the next chapter you can carry on with the task of building a tentative personal theory of counseling; this is a process that will continue throughout the balance of your life.

# SELF-GUIDED EXPLORATIONS

1. Describe a time in your life in which insight was not enough: You understood what the problem was all about, you even had some idea of how it evolved, but you felt powerless to make needed changes. What would it (or did it) take to help you make needed changes?

2. Use a behavioral contract to commit yourself to making some desired change in your life. Make sure your goals are specific, measurable, and, most of all, realistic given your time parameters and track record.

   Goals:

   Procedure to reach goals:

   Consequences:

   Daily reward:

   Contract reward:

3. Use rational emotive behavior therapy (REBT) to dispute the irrational beliefs that underlie a current situation you find upsetting. Hint: A common issue for counseling students is a fear of failure and overstriving for perfection.

4. Consider an aspect of your life that feels stuck. Applying a problem-solving strategy, make a list of all the things you've tried to resolve the difficulty that have not worked. Promise yourself not to do those things

anymore (unless you are convinced that if you try just one more time, maybe one of these might work—in which case, remove it from your list).

5. Now make a list of other alternatives that might work. Start with the exact opposite of things you have already been doing. Make the list as creative and exhaustive as possible.

## For Homework:

Based on one of the assignments you completed in this chapter, implement the procedure or strategy that you came up with. Note what you did, what happened, and what you will do next to make needed adjustments.

## SUGGESTED READINGS

De Jong, P. (1998). *Interviewing for solutions.* Pacific Grove, CA: Brooks/Cole.

Ellis, A. (2001). *Overcoming destructive beliefs, feelings, and behaviors: New directions for rational emotive behavior therapy.* New York: Prometheus.

Ellis, A., & Wilde, J. (2002). *Case studies in rational emotive behavior therapy with children and adolescents.* Upper Saddle River, NJ: Prentice-Hall.

Gladding, S. T. (1998). *Counseling as an art: Creative arts in counseling.* Alexandria, VA: American Counseling Association.

Glasser, W., & Breggin, P. R. (2001).*Counseling with choice theory.* New York: Quill.

Haley, J., and Zeig, J. (2001). *Changing directives: The strategic psychotherapy of Jay Haley.* Phoenix, AZ: Zeig, Tucker.

Lazarus, A. A. (1997). *Brief but comprehensive therapy: The multimodal way.* New York: Springer.

Littrel, J. M. (1998). *Brief counseling in action.* New York: W. W. Norton.

Presbury, J., Echterling, L. G., & McKee, J. E. (2002). *Ideas and tools for brief counseling.* Upper Saddle River, NJ: Prentice-Hall.

Spiegler, M. D., & Guevremont, D. C. (1998). *Contemporary behavior therapy* (3rd ed.). Pacific Grove, CA: Brooks/Cole.

# 7 INTEGRATING THEORY AND COUNSELING SKILLS

KEY CONCEPTS

Theoretical integration

Eclecticism

Tribalism

Personal theory building

Mentorhood

Pragmatism

Generic skills

Counseling stages

Validity

Reliability

Intentionality

Attending skills

Reflective skills

Immediacy

Directives

# INTEGRATING THEORY AND COUNSELING SKILLS

# CHAPTER 7

After a brief (or even prolonged) study of the various counseling theories, a reasonable reaction is to be both impressed and confused. Each theory seems to be useful in understanding people and behavior and appears helpful in promoting lasting change. Yet the theorists seem to contradict one another, and each stands on propositions that directly refute what another holds as sacred. How is it possible that Rogers helps people when he is actively listening, whereas Ellis is aggressively disputing, Freud is wisely interpreting, Perls is integrating, Haley is problem solving, and the rest are analyzing, diagnosing, and counseling in their own unique ways? It is clearly difficult for the practitioner, much less the student, to make sense of the conflicting opinions and the passionate dogma presented by the various theorists.

In this chapter, you will be helped to pull together the discrepant elements in the various theories, as well as to understand the generic process and skills favored by most practicing counselors. Although there is considerable disagreement in the field about which theories are best to use, there is actually remarkable consensus regarding the basic process and skills involved.

## A PERSONAL JOURNEY

In my first introduction to counseling theory, perhaps like your own, I was exposed to the idea that many different theories attempted to explain the human condition. It was comforting to learn that I was experiencing developmental growth and that my confusion was to be expected. According to Erik Erikson (1950), crisis and the resolution of opposing polarities are central to personal and social development. This principle is no less true for the development of a personal theory of counseling than it is for life span development. I really appreciated the support from my first instructors who reassured me that it was normal to be confused and to feel overwhelmed.

In the next phase of professional development, I became personally involved as a client in counseling. Reflecting the spirit of the times, the counselor I selected was sensitive, helpful, and Freudian. It made sense, therefore, that Freud's theory would become the next one I would explore. This was actually quite an exciting introduction to the field: Freud was such a wonderful writer. His ideas lent themselves to immediate application to my own life. Furthermore, the psychoanalytic model offered many interesting possibilities. A Freudian analyst can be detached, knowledgeable, mysterious, and, best of all, omnipotent. Joining the Freudian theory group was like being part of a club, or perhaps even a religion. People were zealous in their belief in Freud, his theory, and his teachings. At that early point in professional development, however, it seemed to me too confining to choose such an encompassing theoretical model. I also noted that for a budding counselor-to-be, psychoanalysis didn't exactly fit the job requirements of my work settings at the time—a half-time preschool teacher and half-time college career counselor.

Next I discovered Carl Rogers as a refreshing change. I wondered what kind of scrooge wouldn't like Rogers. He was kind, he was sensitive, he was the grandfather I always wanted (and now hope someday to be). During this time (the 1970s), practically all counselors were prepared in a client-centered model, even if there were some rumblings from the behaviorists. As a Rogerian counselor, I was instructed to be kind, to smile, and to develop an accepting environment for clients. Reflecting feelings was certainly effective, but the way I was working felt stale and restrictive, especially for some of the clients I was now seeing who had major substance abuse problems.

By the time I graduated I was practicing as a crisis counselor. I felt impatient with some of the limitations of dealing only with feelings and staying only in the present. I also felt that even after attaining a master's degree I still didn't know nearly enough to help people the way I wanted. I still felt like a fraud, obsessed with all the things I didn't understand and all the skills I still couldn't practice as fluently as I preferred. Perhaps a doctorate would do the trick.

Indeed, in my doctoral training I was exposed to other theories that had an impact on me (and my clients) in profound ways. Rational-emotive and behavioral approaches seemed especially attractive to me at the time, theories that seemed to lend themselves quite well to the hospital patients I was now working with. Still, this was hardly enough.

Next I became a workshop junkie, starved for definitive answers about the best theory to help my increasingly desperate clients. I felt lost, but now that I was a new professor and supervisor, I felt it would be in the best interests of my students to hide the fact that I was still struggling to understand how the process of counseling really works. I tried all the new approaches on the market at the time—neurolinguistic programming, strategic therapy, Ericksonian hypnosis, Satir family therapy, reality therapy, to mention just a few. After each of these workshops, I would return to my work reenergized and excited that I had finally found "The Answer." Alas, this confidence usually lasted only a few months before there was a new announcement that whatever I had been doing was now obsolete and if I really wanted to be cutting edge, I had better learn the latest addition to the professional scene.

Feeling restricted once again by an overly technical approach to helping people, I moved on to existential theory, an approach that added some new understanding to my base of knowledge. Unfortunately, this also aided my tendency to intellectualize. I next welcomed the relief of Gestalt theory's apparent simplicity but then realized that it was a lot more complex than I had patience for.

In the years since this formative stage in my development, I continued to evolve in my own understanding and practice of theory. I grabbed every new book on the scene and attended as many presentations as I had the money and time for. By that time I had begun to integrate meaningful parts of the various theories and refine techniques through my work with clients. There is nothing like actually trying out a theory to find out what works best for you, for your clients, in your clinical situation, with your way of operating, with your interpersonal style, and with your support group of colleagues and supervisors.

By about this time I began work in private practice full time. All of a sudden, the criteria for success seemed to change overnight. Symptomatic relief was no longer enough, as it had been with the clientele I had seen earlier in my career. Good counseling, as defined by private practitioners I worked with, cannot possibly take place in less than a year. Now that my livelihood depended on my ability to fill time slots, I became more intrigued with new theories that emphasized longer-term treatments.

Along the way, I also began to teach counseling theory classes and help students to work toward integration. In the struggle to develop my own opinions, I had to sort through everyone else's, saving what seemed useful and fit my personality and style. It is at this stage that you are now encountering me. I am still exploring new ideas and developing models to help my clients. And I am sometimes still confused.

## MOVEMENT TOWARD INTEGRATION

The preceding autobiographical case study typifies the progression of professional development for many counselors as they develop a personal theory. Initially, it is easy to imitate and follow specific rules; later, it is important to integrate these methods into a style that is personally congruent.

Most of the theories mentioned in the previous chapters, and those you will study more closely in later courses and chapters, are not meant to represent a finite selection of absolute approaches; rather, they may be viewed as historical referents that form the basis for effective clinical practice. Our

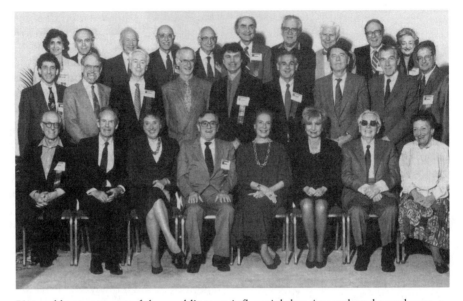

Pictured here are some of the world's most influential theorists gathered together to exchange ideas and reconcile their theoretical differences. Courtesy of the Milton H. Erickson Foundation, Inc.

profession is clearly headed in the direction of theoretical integration rather than allegiance to a single approach (Bradley, Parve, & Gould, 1995; Hubble, Duncan, & Miller, 1999; Kottler, 1991; Mikulas, 2002; Preston, 1999; Prochaska & Norcross, 2003; Young, 1992). It is also encouraging to realize that, in several surveys of counselors and therapists, over half describe themselves as eclectic in orientation and refuse to affiliate themselves with any single theory of practice (Norcross, Prochaska, & Gallagher, 1989; Smith, 1982; Watkins, Lopez, Campbell, & Himmell, 1986). Other estimates place the number of professionals who call themselves eclectic as closer to 70 percent (Jensen, Bergin, & Greaves, 1990). Eclectic, by the way, means that a practitioner is flexible enough to use a variety of approaches, selecting the best available and appropriate, depending on what is called for for a given client and situation.

Some writers, such as Simon (1991), believe it is a professional obligation to pursue an individualized form of theoretical eclecticism. This means that the movement toward developing a personal style of counseling will only continue to flourish, requiring you not only to be intimately familiar with several counseling approaches but to integrate them in an individually designed way that is best suited to your personality, clients, and setting. Lazarus and Beutler (1993) prefer to call this approach a form of "technical eclecticism" in which the counselor selects any number of interventions from a variety of theories without subscribing to their beliefs. Indeed, the future of the profession seems to be moving toward this path of choosing what should work best for a given client in a given situation, depending on our prior experience and the research literature available.

# GRABBING TRUTH BY THE TAIL

The past century in psychology, since the days in Wilhelm Wundt's laboratory, William James' classrooms, and Sigmund Freud's consultation chambers, might well be called the "Hundred Years' War." There is no doubt that the proliferation of significant research, the advances in theory, the development of technology, and the growth of therapeutic counseling as a profession have been spectacular during modern times. The scholarly debates, roundtable discussions, and controversial dialogues in the literature are in fact necessary for the continued progress of any field. Only through dispassionate analysis of conflicting points of view may we ever hope to improve the quality of our theories in explaining complex phenomena and the effectiveness of our interventions in promoting constructive change. In many ways, however, the history of counseling theory shows a spotted record of petty skirmishes, insignificant fights, and self-serving platforms.

Professional counselors who, above all else, stand for the values of flexibility, openness, genuineness, sensitivity, and aggressive truth seeking have often been guilty of levels of rigidity and resistance to change that would make even our clients blush in embarrassment. The field of counseling, which is after all the perfect marriage of philosophy and science, has actually evolved into forms of tribalism, denominationalism, and parochialism. We have different sects under the guise of scholarly theories. Each therapeutic approach, whether psychoanalytic, behaviorist, Gestalt, rational emotive, nondirective, existential, strategic, or whatever, has developed a passionate following of disciples. Each theory claims to be the heir to "truth" and has an impressive body of evidence to support that belief.

Unfortunately, the main attribute of tribalism, in Borneo or academia, is a single-minded determination to preserve the status quo and repel outside agitation. With all his wisdom and farsighted perspectives, Freud set this precedent by ostracizing those of his disciples who were troublemakers—independent thinkers—expelling the apostles who dared question the sacred word of the master. Thus Carl Jung and Alfred Adler, to name but two, left the camp in exile, only to begin their own tribes.

Freud set up a brilliant psychological defense mechanism to protect his ideas—his children—from mutilation. To legitimately criticize his theory, Freud felt, one first had to undergo psychoanalysis. If, after completing the treatment, the critic still persisted in attacks, obviously the psychoanalysis was unsuccessful and further work was indicated. The intent here is not to criticize Freud, who unfortunately has been the scapegoat for a century of attacks, but rather to point out the precedent he established as the protective creator of ideas he did not wish to see deviate from his intent or control.

## VOICE FROM THE FIELD

I can't tell you how ridiculous it looks at conventions I go to. Some of these famous personalities in the field walk around like gods. They seem more interested in furthering their own recognition than they do helping to advance the state of knowledge in the field. When a bunch of them, or their disciples, get together, they talk such different languages they don't even understand one another.

When you've been in the field long enough, you've seen it all. Every time they come up with a new theory, when you really study it, it seems like old stuff that's just been repackaged so that somebody else can make a name for himself.

I know this sounds cynical, but I gotta tell you, I'm just so tired of being judged by some colleagues in the field who have such a firm idea about the best way to do this work, and that anybody who doesn't do it like them is somehow stupid or incompetent.

---

The history of counseling, which is the applied study of personality, is itself a chronicle of the influences of a number of formidable personalities. New schools of counseling are generally not discovered in the laboratory, nor are they usually the result of formal experimentation; they are, rather, the insights and conclusions of a single clinician or a small group of practitioners who have found a particular set of assumptions and techniques to be reliably helpful with clients. In each case, the theory is the result of a life's unique experience and a personality's individual expression. It can be no coincidence that traditionally trained former psychoanalysts such as Albert Ellis, Eric Berne, and Fritz Perls branched off to create new approaches that reflect their unique attributes and values. Carl Rogers, the embodiment of a congruent, genuine, warm human being, constructed a theory that was an extension of his personality. Similarly, Albert Ellis, a logician, a clear thinker, a convincing debater, developed an approach branded with his unique assets. Can we do less for our clients, who are our responsibility and respond to our unique personalities, than to construct a personal theory of action that has been pragmatically designed for our their particular situation?

As Ivan Turgenev explained to Leo Tolstoy in 1856, "The people who bind themselves to systems are those who are unable to encompass the whole truth and try to catch it by the tail; a system is like the tail of truth, but truth is like a lizard; it leaves its tail in your fingers and runs away knowing full well that it will grow a new one in a twinkling" (Boorstein, 1983, p. 81).

# A PERSONAL THEORY

## Criteria of Effectiveness

Theories are not always designed to help clients; rather, they are developed to reduce *the counselor's* anxiety in dealing with the complexities, the ambiguities, the uncertainties of the therapeutic process (Yalom, 1989). In exploring why a particular counseling theory may or may not be helpful in your work with clients, Boy and Pine (1982) identified several influential factors. The effectiveness of any such model will depend on the following:

1. *The quality of the therapeutic relationship.* Any theory is functionally impotent without the cooperation, trust, and motivation of the client—circumstances that can be created and maintained only by a supportive, respectful relationship.

2. *The perception of shared power.* Without approximate equality of responsibility between counselor and client, the encounter is likely to be devoid of commitment, freedom, and independence.

3. *The counselor's understanding of theory.* Before you can use an idea effectively, you must understand its subtle complexities. Far beyond imitating your professors, mentors, supervisors, or colleagues, the counselor should explore the body of knowledge, research, and skills associated with the chosen theory—its history, influences, antecedents, process, goals, outcomes, strengths, and weaknesses.

4. *Intellectual and attitudinal commitment.* Credibility and enthusiastic application depend, to a large part, on the counselor's personal commitment to the theory. This loyalty springs from more than either an emotional allegiance of your beliefs or an alignment of your intellect. A balance is necessary between the two so that the counselor may believe in the power and value of a theory—but as a passionate scholar rather than as a zealot.

5. *Flexible integration within institutional requirements.* The final criterion for effective theory application brings in an important aspect of reality: Counselors do not work in a vacuum. There are powerful pressures from administrators and colleagues, diluted roles, and institutional policies that often make pure application of your theory impossible. A theory should look good not only on the drawing board or when a counselor is functioning in a pure, unencumbered way but also when the counselor is conflicted, distracted, hurried, and pressured. The theory should be useful in reality.

## Guidelines for Usefulness

The criteria just listed are optimally useful when adapting an existing theoretical structure for personal use. For those who are motivated (by growth, curiosity, or the desire to be more flexible and effective) to construct their own theory from the abundance of diverse ideas, there are many other guiding concepts to consider. For instance, one helpful approach is to identify potentially valuable ideas in existing theories. The key to progress is to improve on what has already been done rather than starting over and over again. The impetus to create a new theory comes from the rebellious internal drive to wear your own clothes instead of hand-me-downs from an older sibling. The critical attitude of doing it yourself can lead you to overreact to the limitations of the status quo and thereby reject everything, instead of just those parts that are inhibiting. Freud, Adler, Rogers, Perls, Ellis, and all the rest had something valuable to say, some idea that is salvageable for a new theory, some concept or technique that could still be useful in a slightly altered form.

Often the complaint of the counseling student is that theories tend to be needlessly complex, with jargon and language that are abstract, ambiguous, and incomprehensible. Considering for a moment how difficult it is to explain and understand a phenomenon as complex as the human organism in its process of psychological change, you can see that a simplistic theory is unlikely to suffice. Nevertheless, that is not to say that in your own theory building you cannot work toward clarity, precision, and simplicity of language without sacrificing utility.

## STAGES IN DEVELOPING A PERSONAL THEORY

The process of developing a personal theory of counseling can seem overwhelming, especially to the beginning student, but it is more manageable when broken down into steps. Each of the stages describes a plateau on the road to developing a personal theory and represents a series of questions that can be answered on a personal level and from which generalizations must emerge. A personal theory evolves ultimately from two major sources of knowledge: the techniques and theories of counseling and the richness and realities of life itself. Minuchin and Fishman (1981), two leading family therapists, admonish the beginner to "disengage from the techniques of therapy and engage with the difficulties of life" (p. 10). Developing a valid and useful personal theory of counseling depends on knowing yourself well and participating in the experience of life. Such evolution in your thinking may follow a series of progressive stages (see Figure 7.1).

### Entry

The counseling student begins the task of theory building by learning an overview of theories. Even those students with substantial practical experience choose a formal counselor education program to legitimate their status, as well as to refine skills and acquire additional knowledge. The course of study normally begins with an introductory course, using a text similar to the one you are reading.

The first stage of professional theory development is usually confusing. Within a short period of time the beginning student is exposed to a variety of approaches to counseling. Their conflicting points of view can be disorienting enough, but the student is also learning about relevant theories in other courses. Just when the names and terms of basic theories are beginning to make sense, additional input from these other courses renews the confusion. It is no wonder, then, that the first stage in a beginning counselor's attempts to construct a personal blueprint for guiding behavior is marked by swings from enlightenment to frustration.

**FIGURE 7.1**

**Decision to enter program**

Critical incident, career change

**Formal course work**

Soak in overview and follow progression

**Eclecticism**

Practicum/internship experience leads one
to abandon formal theory temporarily to get
through the experience

**Theory hopping**

Interaction with colleagues leads to greater
flexibility and experimentation

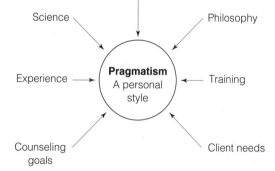

Science          Philosophy

Experience →   **Pragmatism**
A personal   ← Training
style

Counseling
goals          Client needs

Increased flexibility, variability, and work demands encourage many counselors to integrate their training, supervisor feedback, and previous experiences with client
needs and counseling goals. The result becomes a personal style of practice that is grounded in theory and research but reflects one's own personality, beliefs, and
preferences in such a way that client differences may
be honored and individual needs may be addressed.

Eventually most new students, out of a sense of self-preservation, decide to suspend judgment temporarily and try to understand all the theories, deferring evaluation until later. It is difficult, if not impossible, to organize information at this point because all the information is so new that it is hard to know what questions to ask.

The slightly stressful job of the learner is occasionally interrupted by an inevitable question that will push the student onward to the next stage of theory building. The query is, "What are you?" Students' responses reveal the first of their many alliances to a particular theory.

## Mentorhood

When you attempt to answer that deceptively simple question, consider the consequences of declaring your primary theoretical affiliation. Because "I don't know," "What do you mean?" and similar responses may make you appear nonstudious or less mature than your classmates, you will probably prefer to name a particular theory that sounds good and that you understand to some degree. Now you have catapulted yourself into the second stage of theory construction and will experience added pressure to find a label to describe the way you think (even though you are not yet certain about your choice).

During this phase a student is sometimes impressionable and susceptible to hero worship. Professors or supervisors who are good at their work and skilled at helping others learn are good candidates for this role. These mentors and modeling influences are particularly important to later development, for they provide guidance and a behavioral model. It becomes relatively easy to affiliate yourself with the point of view of a model that you admire and even to convince yourself that this is the model that will work best for you.

You now have reason to study one theory thoroughly and intensively. An unfortunate side effect of concentrated interest can be a mental block to examining other theories that increase cognitive dissonance. Some practitioners never progress beyond their allegiance to one counseling approach. Many of them become extraordinarily knowledgeable and skilled at applying its concepts; they can devote time and energy toward improving themselves as specialists in a particular style. With such a commitment comes an increased acceptance of your mentor and of the support system of other like-minded practitioners. There are special books, journals, meetings, and conventions, all intended to help counselors grow in their chosen affiliation. The result can be immunization against others from outside the "club" who could lead a confused sheep astray.

For many students, participation in the practicum or internship helps to shatter the illusion that only one theory works. Taking a class in techniques also helps because it is there you learn the generic skills practiced by almost all counselors. The temporary sanctuary of mentorhood is left behind as the student continues on to the next stage.

## Eclecticism

Held (1984) distinguishes between *technical* and *prescriptive* eclecticism. In the former, the counselor is a technician, a skilled master of technique who may be successful on a practical level without a well-articulated guiding philosophy. Prescriptive eclecticism rests more firmly on a solid theoretical base and places more emphasis on prediction and explanation of phenomena. Flexibility is the hallmark of both eclectic approaches, in which professionals subscribe to parts of many different theories.

Renewed flexibility is the logical result of your first actual experience as a counselor. You soon realize that imitating a mentor is hollow without an integrated understanding of the theory. You may have temporarily abandoned organized theory in your attempts to get through the practicum experience, experimenting with a variety of ideas to alleviate personal anxiety while helping a client. Adventurous students will even try out a few of their own ideas, but such behavior may be risky unless it is successful. You are wise to be conservative and cautious in trying out the range of theories as you have personally interpreted and integrated them. When in doubt, you can always fall back on the ideas of your mentors—who, after all, have spent decades developing and practicing the techniques—or revert back to a previous theory of your own. When not under pressure, you can find another favorite to study. Ever so slowly, your own personality and preferences begin to demonstrate a unique style.

## Experimentation

School is over. As an employed professional, you now have the opportunity to test the theories and techniques that were presented in the classroom. Refinement of theory is encouraged by colleagues and supervisors who have firm ideas of their own regarding the best ways to help clients. The fundamental concepts favored in the textbooks and classroom are sometimes downplayed by the seasoned professionals, who warn: "Forget relying on theory. Around here we do things our own way." Of course, the supervisors are really presenting theories of their own choice.

This particular stage of professional development is often marked by experimental theory hopping, trying out attractive concepts, listening to more experienced peers, and remembering the wise words of mentors. Books play an influential role as the ex-student revels in new freedom while feeling eager for the excitement of new ideas. Because there is so little time and structure to reinforce learning, classic books become the mainstay of further theory development.

## Pragmatism

Not all counselors reach the stage of pragmatic flexibility—nor do they want to. Many practitioners remain satisfied and quite effective at applying the

## VOICE FROM THE FIELD

Early on, I really found that narrative counseling fit me like a glove. Perhaps even better, it seemed to fit my clients who are mostly members of oppressed minority groups. I like the way it can be applied so efficiently. I like the way it looks at the world. I just like it! Maybe sometime I may move on to other things, but for now I like the comfort of learning this one approach as well as I can. And there is so much more to learn! I just can't imagine trying to juggle several different theories. And what's the point? People a lot smarter and more experienced than I am have gone to a lot of trouble to develop this stuff. That's good enough for me.

---

concepts of their favorite theory. The principal advantage is a sense of comfort and familiarity with the theory and its accompanying techniques. The counselor becomes increasingly more experienced and eloquent at personalizing and adapting the preferred theory in his or her work with clients.

For others, single-theory allegiance feels conforming, limiting, boring, and routine. Some choose to move beyond mere eclecticism—a stance of technical proficiency in many techniques—to a philosophy of pragmatism.

As originally conceived by the first psychologist, William James, "Pragmatism unstiffens all our theories, limbers them up, and sets each one at work" (James, 1907, p. 46). The pragmatic counselor is concerned with integrating the body of knowledge from all relevant disciplines into a personalized and pluralistic philosophy that is empirically based and can be practically applied to specific situations.

One of the hallmarks of a pragmatic approach is that prior to any therapeutic action, a counselor asks several internal questions:

1. What appears to be happening?
2. What do I wish to accomplish?
3. How will this intervention meet the desired goal?

If the counselor is unable to answer these questions in a clear and cogent manner, depending instead on intuitive hunches such as, "I have a gut feeling that this will work," then it may be necessary to examine personal motives. A detailed analysis of "gut feelings" will aid the counselor to understand more precisely the underlying rationale for intervention choices and will also help to stifle counselor self-indulgence. Before using confrontation, for example, the counselor can ask internally: "Am I confronting this client because he is genuinely disrupting the process or because he is irritating to me?" Beyond eliminating inappropriate verbalizations, defining the rationale for actions helps the counselor to develop for future use a repertoire of strategies that have been found to be effective in similar circumstances.

Pragmatism is a useful philosophical stance for counselors because it encourages them to view the profession in a broad interdisciplinary context, integrating approaches and techniques from a variety of theoretical perspectives. It also encourages the counselor to avoid an overdependence on a single theoretical construct as heir to truth and facilitates the mechanisms of personal theory building so that relevant principles may be systematically collected from the universe of available knowledge. Perhaps Pablo Picasso best summarized the simplicity of a pragmatic philosophy: "When I haven't any blue, I use red."

# HOW ARE YOU DOING SO FAR?

In spite of feeling a degree of confusion, or even being overwhelmed, by the sheer volume of information contained in the theories presented in these chapters (and the ones to follow), you have already been sorting and organizing things to the point where your options are becoming more manageable. Some theories you've read about you feel immediately drawn to, just as others are not quite your cup of tea. This attraction you feel toward certain theories, and the rejection of others, is not based solely on the pure intellectual and logical analysis of merits and limitations. Your personal values and core views of the world also play an important role, although many of these are likely to change as your counselor education unfolds.

You might find it interesting to take an inventory at this point as to where you stand in terms of the most basic theoretical dilemmas of the profession. For each of the following ten categories, you are presented with three possible positions that might be taken legitimately. There are no correct answers. In fact, among successful practitioners, there are those who feel quite strongly about each of these points of view. I encourage you at this point to go through each of the items and select the choice that most closely fits with the way you think about the world, about other people, about yourself, and about the ways that people change.

You will find at the end of this exercise that a pattern will emerge for you in terms of what it is that you think, feel, and believe about counseling. Many of your opinions will be supported by some of the theories you have read about, perhaps even one or two of them that most closely parallel your own beliefs. As you continue your study of the literature in the field, you will probably discover that other opinions you hold are not supported by research that has been completed to date. In fact, there may be more quantitative and qualitative evidence to support one position over others, but those debates are better left for another time. This Theoretical Dilemmas Inventory is only a starting point.

## THEORETICAL DILEMMAS INVENTORY

Directions: For each of the following items, select the one position that most clearly articulates your own beliefs. Be prepared to defend your position with some evidence based on your experience.

## VIEWS OF PEOPLE

_____ People are born basically good.

_____ People are born basically evil.

_____ People are born basically neutral.

## RESPONSIBILITY FOR OUTCOMES

_____ Clients have primary responsibility for counseling outcomes.

_____ Counselors have primary responsibility for counseling outcomes.

_____ Responsibility is shared equally.

## LEGITIMATE FOCUS

_____ Counseling should focus primarily on feelings.

_____ Counseling should focus primarily on thinking.

_____ Counseling should focus primarily on behavior.

## CONTENT

_____ Counseling content should deal with the past.

_____ Counseling content should deal with the present.

_____ Counseling content should deal with the future.

## SCOPE

_____ Counseling should concentrate on specific goals.

_____ Counseling should concentrate on broad themes.

_____ Counseling should concentrate on the process of what takes place.

## SKILLS

_____ The most important counselor skill is structuring.

_____ The most important counselor skill is interpreting.

_____ The most important counselor skill is reflecting.

## COUNSELOR DIRECTIVENESS

_____ Counselors should be active.

_____ Counselors should be nondirective.

_____ Counselors should allow the client to decide what is best.

## COUNSELOR ROLE

_____ The counselor should be an expert.

_____ The counselor should be a friend.

_____ The counselor should be a consultant.

Theory

    _____ Counselors should become experts in one theory.

    _____ Counselors should become proficient in several theories.

    _____ Counselors should combine several theories.

Criteria for success

    _____ The most important predictor of good counseling is knowledge of theory.

    _____ The most important predictor of good counseling is mastery of core skills.

    _____ The most important predictor of good counseling is a healthy personality.

To compute your score, just take the number of items and multiply by your age, then divide by the course number . . . just kidding! There is no score—but there is a result that may be meaningful to you. As you look over your responses, you will note that you do indeed have some strong opinions about some of these issues, whereas others you are hesitant about until you collect more information and accumulate more experience. That is exactly as it should be.

In asking you how you are doing so far, I hope you recognize that it is normal and appropriate to feel a degree of confusion. It is also useful to realize that you do have some well-articulated beliefs that are already becoming part of a theory of your own that you are in the process of creating at this moment.

## Generic Counseling Skills

While it is true that there is considerable debate about the best theoretical approach to helping people, there is a reasonable consensus about which skills you need to learn in order to be helpful to someone. Many of these skills emerged from specific theories. For example, reflecting feelings is associated with client-centered counseling, disputing beliefs with cognitive therapy, and goal setting with a behavioral approach. Nevertheless, in spite of their origins, many helping skills are now in such wide use across the spectrum of specialties and settings that they are virtually universal. The same can be said for the general stages of counseling.

## Stages of the Counseling Process

Just at a time when you may be feeling somewhat anxious by the lack of agreement about which counseling theory is best, you should be relieved to know that most practitioners share a similar view of the process involved, if not the progressive stages that are followed. Most counselors, whether they are insight or action oriented, whether they favor theories that focus on the past or present, cognitions or affect, still subscribe to a five-stage model that relies on several skills to move forward (Doyle, 1998; Hackney & Cormier, 1996; Okun, 2002; Patterson & Welfel, 1999).

**Assessment**   In the first stage, counselors use both written instruments and clinical observation skills to formulate ideas about the client's presenting complaint. A working diagnosis is usually created that helps the practitioner to make some decisions with the client as to what treatment plan might be best—individual, group, or family counseling, short- or long-term sessions—and how things will be structured. During this initial stage, counselors make use of attending, listening, focusing, and observing skills to help them decide exactly how they will proceed. Some clients, for example, respond better to some approaches than others. A kind of contractual arrangement is negotiated in which both parties are satisfied with the intention and means to reach those goals.

**Exploration**   During the exploration stage, reflections of feeling and content, as well as questioning and probing, are used to help clients clarify issues in the present and past. Efforts are also devoted to building a solid therapeutic relationship. Clients are helped to tell their story, in other words, to describe the circumstances that led them to their current predicament. There is a catharsis, or release of tension, in being able to explore more deeply what is going on. Typically, exploration is also undertaken to collect background information related to family-of-origin issues, health and emotional history, and other relevant areas that may be helpful in the case.

**Understanding**   Whereas not all practitioners believe that promoting insight is sufficient to produce lasting changes in behavior, most agree that there is some benefit to helping clients understand how their troubles developed and how they are connected to other issues in their lives. Through the use of empathic listening, interpretation, confrontation, and other helping skills mentioned later, the counselor works to promote some degree of insight as a bridge to taking constructive action.

Insights can take a number of forms, depending on the theoretical orientation of the counselor. Promoting understanding can focus on issues in the past, current family interactions, dysfunctional thinking, behavioral inconsistencies, or even functional aspects of continuing to act self-destructively. Regardless of the emphasis, the intent of this stage is to help clients understand what they have been doing, why they have been acting in those particular ways, and other options that may be available to them.

**Action**   Just as some counselors prefer to spend most of their time working in the previous stage, others are more action oriented and like to help clients work toward observable changes. Nevertheless, most counselors would agree that some form of action is helpful, whether it involves completing specific homework assignments or, more subtly, simply asking what the client intends to do based on the insights that have been generated.

Skills that are most often a part of this stage include goal setting, role playing, paradoxical interventions, and other strategies that help clients translate what they have been working on in sessions to their lives outside of sessions. Typically, this may be communicated to clients with the following statement: "It isn't what you do with me that matters most; rather, what really counts is how you apply what you've learned to your own life."

**Evaluation**   As with any planned activity, it is helpful to assess the degree to which efforts have reached desired goals. Counselors use all the previously mentioned skills, as well as their knowledge of assessment, evaluation, and research methods, to help clients determine the extent to which they have reached desired goals. Adjustments may need to be made to recycle the process back to previous stages as needed.

# PIVOTAL COUNSELING SKILLS

Many things influence what a counselor does in a session with a client. Certainly many of the previously presented theories on the practitioner's personal philosophy and style of practice play a significant role. The counselor's personality or mood on any given day, as well as the client's concerns and goals, influence the choice of interventions. Nevertheless, most counselors have a core of skills that they use on a regular basis, and a fairly solid research base exists to support their effectiveness. Because of the research support for the core skills, educators of counselors at different institutions across the world teach basically the same skills. Increasingly, however, it is being recognized that these skills must be adapted to fit the cultural, ethnic, and gender differences of each client.

This section will introduce a group of pivotal skills that describe what counselors do during the counseling process and the various stages previously described. First, you are reminded that the overall goal of therapeutic counseling is the development of new behavior that is more adaptive, self-enhancing, and personally fulfilling. Self-exploration is the first goal of helping, and subsequent steps follow a pattern that employs the skills of attending, responding, initiating, and communicating, eventually leading to constructive action.

The process of exploration, understanding, and action is continuously recycled in the helping process. Action provokes feedback, which provides a stimulus for further self-exploration, which in turn facilitates increased and more accurate self-understanding. Real understanding is often the result of learning that follows action. Finally, action is further modified in accordance with a more accurate understanding of self.

Until now, we have focused on how counselors think. We will now examine what counselors *do* in their sessions—the specific interventions that are often used to facilitate client self-exploration, self-understanding, and desired changes in behavior, feelings, and thoughts.

## Being Intentional and Reliable

Developing skills, techniques, and procedures that are valid and tend to influence clients to experience constructive change is a primary concern of counselors. The discussion of validity is complex. Everyone claims validity for his or her chosen approach—and to some extent, each is right. Everything is valid. All techniques, approaches, and styles (even the most bizarre) work—with some clients at some times. Because validity is a measure of whether the technique or process does what it claims to do, most practitioners and theorists can demonstrate validity.

The debate over whether or not something works can often be better replaced with an exploration of *when* it works. Kagan (1973) has stated it succinctly: "The most important issue for our field is not if counseling works but rather what methods work consistently" (p. 234). Reliability is a measure of consistency of valid treatment effects with a wide range of client types. In other words, do your basic counseling/human relations skills influence positive change in most clients with whom you have professional contact? Consistency of effects is the trademark of the intentional counselor. Achieving reliability in counseling is a function of several factors: selection of valid and appropriate techniques, careful training, and integration of one's personal style into a systematic counseling approach. In a sense, being intentional and reducing the impact of chance effects maximize the potential for delivering valid and reliable counseling services. Such is the essence of professionalism and integrity.

Achieving reliability in counseling—that is, reducing the impact of chance on counseling relationships—is often related to the counselor's being consistent. Intentionality refers to the development of a cognitive flexibility integrated into an open and dynamic worldview. An intentional person will clarify choices, focus priorities, and implement goals and action. In a sense, an intentional person is the opposite of those who come for assistance or counseling. Often clients lack direction in their lives, evidencing immobility and the inability to see choices.

As a counselor, your goal, naturally, is to help clients create more options and to do so with methods demonstrated to be reliable and valid. This task is more difficult than it seems, for many counselors can feel successful without really being able to prove they have made an impact. This problem has, not surprisingly, received some attention in the literature and is often an unspoken client concern. Counselors have a responsibility to answer the question for themselves and their clients and to know how and why they believe counseling actually works—and works consistently.

## Significance of Attending Skills

Perhaps the basis for all therapeutic interventions is the physical and psychological attending to persons in need of help (Carkhuff & Anthony, 1979; Claiborn, 1979; Ivey & Authier, 1978). It is through posture, body position, head nods, facial expressions, eye contact, gestures, and verbal encouragements that the counselor communicates intense interest in everything a client says and feels. And it is through such active attending that the counselor can also observe the nonverbal cues evident in the client's behavior. A quivering lip, clenched hand, or furrowed brow provide evidence that is helpful in understanding what the client is experiencing. This focused attention is highly important in all stages of the counseling process, but it is especially critical during the assessment and exploration stages when you are first establishing a relationship.

Effective listening, the core of attending skills, involves the following elements:

1. *Have a reason for listening.* Know what to listen for and how it will be important to the client's exploration, understanding, and action.
2. *Be nonjudgmental.* To listen effectively, you must suspend temporarily the things you say to yourself. Let the client's message sink in without making decisions about it.
3. *Resist distractions.* Resist both internal and external distractions so that your attention and listening focus will not be disturbed.
4. *Wait to respond.* Give yourself time to respond fully and deeply to the client's statements, avoiding hasty and possibly superficial responses.
5. *Reflect content.* Reflecting back to the client what you hear him or her saying communicates understanding and provides an opportunity to check out the accuracy of your perceptions.
6. *Look for themes.* Be selective with all the stimuli presented, and attend to only the content that is relevant and meaningful. Identifying themes will help you to understand where the client is coming from and how the client perceives his or her relationship to the world.

**Listening Skills**   Several response options tend to promote verbal expression and convey interest:

1. *Passive listening*: The use of verbal encouragement and nonverbal attending to acknowledge messages communicated by the client.

   EXAMPLES:
   "I see."
   "Uh-huh."
   "Go on."
   "Yes."

2. *Parrotting*: Repetition of the client's words to indicate interest, demonstrate accuracy of listening, or stall for time until a more elegant response can be formulated.

   EXAMPLE:
   CLIENT: Boy, am I upset.
   COUNSELOR: You're really upset.

3. *Paraphrasing*: Restatement of a message's content to clarify or to focus the client's attention.

   EXAMPLE:
   CLIENT: My life feels useless. My job is a dead end. I don't have any friends. And my parents are always on my case.
   COUNSELOR: You are isolated, trapped, badgered, and don't see a way out.

4. *Clarification*: Confirmation of a message's accuracy or encouragement of further elaboration of an idea.

   EXAMPLE:
   COUNSELOR: You are saying that this issue of feeling vulnerable and getting hurt when you trust others has been a lifelong theme.

5. *Reflection of feeling*: Focus on affect to promote catharsis and self-expression.

   EXAMPLE:
   CLIENT: I don't know. Maybe this marriage isn't worth holding together any longer. We've already tried just about every option.
   COUNSELOR: You feel so frustrated and overwhelmed trying to resolve your conflicts without help from your wife. It's as if she had already given up on your relationship and now you are feeling hopeless and helpless.

6. *Summary*: The linking of several ideas together in a condensed way to promote insight, cut off rambling, identify significant themes, or draw closure.

   EXAMPLE:
   COUNSELOR: So far you have talked a lot about the ways you keep people at a distance. You tend to hang back whenever you feel a potential for a friendship, and those who approach you are quickly discouraged by your reluctance. You have also mentioned that you might have learned your aloofness from your parents, who never seemed to have much time for you.

**Exploration Skills**    There is a set of counselor behaviors that can be especially helpful in drawing out client concerns, facilitating insight, and exploring thoughts and feelings. Most use these skills as the staple of their therapeutic efforts during the first few stages of the process:

1. *Probe*: Questioning in an open-ended manner to gather relevant information or to encourage self-examination.

   EXAMPLE:
   "What are the things you've tried to do throughout your life when you have faced similar struggles?"

2. *Immediacy*: Attempting to bring the focus to the present, to comment on the style of interaction in the session, or to give feedback.

   EXAMPLE:
   "Right this very moment you are deferring to me in just the same way you back down from your boss."

## ◼ VOICE FROM THE FIELD

I remember when I first learned reflective listening skills. I came home that first night all pumped up, just dying to try out what I learned with my family. It just blew me away how powerful this stuff was. At the time, I was so awkward. I probably just repeated whatever anyone said to me. The thing is, though, that it's just so rare that people feel really listened to that when I started to give my full attention to whomever was talking, they just loved it. At first, they weren't even aware of what I was doing; they were just so delighted to be getting my attention. Nowadays, though, they tell me to cut out that counseling crap if they think I'm trying to manipulate them or something.

---

3. *Self-disclosure*: Sharing personal examples from your life to build trust, model personal effectiveness, or capitalize on identification processes.

   EXAMPLE:
   "I can recall the time in my life, at about your age, when I would see someone I liked. I finally swallowed hard and started taking risks. Although I felt rejected a lot, eventually I started meeting new people."

4. *Interpretation*: Promoting insight by pointing out the underlying meaning of a behavior or pattern.

   EXAMPLE:
   "So to compensate for the lack of attention you got from your father, you have constantly searched out relationships with men who are nurturing and dependent."

5. *Confrontation*: Diplomatically identifying discrepancies among (a) what a client has said in the past and is saying now, (b) what a client says versus what she or he does, and (c) what a client describes about herself or himself and what you actually observe.

   EXAMPLE:
   "Whereas you have repeatedly called yourself shy, withdrawn, boring, and a loser, I notice that in our sessions you are usually quite animated, outgoing, and assertive in getting what you want."

**Action Skills**    Most counselors rely on several action responses to move the client beyond self-understanding to constructive life changes:

1. *Information giving*: Providing concise, accurate, and factual information to dispel myths, pique client interest, or create structure.

   EXAMPLE:
   "One of the reasons why you may be having difficulty initiating sex with your girlfriend is that you are not beginning a series of pleasurable activities

called 'foreplay' that slowly lead to lovemaking. Instead, you just rip off your clothes and jump into bed.

2. *Advice giving*: Offering interventions designed to provide practical suggestions or motivate the client to action.

   EXAMPLE:
   "Perhaps the next time you go out on a job interview you might want to give more attention to your appearance and the impression you give."

3. *Goal setting*: Structuring a direction, planning for the future, providing a basis for measuring progress, and obtaining the client's commitment to make needed changes.

   EXAMPLE:
   "You are saying, then, that in the next week you would like to concentrate on being more open with your friends and that, on at least three occasions, you will tell people something that they don't already know about you."

4. *Reinforcement*: Giving support and encouragement to increase the likelihood that desirable behaviors will continue.

   EXAMPLE:
   "The more risks you take, the more courageous and confident you feel. After the great week you have had, I can hardly believe you are the same person."

5. *Directives*: Giving instructions designed to change the structural patterns of interaction or communication by specific means.

   EXAMPLE:
   "Since you aren't having much success by urging your husband to come in for counseling, I think it would be best if you tried a different approach and let him know you'd prefer he didn't come in."

The listening, exploration, and action skills just described will be covered in great depth throughout later courses. You have plenty of opportunity to practice the skills, at first with classmates, and later with clients. They form the foundation of what many counselors do in their sessions, regardless of their espoused beliefs and theories.

In addition to these behaviors that occur mostly in individual sessions, there are also skills that are part of counselors' other roles as negotiators (McRae, 1998), consultants (Parsons, 1996), group leaders (Johnson & Johnson, 2003), and family specialists (Carlson, Sperry, & Lewis, 2003). Other chapters and future courses will prepare you for these varied tasks, even though the bread and butter of what you will do in most settings and situations is to rely on basic listening, exploration, and action strategies within the context of your own preferred theoretical framework.

## VOICE FROM THE FIELD

Goal setting is a dynamite skill. And so easy to learn and apply in many situations. When I first learned it, it was from a behaviorist guy who was just in love with defining, specifying, and measuring things. He taught us this mnemonic device, SPAMMO, in which each letter stands for a different criterion of effectively set goals. So good goals should be specific, pertinent, attainable, mutual, and, of course, measurable, and observable. He just loved that part. Ever since I learned this years ago, I've tried to apply it to my own life. Clients just eat it up too, because they can see progressive steps they are taking toward their ultimate goals.

## SUMMARY

Theory is not the enemy. It should not constrict your freedom and movement. In the words of Leona Tyler, one of our profession's most eminent theoreticians, "If by theory one means a tightly organized set of postulates from which rigorous inferences can be drawn, I certainly do not have one. Furthermore, I do not even want one. . . . If by theory, however, one means simply the organized set of concepts by means of which one attempts to fit experience into a meaningful pattern, then I may call myself a theorist" (Tyler, 1970, pp. 298–299). To Tyler, theory is no more and no less than the search for personal meaning, the organization of ideas, and a way of thinking about a part of the world.

The preceding chapters on theory have given you a foundation to understand the variety of approaches to counseling. Study the concepts exposed to you in class and in books, to practice new skills you see demonstrated, and to learn the techniques described in the various theoretical orientations. But only after you have mastered, summarized, and mimicked these approaches should you then strive to personalize them.

## SELF-GUIDED EXPLORATIONS

1. You have been briefly exposed to a number of counseling theories such as the following:

| | |
|---|---|
| Client centered | Rational emotive |
| Behavioral | Psychoanalytic |
| Existential | Adlerian |
| Gestalt | Multimodal |
| Reality | Strategic |
| Narrative | Feminist |

You may already feel yourself gravitating toward some of these approaches, while eliminating others. Of the theories that are listed above, circle a few that you especially like and cross out a few that you have rejected. Talk to yourself about why you feel drawn to the choices you have circled. What is it about your personality, values, and experiences that has influenced your choices?

2. Critically evaluating, developing, integrating, and applying theories is crucial to the work of counseling practitioners, especially with regard to how people learn, grow, and change. Based on your limited experiences thus far, what is *your* theory to explain how you have made changes in your life?

3. Use the following self-assessment instrument to rate your current functioning in several areas:

RELATIONSHIP SKILLS RATING SCALE
(5) All of the time  (4) Most of the time  (3) Sometimes  (2) Rarely  (1) Never

SELF-AWARENESS

_____ I am in touch with my inner feelings.

_____ I am comfortable with myself.

_____ I am aware of my fears, anxieties, and unresolved conflicts.

SELF-DISCLOSURE

_____ I express my feelings honestly and clearly.

_____ I am concise and expressive in my communications.

_____ I am open in sharing what I think and feel.

ACTIVE LISTENING

_____ I can focus intently on what others are saying and recall the essence of their communications.

_____ I show attention and interest when I listen.

_____ I am able to resist internal and external distractions that may impede my concentration.

RESPONDING

_____ I am perceived by others as safe to talk to.

_____ I can demonstrate my understanding of what I hear.

_____ I reflect accurately other people's underlying thoughts and feelings.

INITIATING

_____ I have the ability to put people at ease.

_____ I am able to get people to open up.

_____ I am smooth and natural in facilitating the flow of conversation.

ATTITUDES

_____ I am nonjudgmental and accepting of other people, even when they have different values and opinions than I do.

_____ I am trustworthy and respectful of other people.

_____ I am caring and compassionate.

MANAGING CONFLICT

_____ I can confront people without them feeling defensive.

_____ I accept responsibility for my role in creating difficulties.

_____ I am able to defuse explosive situations.

Based on this honest self-inventory, as well as consultation with instructors and peers, what would you describe as your current strengths and weaknesses? Describe your plan for improving in areas that you wish to upgrade.

## For Homework:

Team up with two or three partners. Each of you take on the role of passionately arguing one of the theoretical positions presented in the chapter. Afterwards, discuss your respective opinions, supporting them with your own experience.

## SUGGESTED READINGS

Corey, G. (2000). *Theories of counseling and psychotherapy* (6th ed.). Pacific Grove, CA: Brooks/Cole.

Cormier, W. H., & Cormier, L. S. (2003). *Interviewing and change strategies for helpers* (5th ed.). Pacific Grove, CA: Brooks/Cole.

Egan, G. (2003). *The skilled helper* (7th ed.). Pacific Grove, CA: Brooks/Cole.

Erikson, E. (1950). *Childhood and society*. New York: Norton.

Evans, D. R., Hearn, M. T., Uhlemann, M. R., & Ivey, A. E. (1998). *Essential interviewing: A programmed approach to effective communication* (5th ed.). Pacific Grove, CA: Brooks/Cole.

Heaton, J. (1998). *Building basic therapeutic skills*. San Francisco: Jossey-Bass.

Kottler, J. A. (1991). *The complete therapist*. San Francisco: Jossey-Bass.

Mikulas, W. L. (2002). *The integrative helper: Convergence of Eastern and Western traditions*. Pacific Grove, CA: Brooks/Cole.

Okun, B. F. (2002). *Effective helping: Interviewing and counseling techniques* (6th ed.). Pacific Grove, CA: Brooks/Cole.

Preston, J. (1999). *Integrative brief therapy: Cognitive, psychodynamic, humanistic, and neurobehavioral approaches*. New York: Impact.

Prochaska, J. O., & Norcross, J. (2003). *Systems of psychotherapy: A transtheoretical approach* (5th ed.). Pacific Grove, CA: Brooks/Cole.

Young, M. E. (2001). *Learning the art of helping: Building blocks and techniques*. Upper Saddle River, NJ: Merrill.

# 8 CHAPTER

# ASSESSMENT, TESTING, AND THE DIAGNOSTIC PROCESS

## KEY CONCEPTS

Assessment process

Standardized measures

Nonstandardized measures

Test reliability

Test validity

Norms

Stanford-Binet

Wechsler scales

Aptitude tests

Achievement tests

Personality tests

Interest inventories

MMPI clinical scales

Projective tests

Test usability

Observational assessment

Self-assessment

Functional diagnosis

Medical model

Developmental model

Behavioral model

Phenomenological model

Systemic model

DSM-IV

# ASSESSMENT, TESTING, AND THE DIAGNOSTIC PROCESS

CHAPTER 8

Whether therapeutic counselors subscribe to insight-oriented theories, action-oriented approaches, or individually designed personal models, there is virtually universal endorsement of an assessment process in helping. This can take the form of an elaborate set of testing instruments and procedures, or it may simply involve an informal conversation about what is currently going on (and has occurred) in the client's life.

How, after all, could you ever expect to help someone if you don't have a clear idea about what exactly is going on? Assessment, testing, and the subsequent diagnostic process allow both client and counselor to proceed in an organized way. Imagine, for example, that a young woman tells you that she is feeling depressed and would like your assistance in regaining her composure. Before you could jump in and expect to be useful, a number of questions would come to mind.

- What does she mean by "depressed"? Depression to one person could mean incapacitating despondency; to another, it could mean simply a sad feeling.
- What else is going on in her life? What is the context for her present predicament? Was there a precipitant to this present episode? If so, what are the contributions of her family situation, developmental stages, social adjustment, and other relevant variables?
- What would it mean for her to regain her "composure"? What was she like before this current predicament? What is her usual state of functioning?

## VOICE FROM THE FIELD

There's always this moment of panic I feel when a new client walks in the door. Will I be able to help this person? Will I even know what the heck is going on? As I sit there trying to listen during the first few minutes, I feel such urgency to get a handle on the "problem." I know that as soon as this person walks out the door, I'm expected to fill out a treatment plan in which I specify the presenting complaints, the therapeutic goals, and the diagnosis. It strikes me as so stupid that I'm supposed to know all this after a single interview. No matter how much experience I gain and how much I practice doing intakes, I am still humbled by the complexity of each and every human being.

I know that whatever assessment I do—and whatever diagnosis I come up with—is just a starting point. As I get to know the person better, I will have a much better idea of what is going on. The hard part, though, is taking a deep breath and reminding myself to be patient.

- What are her expectations about what you can do for her? What would it take for her to feel as though counseling was successful?
- What has worked for her before when she has experienced similar symptoms? What sorts of interventions have proven to be most and least effective in the past?

This is just the merest sampling of the questions that might run through your mind as you first listen to her tell you about her struggle. Many others may also come to mind: Why she is seeking help now? What was she like before this problem began? What effects is the problem having on other aspects of her life? What benefits is she enjoying as a result of having this problem? What would be the consequences of solving the problem? Who else is invested in having her change in a particular direction? What is her support system like?

It is not that you are procrastinating when you hesitate to answer her query about how you will help her; it is just that you would be foolish to attempt any intervention without fully understanding what you are attempting to accomplish. It would be as if you went to see a doctor complaining of a stomachache and she immediately scheduled you for surgery without running appropriate tests to determine what might be wrong.

In whatever form it is structured—as paper-and-pencil tests, detailed background questionnaires, structured interviews, or lengthy conversations—an assessment process is crucial to accomplishing several important tasks:

- Familiarizing yourself with the client's world and characteristic functioning.
- Learning about past events and developmental issues that have been significant.
- Studying family history and the current living situation.
- Assessing the client's strengths and weaknesses with regard to intellectual, academic, emotional, interpersonal, moral, and behavioral functioning.

- Checking out risk factors related to substance abuse, suicide, or harm to others.
- Identifying presenting problems.
- Formulating a diagnostic impression.
- Developing a treatment plan to reach mutually agreed-on therapeutic goals.

With any situation in which you are faced with the prospect of doing something therapeutic, you must conduct a thorough investigation of the present situation, its current context, and its past history. Care must be taken not to jump to conclusions with too little information because we often have a tendency to seek data that support our preexisting notions about clients (Stevens & Morris, 1995). And most important, you must follow the usual standards of care for someone who may be acutely suicidal or dangerous to others (Bongar, 2002).

## WHAT IS ASSESSMENT?

Assessment is a multifaceted process that involves a variety of functions, such as testing and evaluation, in an effort to determine an individual's characteristics, aptitudes, achievements, and personal qualities. Assessment can be viewed as an integrative process that combines a variety of information into a meaningful pattern reflecting relevant aspects of an individual. It never depends on a single measure, nor does it emphasize one dimension at the expense of another. For an assessment profile to be meaningful and useful, it must provide a means of understanding the individual from as broad and integrative a perspective as possible.

Only with the most accurate information can an assessment be appropriately used in counseling. Consider the challenge, for example, of evaluating a candidate's suitability for entrance into a counselor training program. Let's say we are looking for people who have shown a degree of academic success in the past, who are reasonably intelligent, who write and speak well, and who have high motivation to help people. Furthermore, we might be looking for those who present themselves well in human interactions and who are perceived as likeable and compassionate. We also wish to search for people of high moral character, who take feedback well, and who are inclined to be both introspective and analytic about others' behavior. Finally, we want people who are reasonably healthy emotionally, who will not harm others because of their own unresolved issues that may get in the way.

We are also faced with some practical concerns. We have limited time and resources to screen a number of applicants. In an ideal world, we could spend weeks investigating each of several hundred applicants; in actuality, we need a shortcut method that might at least give us rough indications of predicting success in our program and in a career as a counselor.

We might wish to include a standardized test score—a measure of past academic performance—in our assessment process. With this score, we might weigh those aspects that seem most relevant to our purposes—say, verbal over

## VOICE FROM THE FIELD

When I first started using assessments with children in the school system, I was very rigid and focused a lot of energy on making sure that I administered tests exactly as per the standardized protocol. I looked exclusively at the numbers and the standard deviations of the child's scores and paid little attention to other important aspects of test administration such as rapport, motivation, attention level, and other stuff. But, after I became more experienced in using tests, I began to understand the merit of observation during the assessment process. I began to document in my reports more information regarding how the children responded, their affect, their general demeanor, and their level of interest. I found that these bits and pieces of information were as important as simply looking at the numbers.

I also found that using more than just one instrument helped immensely in painting a more vivid portrait of who the person really is. I believe fully that for this very reason, many agencies and schools rely on a battery of tests and assessments rather than just a single instrument to gain a clearer understanding of the client's personality, achievement, aptitude, strengths and weaknesses, and overall functioning. I also believe that the assessment process in itself can be therapeutic as well, because the clients learn so much about themselves. This new information gives clients an additional mirror to reflect on and evaluate themselves.

---

quantitative ability. We would probably wish to review past experiences most similar to the present challenges, that is, performance in school and previous jobs. Recommendations from knowledgeable observers, certainly previous supervisors, would be helpful in this regard. We would wish to see a writing sample, perhaps one that discusses personal and professional goals. Finally, if all these data seem to fit with what we are looking for, a structured interview would provide additional information that might be useful.

Each of these segments would provide information from which to construct an integrated portrait. Assessment thus attempts to build a comprehensive composite of an individual's characteristics, qualities, or aptitudes from as broad a vantage point as possible, sampling several pertinent sources of information.

Conducting an assessment requires that a wide range of information be gathered to illuminate as many relevant aspects of the person as possible. Information sources can be divided into two general categories. *Standardized measures* include tests that have been designed to ensure uniformity of administration and scoring and for which norms are generally available. *Nonstandardized measures,* which do not ensure uniformity of measurement and tend to be subjective, take a more general and diverse approach to gathering information.

## THE ROLE OF TESTING IN THE ASSESSMENT PROCESS

Although it certainly is not the only way to collect useful information and assess client functioning, testing is one of the most common methods that coun-

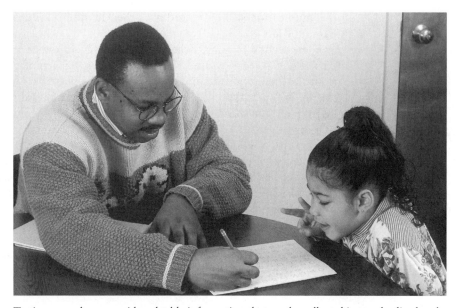

Testing procedures provide valuable information that can be collected in standardized and consistent ways so that results may be compared to others' performance. Skilled counselors pay attention not only to the objective results but also to the very human process involved. © Laura Dwight/PhotoEdit.

selors employ. The history of our profession is very much interwoven with the parallel evolution of the testing movement.

At the beginning of the twentieth century, James Cattell, one of the first experimental psychologists, coined the term *mental test* to describe his attempts to measure the intellectual ability of students. Building on the work of Sir Francis Galton and his development of rating scales, questionnaires, and statistical methods, Cattell began the science and industry of testing, along with researchers in Europe—Kraepelin, who made assessments of the mentally ill, and Alfred Binet, whose scales measured children's mental abilities. Although Binet's intelligence tests for screening schoolchildren were the first widely accepted tests, it was the development of group intelligence testing during World War I that gave real impetus to psychological and educational testing as we know it today. The U.S. Army Alpha and Beta were the first group intelligence tests used to screen those who might be unfit to serve. Army psychologists also worked to develop group personality tests to screen recruits for potential problems.

The army's experience with group intelligence and personality testing provided the basis for a significant expansion of the assessment process in the 1920s. Between 1920 and 1940, many other tests were developed to measure a wide range of characteristics, including intelligence, aptitude, ability, attitude, personality, and interests. The number of tests expanded to the point at which a catalog of instruments was needed just to familiarize the practitioner with all the options that were available. Originally published by Oskar Buros, this publication still exists today as the *Mental Measurements Yearbook* (Impara, 2001).

The second major acceleration in the development and use of testing occurred in the years around World War II for many of the same reasons mentioned earlier—to find more efficient ways to screen personnel and to use their talents in optimal ways. Tests such as the Wechsler Adult Intelligence Scale (WAIS) and the Minnesota Multiphasic Personality Inventory (MMPI-2) were first developed and extensively used during this time.

In spite of whatever advantages testing might offer, it has come under increased criticism, primarily because of concerns that the instruments are culturally and ethnically biased, reflecting the values of the majority culture to the disadvantage of others who are exposed to a different set of educational experiences growing up. These problems have led to a number of restrictions on the use of tests and to some professionals' disenchantment with them. In spite of these concerns, recently there has been an increased use of testing for a variety of purposes because of its economical way of helping decision makers predict future behavior (Watkins, 1994).

## Technology and Assessment

Computers have greatly simplified the general process of assessment, as well as test development, scoring, and interpretation. Counselors now routinely use the Internet, specialized diagnostic software packages, videoconferencing, and web-based sites to conduct their client assessments and to consult with various sources during this procedure (Hohenshil, 2000). Counselor-generated reports will play a significantly more important role in the future, not so much as a substitute for your own clinical judgment but rather as an aid to help you make sense of client experiences and plan effective treatments (Butcher, Perry, & Atlis, 2000).

These recent developments and innovations certainly enhance our ability to select appropriate instruments, score and interpret them, and to make sense of the data, but also at some cost. Concerns continue to be raised about compromised privacy and confidentiality (Garb, 2000; Sampson, 2000). How safe do you feel, for example, that any government agency—or even a meddling computer hack—can access the most personal data about your life without you even knowing about the invasion of privacy?

## Why Study Testing?

Perhaps a useful way to begin a study of testing and assessment is to explore why it is important in the first place. The process of counseling involves decision making at many levels to help the client resolve concerns, effect change, and plan for contingencies and opportunities. For decision making to be maximally effective, it must be based on self-understanding, awareness of various options and alternatives, and a fund of relevant information. We have already examined a number of widely accepted techniques used in therapeutic counseling to provide information for decision making.

Verbal and nonverbal techniques, in particular, have been presented as basic counselor-offered conditions that facilitate counseling and help the client integrate a variety of information about self and relevant counseling issues. Testing, as part of an appraisal process, is an additional source of useful information about clients that can affect the decision-making process. In fact, tests offer a type of information not readily available through nontest methods: They gather information that highlights the ways in which clients are alike and different. The results of a test or series of tests can provide clients with information about themselves and illustrate how they compare with others who are similar to them. This information can help clients understand themselves and can be an asset in exploring alternatives during decision making.

The information provided by testing is not always consistent; therefore, the counselor must be skilled in appraisal technology so that discrepancies in test data can be resolved in an exploration of the information. To help clients have the broadest possible source of information about self, the counselor must be knowledgeable about the selection, use, and interpretation of tests. To be uninformed about testing and assessment is to arbitrarily delete a potentially valuable source of data that could improve the quality of decisions about change of lifestyle, work, or behavior patterns. It is fascinating, if not downright useful, to know how well we perform in a particular area when compared to others who have attempted the same task.

Your clients may have experienced some type of trauma as a result of test abuse. Without the ability to make sense of the raw data to judge the suitability of the particular test, you will never be able to challenge its appropriateness in a given situation. Thus, even if you were never going to administer tests yourself (a highly unlikely situation), you must be familiar with norms, reliability, validity, clinical versus statistical significance, and other relevant concepts so that you can help your clients make sense of their own testing experiences. This knowledge is not only crucial to collecting meaningful information from the client but also helpful in formulating a plan with which to begin therapeutic efforts.

## STANDARDIZED MEASURES

A test is nothing more or less mysterious than an attempt to measure a sample of behavior objectively and consistently. Whether the issue is a client's career preferences, mathematical skill, verbal reasoning ability, personality characteristics, or potential for success, tests are a convenient basis for judging the strength, utility, or desirability of various human qualities.

Tests are used to match the most capable and well-suited individuals with a particular program, position, or job. They have value as predictive devices for hypothesizing about a person's future performance or action. And certainly tests help counselors in their overwhelming task of understanding clients—their characteristic behavior patterns; their strengths, deficiencies, values, aptitudes, and mastered skills; and, most important, their potential and capacity for growth.

For a test to be useful, it must be a *reliable* and *valid* measure of behavior. *Reliability* refers to the consistency or accuracy of a test score, whereas *validity* refers to the extent to which tests actually measure what they purport. Although no test is perfectly reliable or absolutely valid, any assessment instrument or methodology that a counselor uses must meet these criteria for the specific group and context in which it is employed. One other consideration is that certain personality and intelligence tests may only be administered and interpreted by professionals who hold particular licenses in that discipline.

Despite being scientifically designed to be fair, objective, reliable, and appropriate, testing procedures have many problems. In an effort to sensitize counselors to these issues, Prediger (1993) has developed a set of multicultural assessment standards that can be used to evaluate testing materials from a multicultural perspective. Wagner (1987), in his review of the Standards for Educational and Psychological Testing, encourages counselors "to go beyond traditional roles in testing and advisement and to consider client backgrounds in terms of age, sex, and ethnicity in determining the appropriateness of tests and the interpretation of results" (p. 203).

There are several other criticisms and cautionary factors involved in testing procedures:

1. Tests create classificatory categories that are potentially harmful to clients. Application of labels such as "retarded," "mentally ill," "underachieving," and "passive-dependent" often follows test interpretations. And even though sticks and stones will break your bones, names will also hurt you.

2. Test construction is an imperfect science leading to results not necessarily accurate or useful. Test validity and reliability statistics are not impressive. For instance, when a mother brags that her son has an IQ of 116, she is certainly exaggerating appropriate levels of confidence in that magical number. To be honest, she would actually have to state the result in a considerably more cautious way: "There is a 68.4 percent probability that my son's real IQ falls somewhere between 112 and 120."

3. Charges of sexual and racial bias have been directed against many standardized instruments because the questions and norming procedures reflect the language and customs of the white middle-class majority.

4. Testing is often used as an excuse to guide clients in specific directions, often limiting their future vision and potential. A fifth grader who shows early promise as a math wizard may never have the opportunity to develop latent artistic and writing talents.

5. Tests often reveal hidden and disguised information (one of their functions) and therefore may be construed as an invasion of privacy. They reveal aspects of the self that a client may not wish others to know.

Their limitations and ethical problems notwithstanding, standardized tests have several useful functions that cannot be duplicated by alternative assessment strategies, such as the clinical interview and other nonstandardized procedures. First, the fact that tests are standardized means that attempts are made to ensure uniformity of administration and evaluation for all clients. No matter where the test is being administered, at what time, by whom, or to whom, subjective factors will tend to be minimized. Therefore, it is very important that counselors are trained in the use of these standardized tests before actually administering them. Credentials such as licenses to provide counseling services do not necessarily ensure competence in administering these tests. The concept of standardization also refers to the common practice of providing "norms," or measures of normal performance, so that any individual's sample behavior may be compared with that of a large group of others.

Standardized assessment procedures provide a database for making predictions about a client's future behavior. In making clinical judgments about whether a client is a likely candidate for suicide, a good prospect for a particular job opening, or a potentially responsive client for counseling, the interpretation of results from tests is invaluable. Tests can also be used to evaluate the effects of various counseling methods to determine whether supplemental interventions are necessary. They are often used as selection and classification tools as well, helping in the complex process of matching the right jobs with the best people. Finally, tests are simply an additional source of information for clinicians, a concise summary of the client's typical behavior.

Whether administered in groups for the sake of efficiency and economy or given individually, tests come in every conceivable size, shape, and purpose. There are instruments for measuring ability, aptitude, achievement, personality, and interests. Other tests can be used for assessing relationship conflict, marital satisfactions, and a host of other areas in human behavior.

## Tests of Ability

Defining intelligence has been a difficult task, surrounded by controversy and strong debate. Although the dialogue is likely to continue for some time among experts, it is now generally agreed that intelligence consists of several factors: (1) abstract thinking, (2) problem solving, (3) capacity to acquire knowledge, (4) adjustment to new situations, and (5) sustaining of abilities in order to achieve desired goals.

In spite of the difficulty in defining intelligence, a number of instruments attempt to assess an individual's general mental ability or stable intellectual capacity to reason and apply knowledge. Tests that attempt to measure intelligence are most likely to reflect a person's scholastic/academic learning potential, especially with conceptually difficult or abstract material. Most of these tests also include a set of tasks that require a client to demonstrate memory, pattern recognition, decision making, verbal and analytic skills, general knowledge, and the ability to manipulate the environment.

Two of the most popular intelligence tests are the Stanford-Binet, which is considered to be the most accurate measure of verbal intelligence, and the Wechsler scales, which include specific instruments designed for adults (Wechsler Adult Intelligence Scale), children (Wechsler Intelligence Scale for Children), and preschoolers (Wechsler Preschool and Primary Scale of Intelligence). Both the Wechsler Scales and the Stanford-Binet are examples of individually administered intelligence tests that attempt to measure IQ (intelligence quotient) as a general underlying composite of intelligence, often with an emphasis

## VOICE FROM THE FIELD

As an educational diagnostician for a smaller community college, I have tested many college students for learning disabilities. I enjoy testing a great deal and find that the real challenge in assessing intelligence is not how to administer the Wechsler or the Stanford-Binet but what we actually do with the results of such testing. Understanding how each subscale score affects clients in their daily life and how to help them overcome their weaknesses and build on their strengths is the true key in testing of this nature.

I've also learned that discussing the results with the client at follow-up is a very sensitive issue and many times the client is very apprehensive and anxious to find out their results, especially when there are significant weakness areas. It's hard to present the results in such a way that the client doesn't leave discouraged or feeling like a failure.

---

on verbal and nonverbal problem solving. Administering these tests requires special training and often a state license as a psychologist or other mental health professional.

There are also group ability tests, such as the Otis-Lennon Scholastic Ability Test, that tend to measure intelligence as scholastic aptitude and are more dependent on previous learning experiences. These group tests, however, do not have the same administrative requirements as the individual tests and are often used in educational settings.

## Tests of Aptitude

Aptitude tests are concerned primarily with prediction of a person's performance in the future. All of us have, at one time or another, run the gauntlet of tests to determine whether we are good candidates for an available slot. It is likely that you have had experience with the Scholastic Aptitude Test (SAT) or the American College Test (ACT) for admission to college or the Graduate Record Exam (GRE) for entrance to a graduate program. You may also have some rather strong opinions about the validity of these instruments for predicting academic success.

The Law School Admission Test (LSAT) is another example of a test used to predict success in programs of advanced study. At the level of state employment agencies, aptitude tests such as the General Aptitude Test Battery (GATB) are used for job placement, and school systems rely on instruments such as the Differential Aptitude Test (DAT) for assessing academic aptitude and educational placement of children.

## Tests of Achievement

Often called proficiency tests, achievement tests are used to measure learning, acquired capabilities, or developed skills. They are widely used and can be adapted to almost any type of task from measuring course content (a typical exam) to administering the road test for a driver's license. Results can be used as diagnostic tools, as demonstrators of accountability, and, because past performance is the best measure of future performance, as predictors. Commonly used tests in this category are the California Achievement Test and the Metropolitan Achievement Test.

## Tests of Typical Performance

Tests designed to measure an individual's day-to-day behavior or performance are interested not in what a person can do (ability) but in what a person does. Although motivation is important in this type of test, it is less so than in ability testing. Two common categories of typical performance testing are personality inventories and interest inventories.

**Personality Inventories**   These tests are designed to gather information on an individual's preferences, attitudes, personality patterns, or problems. Results are expressed by comparison with a specific reference group. A concern with personality inventories is the possibility of faking responses, but most instruments of this type have a "lie scale" to detect a tendency to present an overly favorable profile. Examples of personality inventories include the Edwards Personal Preference Schedule (EPPS), the Personal Orientation Inventory (POI), and the Minnesota Multiphasic Personality Inventory (MMPI-II) (See Table 8.1).

Another type of personality measure is the projective type, which does not use a pencil-and-paper format but is individually administered (usually by a psychologist). This type of test requires a client to respond to unstructured stimuli such as an inkblot or an incomplete sentence. A qualified examiner then interprets these responses as reflective of underlying personality organization and structure. Examples include the Rorschach and the Thematic Apperception Test (TAT).

**Interest Inventories**   Interest inventories attempt to develop a profile of an individual's career interest areas through a series of questions about preferences, jobs, hobbies, and other activities. The pattern of responses is then compared to the responses of persons successfully engaged in a variety of occupational areas. Profiles are constructed by matching high and low scores in occupational clusters. A limitation of these inventories is that, because interest does not reflect ability, it is possible for a person to dislike a career area in which he or she has earned a high score. Commonly used interest inventories are the Strong-Campbell Interest Inventory and the Kuder Preference Record.

## Selecting Tests

One of a counselor's important responsibilities is to select tests from myriad choices. The selection of a test is complex because a number of competing factors must be analyzed and evaluated. Among the resources frequently

TABLE 8.1 | MMPI-II SCALES AND SIMULATED ITEMS

Unless you are a licensed psychologist, in most states you will probably not be administering and interpreting MMPI tests. Nevertheless, because this instrument is so widely used, you should have some working knowledge of the various clinical scales:

1 or Hs (Hypochondriasis) Items derived from patients showing abnormal concern with bodily functions such as reporting chest pain several times per week.

2 or D (Depression) Items derived from patients showing extreme pessimism, feelings of hopelessness, and slowing of thought and action.

3 or Hy (Conversion Hysteria) Items from neurotic patients using physical or mental symptoms as a way of unconsciously avoiding difficult conflicts and responsibilities.

4 or Pd (Psychopathic Deviate) Items from patients who show a repeated and flagrant disregard for social customs, an emotional shallowness, and an inability to learn from punishing experiences.

5 or Mf (Masculinity-Femininity) Items that distinguish gender differences.

6 or Pa (Paranoia) Items showing abnormal suspiciousness and delusions of grandeur or persecution.

7 or Pt (Psychasthenia) Items based on neurotic patients showing obsessions, compulsions, abnormal fears, and guilt and indecisiveness.

8 or Sc (Schizophrenia) Items from patients showing bizarre or unusual thoughts or behavior, who are often withdrawn and experiencing delusions and hallucinations.

9 or Ma (Hypomania) Items from patients characterized by emotional excitement, overactivity, and flight of ideas.

0 or Si (Social introversion) Items from persons showing little interest in people and insecurity in social situations.

consulted in the effort to evaluate and select tests, here are four important ones:

1. Buros' *Mental Measurements Yearbook* (Impara, 2001) contains reviews of major tests by experts in the field who evaluate them critically, emphasizing shortcomings and strengths. It is a reasonably objective source of information about tests and should be consulted in the process of making selections.

2. Test manuals accompanying published tests compile relevant data on the theoretical base, development, standardization, validity, reliability, and other technical features. This information can assist the potential test user to evaluate a test's suitability for a target population.

3. Test reviews often appear in professional journals and on Web sites, which also publish articles reporting technical data.

4. Tests should be evaluated to determine their compliance with the multicultural assessment standards.

## VOICE FROM THE FIELD

I know a lot about teenagers. Having been a high school teacher in the past, I have seen the best of times and the worst of times in kids. But as a vocational counselor for the past three years, I find my new role in the lives of these kids to be very exciting. I am able to help them through certain aspects of their identity confusion by helping them to find a sense of direction for their future careers.

I find that using interest inventories with them such as the Strong-Campbell or Holland's Self-Directed Search can be a really valuable and enlightening experience for them. Some of them seemed reluctant to sit down and go through all the questions on these inventories. However, once they'd been scored, most of the students are very glad for

such an experience and seem to have a fresh sense of direction.

You shouldn't place too much emphasis on the results of interest inventories but should simply use them as a tool to empower the student with another piece of information about who they are. I have also seen many families drawn closer together from such a testing experience since many of these students take their results home and discuss them with their moms and dads. Sometimes their parents become more involved in their lives as they realize that their children are starting to become adults and are in need of support to make the next transition from school to work or college.

---

Each of these sources can provide useful information to the counselor, who must then relate these data to the characteristics of the population to be tested. Ideally there should be a high degree of correspondence among the test objectives, the standardization sample, and the population to be served. In collecting test evaluation data, the counselor should consider a number of factors:

1. *Validity,* the most important single factor in test selection, refers to the extent to which the test measures what it claims to measure. Evidence supporting validity claims of tests must be carefully analyzed to determine whether the test is appropriate for the ways in which it will be used.
2. *Reliability* refers to the consistency of scores and freedom from error of measurement. Evidence supporting reliability should be carefully evaluated for relevance to the target population.
3. *Usability* takes in factors such as convenience, cost, and ease of interpretation, which need to be carefully considered, along with such things as reading level, suitability of content, design of the booklet, ease of administration, scoring procedures, examiners' qualifications and required training, and reviewers' comments.

When selecting tests, remember that no one test will be ideal for a given task; there are always trade-offs. It is the counselor's responsibility to select tests that have the highest possible relevance for the purposes at hand, recognizing their limitations and imperfections.

# NONSTANDARDIZED MEASURES

Nonstandard assessment tools are widely used to gather information about clients. They represent a "nontest" approach and are especially useful in gathering data that do not lend themselves to numerical reduction. Combining the results of standardized and nonstandardized measures often creates an optimal base for developing a truly multifaceted assessment process. Some of the more common types of nonstandardized measures are discussed here.

## Observational Assessment

Observational measures are commonly used to gather information that is often unavailable through other means. Observational procedures can be classified in a number of different ways, according to type (systematic, controlled, or informal), setting in which they take place (natural or contrived), or methods used (interview, direct observation). For example, one direct and systematic means of observation in a natural setting might involve counting the number of times a client averts his or her eyes whenever an emotional topic is introduced in counseling. Another more contrived and controlled method of observation would be to use a standardized interview technique to ask a series of questions and note responses.

The interview is the most commonly used observational technique in counseling; however, other methods are also used. Anecdotal data, for example, often form the basis for progress notes, and role-playing structures might be seen as situational tests. Observational methods, however, lack the normative data available from well-defined populations, a characteristic of standardized assessment tools, and are therefore more susceptible to biases. They have also been criticized because subjects can change their behavior if they know they are being observed, and the relatively limited range of situations available for observation may not produce an adequate sample of behavior.

Nevertheless, among all the assessment tools available, you will be using your eyes, your ears, your intuition, and all your senses to observe carefully what your clients are experiencing and communicating. You will attempt to decode these cues and make sense of their behavior. And you will coordinate these observations with other data at your disposal.

## Rating Scales

Rating systems provide a common basis for collecting certain types of observational data. They differ from observation in that observation is only the recording of behavior, whereas rating involves both recording behavior and simultaneously making an evaluation of specified characteristics, which are usually tabulated on a scale. The value of ratings depends primarily on the care taken in the development of the rating form and the appropriateness with which it is employed.

When doing a simple observation you note that a client appears anxious. You make this assessment based on several nonverbal cues—a repetitious

## VOICE FROM THE FIELD

The thing I have learned to rely on most during difficult or confusing times with clients is my own intuition about the situation. What does my heart tell me? I listen to my head as well, of course, but it is in my heart that I often find answers—or at least clues—that elude me when I am solely in a thinking mode. I analyze what is going on. I use logic and systematic reviews to try and unravel what is happening, especially with a very challenging, difficult case. Yet when this strategy fails me, or comes up short, I try to listen carefully to whispers inside me.

In order to access the intuitive part of me, I try to disengage as much as I can at the time from what is going on. The client might just see me as quiet and reserved but what I am tapping inside are the hunches, the wonderings, the most subtle guesses about what I sense and what I feel. I am not always right; I may not even be on target most of the time. But I find that approaching a case or situation like this often frees me up to see and hear things that I might ordinarily miss.

tapping of the foot, averted glance, and wringing hands. You check out your assumption by reflecting the feeling you observe: "You are feeling anxious because you aren't sure where to go next." If you attempted to actually measure the degree of anxiety that is experienced, you could ask the person to rate on a 1 to 10 scale just how nervous he really is. Such rating scales, whether administered in verbal or written form, are often useful in getting a more accurate assessment of not only what someone is feeling or thinking, but to what degree.

## Self-Assessment

Self-assessment is a valuable nonstandardized assessment tool that is often underused in appraisal programs. Self-assessment reinforces self-determination and recognizes that the individual is truly the expert on himself or herself. It further enhances the participatory aspect of assessment. Person-centered approaches to assessment particularly emphasize the importance of the client's self-authority in identifying and using assessment information. Portfolios are often used as supporting documentation in which a number of items—including journal entries, videotapes, photographs, and drawings—are included.

There is actually a parallel process involved in assessing the self. Just as you would ask your clients to check out how they are doing, what they are feeling and thinking, and then reflecting on these self-observations, you would be doing the same thing. This becomes the source of your intuition that develops from experience but also your way of monitoring how you are doing at each stage of the process. How are you reacting to this person at this moment in time? What is being triggered inside you by this interaction? Who does this person remind you of? What fantasies are elicited as a result of what is going on? What is your felt sense about what this means? A host of such questions are often reviewed as part of your supervision, but also as an ongoing part of your work during sessions.

# USING ASSESSMENT METHODS IN COUNSELING

Ideally, in conducting an assessment, a counselor would choose options among both standardized and nonstandardized measures to ensure the broadest possible base of information on which to plan intervention techniques. Although developing a comprehensive base for each client assessment is not always possible, counselors should strive for the fullest range of information and acknowledge the limitations of over-relying on any single measure.

## Test Interpretation

A prerequisite of effective interpretation of tests and other assessment results is a thorough understanding of their technical aspects, including limitations of the assessment data. Further, the ability to integrate information into meaningful patterns, as in the case-study method, is a crucial skill. Undergirding these skills, however, is the necessity of applying counseling methods in both individual and group interpretations. Computer technology is helpful as an aid to the counselor in the process, but it is unlikely to replace the need for trained counselors to work in face-to-face situations with clients exploring assessment results.

The interpretation of assessment data should fully engage the client in thinking about the implications of the assessment results for his or her own problem solving and self-awareness. Clients should not have interpretations done to them but must be directly involved in the process. The following factors should be considered in interpreting test results to clients (Miller, 1982; Tinsley & Bradley, 1986):

1. Engage the client in a discussion of feelings about the test experience.
2. Review the purpose of the testing procedures and discuss how the results will be presented. Ensure that the client understands concepts such as norms, percentiles, stanines, ranks, and other relevant measures, including the use of profiles.
3. Present the test scores and examine the actual test. Discuss what the scores actually mean to the client.
4. Integrate the test results with the client's other self-knowledge, helping the client to see the relationship between the scores and the self.
5. Assist the client to develop a plan for operationalizing the results of the testing experience, using the test scores and other self-knowledge.

## Summary of Assessment Principles

1. Never use an assessment device without having a specific purpose and use for the results.

## VOICE FROM THE FIELD

I think of testing as a kind of consultation—just a way to check out my own hunches and impressions. For instance, if I'm seeing a new client who strikes me as unusually manipulative and gamey, I might use an MMPI—not even so much for the clinical scales as just to see how the person comes out on the "lie scales." Or with a client who seems confused and inarticulate about career preferences, I might use a career inventory to help pin things down. In any of these cases, I use testing as just another source of information to combine with what I already know—or think I know.

One of my favorites is to ask clients to draw themselves with their families. That can say a real lot about relationships and self-image and even give information about alignments in the family. It provides a wonderful stimulus for things to talk about, too.

2. The results belong to the test taker, who has a right to have them explained in understandable terms.
3. The test user is responsible for preparing clients to take the test under optimal conditions (pretest orientation).
4. No set of numerical test results captures the essence of a human being.
   a. It's possible and desirable to describe things nonnumerically.
   b. Numbers have no meaning in themselves; only people experience meaning. Thus there is no such thing as objectivity.
   c. Numbers as labels imply static beings. Humans are dynamic.
5. Things that can be measured precisely tend to be relatively unimportant.
6. Assessment must be carried out with techniques that
   a. Are suitable for the test taker.
   b. Are of high validity and reliability.
   c. Engage the participation of the assessed person as much as possible.
   d. Are supported by multiple observations.
7. Interpretation should focus on strengths, on possibilities, and on remedies. Healthy optimism is a key to helpful interpretation.

## Critical Application of Assessment Principles: Recognizing and Reporting Child Abuse

If there is one clear area that demonstrates the need for reliable, consistent, and appropriate assessment procedures, it is in protecting the welfare of children. Regardless of your professional affiliation, state of residence, or clinical setting, almost all licensing jurisdictions require practitioners to report suspected child abuse or neglect. This awesome mantle of responsibility does not solely fall on your shoulders as many other professionals are also required to report such suspicions including medical personnel, child care workers, teachers, clergy, even animal control officers and film developers. Nevertheless, you are almost certainly going to face situations in which you will have to assess the possibility of abuse. I mention this critical application of assessment skills not only because it is so important to protect children against harm, but also because it represents a fairly uniform and consistent procedure.

Basically, if you have any reasonable suspicion that a child has been (or is currently being) harmed physically, emotionally, or sexually, you *must* report this to authorities. Failure to do so not only continues to put the child in harm's way but also subjects you to possible prosecution for failing to do your duty. You are not, by the way, held responsible for being absolutely correct in your assessment of the situation; merely, that you have some reasonable evidence that abuse *may* be taking place.

So, how do you know that child abuse may be going on? You don't. You can only make your best professional judgment based on the evidence that you have examined. It is then up to the authorities (child protective services and law enforcement) to investigate and make a determination. Nevertheless, this assessment challenge is a very good example of how you apply your clinical skills, knowledge about laws and standards of care, and training in recognizing possible symptoms.

What would you look for as evidence of possible neglect or abuse? First, look for emotional signs such as sadness, guilt, fear, irritability, anger, lowered self-esteem, hopelessness, and a feeling of being "damaged goods." Of course, presentation of these symptoms alone could mean a whole host of possible underlying causes other than abuse. It is when they are seen in conjunction with other factors, that child abuse may be suspected. These factors could include both physical (bruises, chipped teeth, burn marks, broken bones, ligatures) and behavioral (inappropriate sexualized behavior, phobic reactions, regression, detachment) factors (Faller, 1993).

## Applications of Assessment Principles to Other Clients-at-Risk

While I used the assessment of child abuse as one example, there are several other areas that you will also be expected to identify accurately. These areas include recognizing that a client is a suicidal risk or may be likely to harm someone else. Within the landscape of contemporary schools, you may also be required to assess potential threats and inclinations toward violence, which means being able to determine if someone is likely to engage in violent behavior toward others by assessing the person's motivation, previous patterns, mental condition, developed plan, and context (Daniels, 2002). Keep in mind that in spite of our latest technology, advances in training, and best intentions, we aren't all that great at predicting when someone is going to do harm to themselves or others. It is better to be safe than sorry, and to seek consultation with a supervisor whenever you are in doubt.

Within a remarkably brief period of time, you may be called on to form a judgment about whether a client is at risk for some form of harm. Applying a decision pathway model to assessing domestic violence, Miller, Veltkamp, Lane, Bilyeu, and Elzie (2002) provide a framework that is useful in making other sorts of clinical decisions that involve clients at risk.

1. The first step is always that you see some sign or symptom of abuse, whether that is physical evidence (bruises, lacerations), anecdotal evidence, or emotional effects.
2. Next, you screen for a history of abuse by reviewing the situation with the client and the family, as well as informing the client of reporting requirements in your jurisdiction.
3. Next, you *must* comply with all reporting laws and requirements by contacting the appropriate agency.
4. Assess safety considerations of your client, and any others who might be at risk.
5. Make appropriate referrals for medical evaluation and care if needed.
6. Provide support and counseling as needed to focus on the incidents and the consequences of the abuse. Bring in other family members as needed.

You can see clearly that while assessment is a general process of checking out what is going on with your clients, and what they need most, it is also a procedure that can be applied to a number of clinical situations. This is especially the case with people who are at-risk to harm themselves, harm others, or suffer the effects of others' violence or abuse.

# FORMAL AND FUNCTIONAL DIAGNOSIS

A new female client enters the office, furtively glances around for a place to sit, briefly locks eyes with the counselor, and finally, with an inward sigh, burrows deeply into the couch. The mutual assessment process has already begun. While she nervously checks out the furniture, books, and framed diplomas and wonders what sort of image she is projecting, the counselor casually yet systematically makes careful observations. The client's dress, posture, and bearing are noted, as well as where and how she has chosen to sit. Facial expressions, gestures, body language, and other nonverbal behavior also give valuable cues regarding her style.

The interview progresses. Information about the presenting complaint, the solutions that have already been tried, and the current life situation is gathered. The counselor is searching for a summary statement of her problem, a formal diagnosis to describe the general pattern of behavior, and a behavioral label to describe meaningfully and individually what the client is doing, feeling, and thinking. Making these distinctions is important. In the assessment process, diagnoses are significant because they have implications for selecting a treatment strategy and because they are often required by the system. For example, the diagnosis of "cyclothymic disorder" might imply a condition involving dramatic mood swings that have been chronic throughout the client's life and may be bio-chemically triggered, thus suggesting the importance of medical consultations on the case. The diagnosis, however, gives us very little meaningful information about what the client is like as a person. Although useful in the general under-standing of a behavioral syndrome, in formulating goals, predictions, and prog-noses for the case, and in creating a few working hypotheses for designing a treatment strategy, a diagnosis alone is not enough for beginning treatment (Seligman, 1998).

There are many diagnostic decisions that counselors must continuously make, revising them as they gather more information. Imagine, for example, that a severely depressed teenager enters your office. Dozens of diagnostic questions will likely flash through your mind:

- Is he a good candidate for counseling?
- Is he most suitable for individual, group, or family treatment?
- Which counseling interventions are likely to be most helpful?
- Is medication indicated in this situation? Should I ask for a psychiatric consultation?
- Is he actively suicidal?

During an assessment process such as this, there rarely is a single correct diagnosis that accurately summarizes what is happening for a client. That is one reason why you should not rush to judgment but take your time weighing all the complex factors involved (Hill & Ridley, 2001). The question, more appropriately, should not be whether your diagnostic impression is correct but whether it is useful. "A useful diagnosis is one that offers us a treatment plan that is (1) easy, (2) efficient, and (3) effective" (Weltner, 1988, p. 54). By this Weltner means that, when assessing where clients are, what their problems are, and what is causing them, it is important to be pragmatic and flexible. Be-cause there is probably no single correct diagnosis of a situation, Weltner be-lieves, the best counselors can do is generate as many definitions as possible. For each one you can then develop a different treatment plan, systematically trying them all until you get desired results.

For example, suppose you are called on to help a 9-year-old girl who is re-ferred to you by her teacher because she appears withdrawn. Although she is a cooperative and likable young girl, as well as a good student, the teacher has expressed some concerns because she doesn't interact much with other chil-dren. She stays pretty much to herself or clings to the teacher.

The girl, who has only recently moved to the school district, is an only child. After meeting with her for a very brief period of time, you readily agree that she does indeed appear to be unhappy. How, then, would you proceed in your counseling efforts?

There are, of course, a number of directions in which you might head, de-pending on which part of the problem draws your attention. Although you would certainly want to collect quite a bit more background information be-

TABLE 8.2 | DEFINITIONS OF THE PROBLEM AND POSSIBLE COURSES OF ACTION

| Diagnosis | Treatment Plan |
| --- | --- |
| She is lonely and isolated because of a deficiency in social skills. | Provide structured practice for initiating relationships. |
| She is holding in feelings that she has been unable to express. | Reflect her underlying feelings of fear and inadequacy. |
| She is discouraging herself by repeating self-defeating thoughts. | Use cognitive restructuring to help her think differently. |
| She is emotionally underdeveloped due to unresolved issues in the past. | Use play therapy to help her come to terms terms with unexpressed rage and resentment. |
| She is depressed in response to unresolved conflicts between her parents. | Begin family counseling or parallel marital counseling to help the parents. |
| She is going through a normal adjustment and grieving process that is part of a major life transition. | Offer reassurance and support until she acclimates herself to her new situation. |

fore you formulated a reasonable plan, this case illustrates that a number of diagnoses and corresponding treatments are possible. Each of the definitions of the problem and courses of action shown in Table 8.2 is based on reasonable assumptions drawn from the limited clinical data provided and the various theoretical approaches presented in the previous chapters.

The point of this summary is not to overwhelm you with all the options that are possible but rather to acquaint you with the intrinsically elastic properties of the assessment process. Before we move into some of the more traditional forms of diagnosis and assessment that are part of the helping professions, you should understand how subjective this process can sometimes be.

Five major diagnostic models are used by practitioners in the various helping professions. Depending on their professional identity, training, and treatment philosophy, counselors or therapists may rely on a medical, developmental, phenomenological, behavioral, or systemic model. Each of these diagnostic systems is based on different structures, assumptions, and research data and has distinct advantages and disadvantages (see Table 8.3). Although you should become familiar with each of these models so that you may converse intelligently about your cases with a variety of helping professionals, the developmental and medical/psychiatric models are the ones most commonly used by those in the counseling profession. The developmental model has been used traditionally in educational settings and is part of our identity as therapeutic counselors. As opposed to a medical model (described in the

**TABLE 8.3** │ DIAGNOSTIC MODELS

| Model | Primary Structure | Sources of Information | Advantages | Disadvantages | Treatment Implications |
|---|---|---|---|---|---|
| Medical | Discrete categories of psychopathology | Data based on quantitative research | Organization of etiology, symptom clusters, and prognoses | Categories not as discrete and reliable as needed; individual reduced to a label | Application of treatment to diminish symptoms and cure underlying illness |
| Developmental | Predictable stages of normal development | Case studies; qualitative and quantitative research | Ease of prediction; emphasis on healthy functioning | Stages overlap and are difficult to assess; system not universal | Identification of current level of functioning so as to stimulate growth to next stage |
| Phenomenological | Complex descriptions of the person with minimal use of labels | Qualitative research and personal experience | Focus on capturing of essences; flexibility | Model is subjective, subject to biases and distortion | Use of self as instrument to establish relationship and understand client's world |
| Behavioral | Specific description and identification of behaviors and reinforcers | Direct observation and quantitative measurement | Ability to be very specific and descriptive | Misses complexity of human experience | Establishment of specific goals to increase or decrease target behaviors |
| Systemic | Contextual descriptions | Direct observation; family history | Ability to view bigger picture of presenting issues | Negates autonomy and individuality | Work within family dynamics and structures |

next section), a developmentally based diagnosis describes client symptoms and behavior in terms of their adaptive functions and focuses primarily on levels and stages of present functioning (Blocher, 2000; Ivey, 1991). This is also the case with the systemic model favored by marriage and family counselors (see Chapter 10). This is a quite different way of thinking about assessment than the diagnostic system favored by psychiatrists and many psychologists.

# Diagnosis

Therapeutic counselors in community agency settings are expected to have a working knowledge of a diagnostic system. Two models in wide use today are the *Diagnostic and Statistical Manual of Mental Disorders,* 4th edition, revised (DSM-IV-R), and the *International Classification of Diseases, Clinical Modification,* 9th edition (ICD-9-CM). Both of these diagnostic systems have been developed primarily by psychiatrists employing a "medical model" of conceptualizing mental illness. If you look at the list of consultants and contributors who were involved in the creation of these manuals you will notice that the vast majority hold medical degrees.

Currently the DSM-IV is considered to be the "bible" of the mental health professions, containing authoritative information and "official opinions" about the range of mental problems. This latest edition includes a number of changes from its predecessors: It is supposed to be more sensitive to gender and cultural differences, it is more logically organized, and it includes 13 new mental disorders while eliminating eight that are considered obsolete. Counselors rely on the DSM-IV: (1) as a source of standardized terminology in which to communicate with other mental health specialists; (2) for satisfying the record-keeping requirements of insurance companies or credentialing agencies such as the Joint Commission on Accreditation of Hospitals; (3) for classifying clientele in statistical categories, as is necessary for research and accountability; (4) for predicting the course of a disorder and the progress of treatment based on available evidence; and (5) for constructing a treatment plan that will guide interventions (Seligman, 1998).

The actual process of differential diagnosis with the DSM-IV is complex, and mastery of the system requires considerable study and supervised clinical experience. Such a task is very important for counselors entering the field. Wylie (1995) sums up the need for a thorough understanding of the diagnostic process in today's era of managed care: "In short, therapists are expected, as never before, to pass a DSM litmus test for diagnostic legitimacy, to show cause to a stranger sitting in a large corporate office checking off notches on a symptomatic yardstick, exactly why, by what measure and in what way their clients need treatment at all" (p. 24).

Diagnostic information is obtained during a clinical interview that is primarily symptom oriented, focusing on significant behavioral and psychological patterns associated with a presenting complaint. It is therefore very important that the counselor choose a clinical interview (structured or more

## VOICE FROM THE FIELD

Having been a clinician for many years for a mental health agency, it becomes very easy to label and diagnose an individual with very little information. After asking a short series of questions with each response guiding the next question, I can arrive at a diagnosis in a very short amount of time. However, I have to constantly remind myself that this person sitting across the table from me is a human being with real concerns and should not be treated as a "schizophrenic" or a "bipolar" but rather as a person with symptoms of schizophrenia or bipolar features. I have often seen instances in which a fresh new counselor is more sensitive and empathetic than the more well-seasoned clinician that is supervising the newcomer. I suppose that the moral of the story is to continue to work with people and not focus so much on constructed labels. These clients that I diagnose usually have some understanding of their issues and often feel inadequate in certain ways. To brandish a DSM and throw labels at them can leave them feeling even more inadequate.

informal) that provides the most meaningful information to guide treatment (Vacc & Juhnke, 1997).

One example of the criteria used in the DSM-IV for making diagnostic decisions is illustrated in Table 8.4. You can see from examining this chart that each psychological disorder (in this case, "Generalized Anxiety Disorder") is described in terms of specific symptoms that can be compared to a client's presenting complaints and behavior.

In addition, information is provided about the disorder's essential characteristics, frequency of occurrence, predisposing factors, and suggestions of other problems that have similar features.

The process by which the interviewer uses the DSM-IV involves making a series of decisions about the client's functioning in five different areas called *axes*. These are described as follows:

Axis I:   Clinical Disorders

Axis II:  Personality Disorders

Axis III: General Medical Conditions

Axis IV: Psychosocial and Environmental Problems

Axis V:  Global Assessment of Functioning

The major strength of this diagnostic system is that it captures the essence of the client's symptomatology, personality style, and functioning in a brief descriptive summary. It allows the counselor to communicate information about clients in a standardized format. For example, in a case suggested by Spitzer, Skodol, Gibbon, and Williams (1994), we look at how the diagnostic process would be applied to a young woman.

TABLE 8.4 | DIAGNOSTIC CRITERIA FOR 300.02 GENERALIZED ANXIETY DISORDER

A. Excessive anxiety and worry (apprehensive expectation), occurring more days than not for at least six months, about a number of events or activities (such as work or school performance).

B. The person finds it difficult to control the worry.

C. The anxiety and worry are associated with three (or more) of the following six symptoms (with at least some symptoms present for more days than not for the past six months).

   Note: Only one item is required in children.
   1. restlessness or feeling keyed up or on edge
   2. being easily fatigued
   3. difficulty concentrating or mind going blank
   4. irritability
   5. muscle tension
   6. sleep disturbance (difficulty falling or staying asleep, or restless unsatisfying sleep)

D. The focus of the anxiety and worry is not confined to features of an Axis I disorder; for example, the anxiety or worry is not about having a Panic Attack (as in Panic Disorder), being embarrassed in public (as in Social Phobia), being contaminated (as in Obsessive-Compulsive Disorder), being away from home or close relatives (as in Separation Anxiety Disorder), gaining weight (as in Anorexia Nervosa), having multiple physical complaints (as in Somatization Disorder), or having a serious illness (as in hypochondriasis), and the anxiety and worry do not occur exclusively during Post-Traumatic Stress Disorder.

E. The anxiety, worry, or physical symptoms cause clinically significant distress or impairment in social, occupational, or other important areas of functioning.

F. The disturbance is not due to the direct physiological effects of a substance (for example, a drug of abuse, a medication) or a general medical condition (as in hyperthyroidism) and does not occur exclusively during a Mood Disorder, a Psychotic Disorder, or a Pervasive Developmental Disorder.

*Source:* Reprinted with permission from the *Diagnostic and Statistical Manual of Mental Disorders.* Fourth Edition. Copyright 1994 American Psychiatric Association.

Misty is a 17-year-old high school junior who became agitated during the funeral of her father, who had died suddenly of a heart attack. She complained of stomach problems that turned out to be stress-related gastritis. She also developed bizarre delusions that the devil was coming to get her and spent hours each day rocking in the corner of her room. She had no previous psychiatric history, and Misty was well adjusted before her father's death and a good student in school. Sometimes she was described as "overreacting" to things in her life.

DSM-IV DIAGNOSIS FOR MISTY:

Axis I: *Brief psychotic disorder*

Psychotic symptoms of less than two weeks in reaction to father's death.

Axis II: *Histrionic traits*

Her personality style is prone to "overreacting."

Axis III: *Gastritis*

She developed physical symptoms in response to her father's death.

Axis IV: *Severity of stress:* 5, Extreme

A father's death is a fairly severe incident in an adolescent's life.

Axis V: *Highest level of functioning during the past year:* 80, Very Good

Prior to this episode, Misty was generally high functioning.

There is a thinking process that accompanies the use of the DSM-IV in which a client's symptoms are clearly defined and described, compared to and differentiated from other similar kinds of disturbances, and then progressively narrowed in focus from the general to more specific diagnostic categories (Morrison, 1994). In an appendix to the manual, flow charts are presented that illustrate the process of diagnostic decision making. In the case of Misty, for example, the following questions might be asked:

| Diagnostic Questions | Behavioral Evidence |
| --- | --- |
| Is there evidence of psychotic symptoms? | Yes, bizarre delusions. |
| Are there organic factors operating? | No, symptoms appear reactive. |
| Duration of symptoms? | Less than one week. |
| Recurrent episodes? | No, first episode. |
| Major mood disorder present? | No. |
| Ongoing personality disturbance? | A dramatic style but no disturbance. |

This series of questions would then allow the diagnostician to differentiate Misty's brief psychotic episode from other possibilities such as schizophrenia, a schizo-affective disorder, or a mood disorder. Although you may not be called on (or trained) to work with severe emotional disturbances, it is important for you to understand the diagnostic process and procedures that other mental health professionals use in their work.

Counselors also find it valuable to apply differential diagnostic thinking when working with less severe presenting problems such as adjustment reactions. For example, if a client were to come to you complaining about feeling anxious, you should be able to distinguish among an anxiety disorder, an adjustment reaction with anxious mood, a panic disorder, or agoraphobia. There are features common to all these diagnoses, yet the treatment strategy would

Okay, true confession time. I love the *Diagnostic Manual.* I love its illusions of truth, as if these conditions described really do exist. I love pretending that I really can figure out which little box fits which client. I like holding my own with doctors and psychologists. I can talk DSM stuff with the best of them. But best of all, I really enjoy the logical process involved in constructing a treatment plan from be-

ginning to end. It all appeals to my own sense of logic in a world that is essentially pretty chaotic. There it is before me: which personality attributes, organic contributors, clinical syndromes, behavioral indices, and family influences might be involved. All of this helps me to figure out the best way to approach a case and which elements I should include.

---

probably vary with each one. One of the hallmarks of effective practice is adapting what you do with clients depending on their presenting complaints and individual needs.

## Ethical Concerns

Diagnosis, in and of itself, creates its own ethical problems, not through its use but through its abuse and imperfections. First, it has less-than-perfect reliability: When several clinicians view the same client in action, they may be unable to agree on the proper category. Diagnoses are often inconsistently applied and err in the direction of pathology rather than health. Counselors often find this last point to be particularly restricting, because much of their orientation views client symptomatology from a developmental rather than a psychopathological perspective; that is, rather than trying exclusively to find out what is wrong with clients, they attempt to focus on clients' internal strengths, capacity for self-healing, and resources for resolving normal life crises.

Other sources of error that affect the accuracy and validity of a psychiatric diagnosis include the counselor's expectations, theoretical orientation, and observational skills, as well as the client's inconsistent behavior, attitudes toward treatment, similarity to the counselor in basic values, and socioeconomic background. Cultural, racial, and gender differences are also sources of diagnostic error (Malgady, 1996; Paniagua, 2001; Ritchie, 1994; Sinacore-Guinn, 1995). Poor people are more often diagnosed as crazy, whereas rich people are labeled eccentric.

There is nothing magical about the classification scheme currently in use. There is no overwhelming evidence or research data to support the discrete categories that make up the various DSM-IV diagnoses. Kroll (1988) has pointed out that this is especially true with the "personality disorders," which are supposed to be stable, relatively permanent traits that are part of a person's characteristic style of functioning. Although there are an even dozen of such diagnostic classifications—paranoid, schizoid, schizotypical, histrionic, narcissistic, antisocial, borderline, avoidant, dependent, compulsive, passive-aggressive, and atypical—they are not necessarily mutually discrete groups, nor do they represent an exhaustive list. Kroll points out that, although there is no diagnosis for "macho" or "pedantic" personality disorder, he certainly knows people who would fit. Likewise, although borderline, narcissistic, and histrionic personalities are supposed to be different entities, some clients meet the criteria for all three. To complicate matters further, traditional diagnostic systems such as the DSM-IV can be easily abused in that they encourage practitioners to look at people as labels. In one review of the literature on the subject of so-called difficult clients—meaning those who do not meet the counselor's usual expectations—they were called "character disordered," "stressful," "hateful," "abrasive," and even "bogeymen":

> Difficult clients are frightened. Their behavior, which we call resistance, is normally something that we try to prevent or circumvent—an enemy to be defeated. These people are certainly not ferocious barracudas seeking to eat us alive. Difficult clients are often just people with problems that are more complex than those we usually confront, and with an interactive style that is different from what we might prefer. Calling them names only disguises the reality that resistant clients are attempting to tell us about their pain, even if their method of communication is sometimes indirect and annoying. (Kottler, 1992, p. 391)

Application of the medical model to therapeutic counseling has been eloquently and passionately denounced as morally unacceptable by such influential writers as Thomas Szasz, R. D. Laing, Erving Goffman, Theodore Sarbin, and even Chief Justice Warren Burger (Edwards, 1982). Critics warn that the diagnostic scheme developed from the medical model is not useful for therapeutic practice because its concepts are descriptive rather than normative, exhibit physical symptoms instead of behaviors, rely on known physical causes, use physical treatment interventions, and define the client as "sick" or "diseased." Wakefield (1997) believes that the DSM-IV tends to be overinclusive and includes diagnostic criteria that are not necessarily mental disorders.

Moreover, diagnoses can be dehumanizing in that they pigeonhole human beings into slots that can be difficult to escape. Some clinicians are especially concerned with the overuse of terms such as *minimal brain dysfunction, hyperkinetic,* and *retarded* to describe children who are disruptive, active, or easily distracted. Although in some cases these labels denoting disturbances of conduct or organic problems may be justified, in other instances, the child's behavior is the logical response to a teacher's or parent's confusing messages. Meanwhile, the labels remain forever imprinted in the minds of others and in the records that follow the child wherever he or she may go. It is for this very reason that it is so important to use the least stigmatizing label possible that is consistent with accurate reporting. Furthermore, counselors and school counselors alike should collaborate efforts whenever possible with primary care physicians and other appropriate mental health professionals when dealing with clients with severe mental disorders (Geroski, Rodgers, & Breen, 1997).

There are alternatives to diagnostic systems based on the medical model, which equates client problems with pathological processes. Boy (1989), for example, describes a diagnostic method based on a client-centered model that emphasizes a person's individuality and uniqueness rather than trying to put her or him into a particular box. You have also read about how strategic counselors prefer to use diagnoses that are descriptive and phrased in such a way that they imply that a solution is likely. A developmental model of diagnosis is another alternative that allows counselors to assess a client's current functioning levels in terms of cognitive, language, physical, self-perception, social relations, moral, and personality factors (Capuzzi & Gross, 2001). Finally, constructivist/narrative models of diagnosis are less interested in classifying and labeling any disorder than they are helping clients to understand their own struggles within a larger context of their culture and history.

## Behavioral Diagnosis

Functional behavioral labeling is another alternative assessment and diagnostic strategy. In this process, a client's specific behaviors are described in meaningful, illustrative, individualized language, not only to help the counselor to understand exactly which concerns are to be addressed but also to aid the client's understanding of how, when, where, and with whom the self-defeating patterns are exhibited. There are thus therapeutic advantages to functional behavioral labeling:

1. Clients learn the methods of identifying and describing complex, abstract, ambiguous processes in specific, useful terms.

   BEFORE: "Ah, I don't know exactly. I just can't seem to concentrate anymore."

   AFTER: "I have difficulty structuring my study time on the weekends I spend at home, particularly when I allow the distractions of my brother and girlfriend to interfere."

2. Clients understand that they are unique individuals with their own characteristic concerns.

   BEFORE: "I've been told that I'm a drug addict."

   AFTER: "I'm a person who tends to overindulge in cocaine and marijuana when I feel school pressures building up."

3. Clients describe their behavior in such a way that it can be changed. Whereas a personality characteristic is stable, invariant, and permanent, a behavior can be changed.

BEFORE: "I'm shy. That's the way I've always been."

AFTER: "I sometimes act shy when I meet a new guy I find attractive."

4. Clients label their behavior in the specific situations in which they have difficulty.

BEFORE: "I'm depressed."

AFTER: "I feel depressed in situations like my job and marriage, in which I feel powerless to do anything to change."

5. Clients accept responsibility for their destructive behaviors rather than blaming them on something beyond their control, such as bad genes.

BEFORE: "I'm passive. Everyone in my family is. What do you expect?"

AFTER: "I act passively in some novel situations because I have learned to let others take charge. Yet in other situations, in which I feel more comfortable, I don't act passively at all."

Within the context of the assessment process are several methodologies that may be used to collect valuable data, formulate workable diagnoses, and create specific behavioral assignments. Standardized testing is certainly helpful in that regard. However, all assessment efforts and testing practices are effective only in the context of the therapeutic relationship.

# SUMMARY

In this chapter we have presented a brief overview of the major themes involved in testing and assessment. The field is broad, the focus controversial, and the need for technical expertise and cogent thinking great. Assessment cannot ethically be avoided by counselors; it's their job to observe, evaluate, diagnose, and intervene. It is my contention, and I hope your growing awareness, that using as broad a range as possible of relevant assessment devices, including standardized instruments, provides to both client and counselor the maximum amount of potentially useful information. Assessment will be done; the only question is: Will it rest on a defensible base?

# SELF-GUIDED EXPLORATIONS

1. In what ways have particular tests or assessment instruments had an influence in some major choices and decisions you have made in your life?
2. Recount an episode in which you were assessed and evaluated by someone. What was that experience like for you? How do you wish the experience had been handled differently? When you are in a position to assess others, what do you intend to do that is different from your experiences?

3. From what you know and understand about the various diagnostic labels that counselors and therapists use, write a diagnostic assessment of yourself. Include as much professional jargon as you can, as if you were writing up a case report of a client.

4. In addition to the medical model described in the previous question, there are several other diagnostic models (developmental, phenomenological, behavioral, systemic) that are sometimes employed. Describe some aspect of your life in the language of each of these alternative models.

   *Developmental*—current functioning in terms of stage- and age-related norms

   *Phenomenological*—essence of your experience while minimizing labels

   *Behavioral*—specific description of your observable behavior

   *Systemic*—attention to interactive factors in your family and peer group

5. Write three sample test questions that you believe measure accurately what you learned in this chapter about the assessment process. Describe the challenges you experienced in developing some means of evaluating your performance.

## For Homework:

Make plans at the career center, counseling center, or some other agency to take a series of tests including an interest inventory, an aptitude test, a projective test, and an objective personality instrument. Review with the counselor the limitations and most useful information derived from this experience.

## SUGGESTED READINGS

American Psychiatric Association. (2000). *Diagnostic and statistical manual of mental disorders*. Washington, DC: American Psychiatric Association.

Bongar, B. (2002). *The suicidal patient: Clinical and legal standards of care*. Washington, DC: American Psychological Association.

Hoffman, E. (2001). *Psychological testing at work: How to use, interpret, and get the most of out of the newest tests in personality, learning style, aptitudes, interests, and more*. New York: McGraw-Hill.

Hood, A. B., & Johnson, R. W. (2001). *Assessment in counseling: A guide to the use of psychological assessment procedures*. Alexandria, VA: American Counseling Association.

Janda, L. (1998). *Psychological testing, theory, and applications*. Boston: Allyn & Bacon.

Jones, W. P. (1997). *Deciphering the diagnostic codes: A guide for school counselors*. Thousand Oaks, CA: Corwin Press.

Murphy, K. R., & Davidshofer, C. O. (2000). *Psychological testing: Principles and applications*. Upper Saddle River, NJ: Prentice-Hall.

Paniagua, F. A. (2001). *Diagnosis in a multicultural context: A casebook for mental health professionals.* Thousand Oaks, CA: Sage.

Seligman, L. (1998). *Selecting effective treatments: A comprehensive, systematic guide to treating mental disorders* (2nd ed.). San Francisco: Jossey-Bass.

Simeonsson, R. J., & Rosenthal, S. L. (2001). Psychological and developmental assessment. New York: Guilford.

Spitzer, R. L. (2001). *DSM-IV-TR casebook.* Washington, DC: American Psychiatric Press.

Welfel, E. R., & Ingersoll, R. E. (Eds). (2001). *The mental health desk reference.* New York: Wiley.

# COUNSELING
# APPLICATIONS

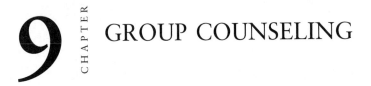

# 9 CHAPTER   GROUP COUNSELING

## KEY CONCEPTS

Group norms

Group modalities

Screening procedures

Spectator effects

Curative factors

Cohesion

Rehearsal

Process stages

High-functioning groups

Intervention cues

Leadership skills

# GROUP COUNSELING

In some ways group counseling is not unlike the therapeutic experience of individual sessions. In both settings, a systematic helping procedure is used to further the work of individual clients toward improving their personal functioning: identifying specific behaviors clients wish to change, understanding the underlying causes of problems, and designing strategies for making constructive changes. Although individual and group counseling modalities share similar theoretical heritages, basic strategies, and desired outcomes, some fundamental differences between them warrant closer inspection. There is no doubt that counseling in groups is more complex, requires more leader training, and has the potential to do more good or harm than similar helping efforts in individual counseling. It is for these reasons that students are given additional training in group modalities, as well as cautioned in their judicious use.

## SURVEY OF GROUPS

We live in a world of groups: social groups, family groups, ethnic groups, athletic groups, fraternities and sororities, neighborhood groups, professional groups, religious groups. The only time we are ever really alone is in the car or the bathroom, and even then we are often invaded by intrusions. There is an ambivalence that most of us feel for being in the groups of our lives: On the one hand, we are resentful of the pressures we feel to conform to others' expectations; yet on the other hand, we appreciate all the support we receive being part of something bigger than ourselves.

One group member describes this all-too-familiar feeling:

> I really do appreciate all of you here in this group. When I'm with you I don't feel so alone. Even when I'm not with you, I carry a part of you inside me. I know that you care about me. I don't exactly like it when you confront me and make me look at ugly stuff, but without your efforts I would forever be stuck where I am.

> Sometimes, though, I feel so stifled by this group. There are things I want to say or do but, somehow, it feels like I would be letting some of you down. I get confused as to whose expectations I am really living up to—yours or mine. There have been many times when I've thought how free I would feel not to come here again.

The composition of any group, whether for social, business, or therapeutic purposes, involves a collection of persons gathered together for compatible goals. Although they may (and usually do) have personal motives and objectives that they wish to satisfy as a result of their participation, group members agree on a set of basic governing principles to guide their collective behavior. These norms and rules implicitly or explicitly specify leader actions as well as appropriate member behaviors.

Groups have many different labels that have been somewhat arbitrarily used, leaving the public as well as some professionals a bit confused. Some of the most common types are illustrated in Table 9.1.

Differences exist not only in the various modes of group work, but also in the myriad of leadership styles that can be applied, each with its own set of goals (see Table 9.2). Corey (2000) asks whether group leaders should best function as facilitators, teachers, therapists, catalysts, directors, or perhaps just as other more experienced members.

Whereas some approaches focus on the group goal of building greater trust, intimacy, and interpersonal openness, other approaches de-emphasize group goals altogether, instead helping each individual member to commit to reaching personal objectives. Just like the varied approaches to individual counseling covered in previous chapters, many theories guide the behavior of group leaders. Some counselors lean toward more directive teaching models favored by cognitive/behavioral theories; others prefer experientially based groups that are patterned after Gestalt, existential, or humanistic philosophy. Recent innovations in a social constructionist approach to group work are also changing the professional landscape in such a way to be more sensitive to issues of power, language, social discourse, and a more humble way of listening to people (O'Leary, 2001).

At some later time, you may wish to consult sources (Corey, 2000; Gazda, Ginter, & Horne, 2001; Gladding, 2003; Kottler, 2001) that introduce you to group counseling theories in greater depth. You may also wish to focus on a more integrative model (Johnson & Johnson, 2003; Kline, 2003; Shapiro, Peltz, & Bernadett-Shapiro, 1998; Yalom, 1995).

## TABLE 9.1 | A Continuum of Group Work Styles

| Discussion Group | Group Guidance | Human Potential Group | Counseling Group | Group Therapy with Neurotics | Group Therapy with Psychotics |
|---|---|---|---|---|---|
| EDUCATIONAL MODEL | | | | | MEDICAL MODEL |
| Cognitively oriented | | | | | Affectively oriented |
| Task oriented | | | | | Process oriented |
| Short term | | | | | Long term |
| For normal functioning persons | | | | For those with problems in reality testing | |
| Identification of goals | | | | | Use of differential diagnosis |
| Focus on upgrading skills or knowledge | | | | Focus on personality restructuring | |
| Use of readings and homework as adjuncts | | | | Use of medication and individual therapy as adjuncts | |

SOURCE: Kottler, J. A. (1984). *Advanced group leadership*. Pacific Grove, CA: Brooks/Cole.

TABLE 9.2 | COMPARATIVE OVERVIEW OF GROUP GOALS

| | |
|---|---|
| Psychoanalytic | To provide a climate that helps clients reexperience early family relationships. To uncover buried feelings associated with past events that carry over into current behavior. |
| Adlerian | To create a therapeutic relationship that encourages participants to explore their basic life assumptions and to achieve a broader understanding of lifestyles. |
| Psychodrama | To facilitate release of pent-up feelings, to provide insight, and to help clients develop new and more effective behaviors. |
| Existential | To provide conditions that maximize self-awareness and reduce blocks to growth. To help clients discover and use freedom of choice and assume responsibility for their own choices. |
| Person-centered | To provide a safe climate wherein members can explore the full range of their feelings. To develop openness, honesty, and spontaneity. |
| Gestalt | To enable members to pay close attention to their moment-to-moment experiences so they can recognize and integrate disowned aspects of themselves. |
| Transactional | To assist clients in becoming free of scripts and games in their interactions. To challenge members to reexamine early decisions and make new ones based on awareness. |
| Behavioral | To help group members eliminate maladaptive behaviors and learn new and more effective behavioral patterns. |
| Cognitive | To teach group members that they are responsible for their own emotional disturbances and to help them identify and abandon the ways they keep their disturbances alive. |
| Reality | To guide members toward learning realistic and responsible behavior and developing a "success identity." To assist group members in evaluating their behavior and in deciding on a plan of action for change. |

*Source:* Corey, G. (1999). *Theory and practice of group counseling* (5th ed.). Pacific Grove, CA: Brooks/Cole.

In addition to the confusion surrounding the different styles of group leadership, each of the different kinds of groups have particular goals, structures, and compositions. Among these various formats, you may be expected to play a variety of consulting or leadership roles.

## Encounter Groups

The most ambiguous category of groups includes names such as Human Relations Group, Human Potential Group, T-Group, Training Group, Encounter Group, and Growth Group. All of these groups developed from the early

■ | VOICE FROM THE FIELD

There are so many different roles you play when you're leading a group. Initially, you try to be a model for group members, demonstrating as many of the important skills and behaviors you can. I'm usually the one who does most of the confronting in the beginning, until others catch on to how to do it without being insensitive or offensive. Then I switch to a more supportive role, cuing other members to do the work whenever I can. For example, if I'm feeling bored or irritated with what's going on, rather than being the one to say something I usually look around the group and find someone else who appears to be feeling what I am. Then I'll say to that person, "What's going on with you? You seem to be feeling a bit antsy right now."

I think in general the best way to lead a group is by playing a supportive role and getting the members to do most of the work. In this working stage, you just kind of act like a referee, making sure that people don't get hurt and that things keep moving along.

---

work of the National Training Laboratory (NTL), the Esalen Institute, and the writings of Carl Rogers and Kurt Lewin. These groups were very popular in the 1960s and 1970s because of their emphasis on creating a learning community built on trust and honesty. They were extremely powerful in their impact on participants; the problem is that they often produced casualties as well as fans because of their uneven quality of leadership (Yalom, 1995).

Although today encounter groups have diminished in popularity, there are still a number of personal-growth types in existence, in some of which you may play a leadership role. They are designed for relatively normal persons and usually have a fairly loose structure. According to Rogers' (1970) original conception, the leader is viewed primarily as a facilitator/participant rather than as an expert.

## An Encounter Group in Action

The silence has lasted four minutes by the clock, but it feels like an hour. Everyone looks to the leader, who merely smiles and waits. Finally, one woman screams out in exasperation, "I'm tired of this crap! When are we going to do something?"

"This is your group," the leader says softly, meeting her eyes. "What do you want to do?"

Another participant chimes in, then another, all voicing their frustration at the aimless direction in which they have been moving: "What are we supposed to be doing here?"

"I feel frustrated too," the leader answers, nodding his head. "But isn't this a bit like our lives? It's up to us to create structure."

The leader looks around the room and notices some puzzled faces; others nodding thoughtfully. "Maybe a good place to start," he suggests, "would be for us to tell each other how we are feeling about being here right now. Who would like to start?"

## Psychoeducational Groups

In contrast to the relatively unstructured format of many growth groups, psychoeducational groups usually have a definite agenda. Furthermore, they tend to be didactic and instructional rather than experiential and focused on feelings. They often have planned, structured activities and fairly definite goals that are identified by the leader, who operates in an instructor/facilitator role. These are the sort of groups that used to be called "guidance" groups in the past in that they were designed in school settings to help students make career decisions.

Among those groups that are organized in school settings, some leaders have combined features of growth groups described earlier with more structure to teach children adaptive skills (Roland & Neitzschman, 1996; Wasielewski, Scruggs, & Scott, 1997). Whether offered in schools or other settings, group leaders attempt to provide relevant information on careers, sex, job possibilities, colleges, and other topics that might be of interest. Generally, they focus on preventing problems in the future by encouraging developmental growth, aiding the decision-making process, teaching valuable life skills, and providing useful information. Psychoeducational groups are particularly well-suited for many structured interpretations that facilitate self-awareness and values clarification. School, rehabilitation, and substance abuse specialists, in particular, will be called on to lead these types of groups.

## A Psychoeducational Group in Action

"You have all had time to study various careers, visit job sites directly, and hear some interesting talks by representatives of various professions. Still, many of you are confused as to which direction to move in and are even more uncertain as to what you are uniquely suited to do. Although just beginning your lives, you already are aware of things you like and dislike as well as those things you can easily do or not do. Perhaps it might be helpful for you to get some honest feedback from your friends in this group who know you so well. Tina, you had mentioned earlier that you could never be in a medical profession because you can't stand sick people. Based on what the rest of you know about her, what careers do you think she'd be good at?"

## Counseling Groups

Group counseling is the modality most appropriate for students using this textbook. The techniques and strategies are all designed to help resolve interpersonal conflict, promote greater self-awareness and insight, and help individual members work to eliminate their self-defeating behaviors. Most often, the clientele have few manifestations of psychopathology; they simply wish to work on personal concerns in daily living. In addition, counseling groups are also designed to be rather brief treatments, often focusing on resolving specific problems (LaFountain & Garner, 1996; Shapiro, Peltz, & Bernadett-Shapiro, 1998).

## VOICE FROM THE FIELD

I gotta tell you: I do groups as much for me as my clients. There is nothing more exciting in my job, more stimulating, more unpredictable. I've been doing groups for a long time and they're always different, every one of them. You just never know what's gonna happen, even when you think you've seen it all before.

The energy in a group is simply amazing. There is so much to track, to watch, listen to, sense, feel. It's exhausting trying to follow it all. One person speaks and you try and give full attention but there's about a dozen other things going on at the same time, each one potentially meaningful. It's like a roller coaster—you just sort of hang on and enjoy the ride. Well, maybe that's not strictly true—as the leader, I'm supposed to be the one driving the thing, but the truth is that sometimes groups just seem to have a life of their own. That's not usually a problem if you've set things up right and created the right norms. But you've still got to pay very close attention so things don't get out of hand.

---

Group counseling is usually focused in the present rather than dwelling on the past. It is relatively short term, spanning a period of weeks or months, and stresses relationship support factors to resolve stated conflicts. For an example, an elementary school counselor might organize a counseling group for kids who are having behavioral adjustment problems at school (Nelson, Dykeman, Powell, & Petty, 1996), or a university counseling center might design a counseling group for students with learning disabilities to talk about their frustrations (McWhirter & McWhirter, 1996), or mental health counselors might organize groups for at-risk adolescents (Wilson & Owens, 2001).

In contrast to some growth and psychoeducational groups led by lay people, as well as self-help groups, counseling groups are always led by a trained expert who is prepared to protect individual client's rights while stimulating constructive interpersonal action. Clients are usually helped to work toward individually designed goals, although there is a common interest in becoming more intimate, trusting, accepting, empathic, and interpersonally effective.

## A Counseling Group in Action

COUNSELOR: Who wants to use group time today? We've cleared up some loose ends from last week and got progress reports on what has happened during the week, so let's move on.

KILE: Well, if nobody else wants—

SARAH: Damn it, Kile! You talk too much. Why don't you give someone else a chance?

KILE: But I was only—

COUNSELOR: Sarah, you seem unusually frisky today. I don't think you're as angry at Kile as at yourself for letting things slide so long. But there's plenty of

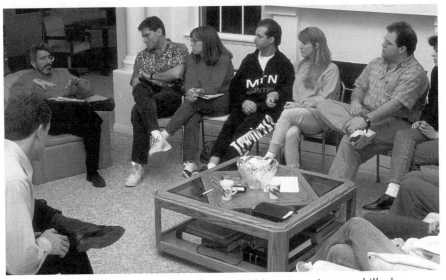

Groups provide support, resources, and opportunities to practice new skills that are not possible in individual counseling. © Michael Newman/PhotoEdit.

time for both of you. And I remember that you, Paolo, had a concern you wanted to work on as well. Let's budget our time accordingly.

KILE: Sarah, I know you're not angry at me and I'm glad you finally want to work on something. I only need about ten minutes anyway. A few weeks ago all of you helped me a lot, and things are much better with my girlfriend. The only thing is that I'm having second thoughts about getting married. I just wanted to get some feedback from the rest of you as to how you felt before you got married and how you feel about your situations now.

## Therapy Groups

In practice, there is often very little difference between group counseling and group therapy, whereas in theory the goals and purposes are somewhat different. Psychotherapy in groups most often takes place in hospital, medical, or clinic settings with patients who are diagnosed as having some form of diagnosable mental disorder. These severe disorders require longer treatment, intensive analysis, and structural personality changes. In addition, therapy groups frequently have participants who act out in dramatic ways (Silverstein, 1997).

The content of most counseling programs does not adequately prepare students to deliver group psychotherapy services because of their emphasis on longer term, more intensive treatment with more disturbed populations. However, often counseling practitioners may find themselves, by choice or circumstances, functioning as group therapists and so often seek to supplement their expertise with further training.

## A Therapy Group in Action

The therapy group has been meeting weekly for two years. The support has been crucial for many of the participants, who include an alcoholic, a spouse abuser, a man with severe depressive episodes, a woman with an eating disorder who indulges in periodic binges, another woman fearful of crossing bridges, a man with chronic anxiety and insomnia, and a man who won't admit he has any problems, although his behavior is passive-aggressive. There are two leaders: a psychiatrist who monitors medication and a psychologist who works with them in testing. Both have a psychoanalytic perspective and have been working to help each patient minimize his or her symptoms, understand past actions, and function more normally in their worlds. The sessions are usually quite emotionally charged, requiring all the skills and training of the two leaders to reduce manipulation, resistance, and game playing and to avoid casualties. The group has acted as a buffer, a transitional step between the members' intensive individual therapy sessions and a gradual tapering off of treatment that will eventually lead to a monthly checkup and support system.

## Self-Help and Support Groups

The self-help movement has become a dynamic force for change over the past twenty years. Self-help books have become huge best-sellers, and self-help authors are commonly visible in the media. The self-help movement touches on a strong chord of independence within the North American character coupled with a desire to improve life conditions. Self-help groups have also proliferated widely and are an essential aspect of this self-help movement.

Self-help groups often do not have a professionally trained leader and, instead, use a more experienced member who has hopefully resolved the issues with which others are struggling. The purpose of self-help groups is to provide emotional and social support, to develop new ideas about coping with a common issue, and to provide constructive direction for members. The membership of self-help groups is open and fluctuates from meeting to meeting. Examples of self-help groups might include: Alcoholics Anonymous, an eating disorders group, a Heart-Smart group for individuals with cardiac problems, a group for people diagnosed with HIV, and many others on almost any conceivable topic or issue.

Support groups are closely related to self-help groups; in fact, the terms are sometimes used interchangeably. Support groups are often developed and sponsored by professional organizations or professional individuals, and they rely on the resources of the sponsoring organization/individual to a greater extent than self-help groups. Examples of support groups might include breast cancer survivors, Parents Anonymous, Parents of Children with Attention Deficit Disorders, and spouse loss/grief groups.

Historically, mental health professionals have had ambivalent or guarded reactions to self-help/support groups; however, these attitudes have become more positive recently. The change has to do with the positive personal experiences on the part of many professionals and the recognition that self-help/

## VOICE FROM THE FIELD

What you learn in school is just the beginning, just the barest basics. In a beginning group class, you learn about curative factors, stages in the process and all. You may even get the chance to be part of a group so you can really feel what it's all about. But like so many aspects of learning this job, once you get into the real world, you have to work like crazy to catch up to what more experienced folks are doing.

In school, I learned this one model for doing groups that probably works pretty well with relatively high-functioning counseling students. Then I get this job working with dual-diagnosed inpatients—that means they're not only pretty crazy but also drug addicted—and I've got to tell you, I had to start all over again. Just imagine trying to lead a group with people who are hallucinating.

support groups will continue to play a crucial role in mental health services (Posthuma, 2001).

Self-help groups are not therapy or counseling groups; they differ in several important ways (Corey, 2000):

1. The goals of a self-help group focus on a single issue, whereas therapeutic groups focus on improving mental health and overall interpersonal functioning.
2. Self-help groups often have a political as well as individual focus. Therapeutic groups tend to de-emphasize political and social issues and focus on individual change.
3. The leaders of self-help groups are not assigned and tend to emerge from the group. The leaders themselves are dealing with the focus issue. Leaders of therapeutic groups are designated and are generally not personally involved with the focus issue.
4. The problem focus of therapeutic groups tends to be broader and inclusive of more pervasive mental health issues, whereas the focus of self-help groups is less pathological and more targeted.

Self-help and support groups can be a viable resource for professional counselors and their clients. You'd be well advised to educate yourself with all the kinds of groups available in your community so that you can make appropriate referrals for your clients and work cooperatively with those who are attending such groups.

## SOME CONSIDERATIONS IN THE USE OF GROUP MODALITIES

There has been considerable debate in the literature about whether group counseling is essentially safe and successful as a treatment modality or whether it produces too many casualties and is a waste of time. Historically, some critics believed that group therapies were faddish and possibly detrimental. Still other writers question whether group counseling is really any different from individual or family counseling because all the treatments make use of essentially the same therapeutic variables (Hill, 1990).

It may therefore be helpful to review some considerations in the use of groups so that you, as a student, may realistically assess the potential and dangers of this helping procedure. If you choose to work in groups—as a leader of a counseling group, as an administrator conducting meetings, as an instructor in the classroom, as a public figure in the media, or as a consultant in the field—study the contraindications of group methods carefully to to prepare adequate safeguards as well as for facing potential criticism. Similarly, you can capitalize on the therapeutic variables that operate in groups only if you are well aware of what can and cannot be effectively accomplished.

The history of group work is checkered with the contributions of many distinguished professionals, as well as the practices of charlatans and witch doctors. Recall that, throughout human history, group hysteria has accounted for more havoc and death than all contagious diseases. After all, what is war but an organized form of group work, in which one team, led by leaders who are masters of group dynamics, attempts to obliterate the other team in the name of abstractions such as territorial boundaries? In recent history, we have witnessed the dramatic influencing capabilities of self-serving group leaders who could induce murder or suicide with their persuasive tongues and intricate knowledge of the power of group forces. Adolf Hitler and Saddam Hussain are but two of the more skilled group tacticians of the last century who could warp group dynamics to suit their own needs.

It is no wonder that therapeutic groups are often viewed with suspicion by the public and by some clinicians. It has only been in the last few decades that standards for acceptable practice have been developed and systematic training programs implemented (Association for Specialists in Group Work, 1992). For these reasons, new graduates sometimes experience frustration when trying to begin group work in their schools or agencies. They get opposition from their clients, who resent the pressure to participate in an uncomfortable setting and who thus resist the coercion. Further, clients are often more inhibited in groups, less willing to disclose because of fears—some of which are justified. How, after all, can confidentiality ever be enforced and guaranteed in a group? Who can promise never to let secrets slip out inadvertently or never to talk about private things outside the group? And who would believe such promises?

There are also complaints from parents and spouses: "What's this? I heard that you stuck my son in one of those touchy-feely groups. I'll not have a child of mine in one of your orgies!" Or, "I notice my wife is different since she's been hanging around with those dingbats in that group. How dare you people interfere in my life!"

Some senior colleagues in administration or counseling who never received much group training may resist implementing group strategies. Many counselor/therapist education programs added their first course in the techniques of group work only in recent years, and the depth and intensity of group work training is a limitation of many counselor education programs. Students may have concerns about dual relationships since they may be expected to share intensely personal issues in classes where instructors are also evaluating them. Many of these issues can be addressed by providing students with informed consent, separating what goes on in class from products that are evaluated, and giving them the opportunity to go only as far as they feel comfortable.

It is very difficult to learn to be a group leader without logging considerable experience as a member. Moreover, it is somewhat hypocritical to expect clients to take risks and share personal concerns when the counselor has been unwilling to do so.

In group work, clients receive less time than they would in individual sessions and have less privacy. Groups require more sophisticated training on the part of leaders and are generally not suited for people who are easily intimidated or manipulative or who talk incessantly.

Why, then, would we ever choose to work in group settings? Why indeed?

## COUNTERACTING POTENTIAL LIMITATIONS

Many of the disadvantages previously mentioned can be controlled, or at least minimized, through sufficient caution and training. Issues such as the suitability of certain personality types (passive-dependent, sociopathic), appropriateness of the group for individual problems, and level of psychological functioning (borderline personality, psychotic) can be handled through screening procedures that would permit participation only by those who are reasonably respectful of others' rights and who seem to be good candidates for groups (however that may be operationally defined).

Other issues may not be so readily dismissed. Confidentiality cannot be strictly guaranteed, and this presents a number of ethical and legal problems for the participants. One other reality is that clients receive less attention than in private counseling. With these limitations in mind, the leader must take extra care to ensure that time is spent equitably and that adequate safeguards are planned to prevent anticipated problems. Taking these conditions as givens, we can more realistically survey some of the powerful advantages implicit in therapeutic groups.

## ADVANTAGES OF GROUP WORK

### Cost Efficiency

A counselor would need two full working days to see a dozen clients in individual sessions; the same number could meet in a single group session for two hours. The counselor is thereby able to reach more prospective clients in a considerably shorter period of time—and at significant savings to the institution and clientele. Most counselors and agencies are already so overburdened with work demands that group modalities allow for the most cost-efficient means to help the largest needy population.

## Spectator Effects

While one person is receiving help in a therapeutic group—struggling, confronting, exploring, growing—a dozen other clients are carefully observing the process. They are internalizing the therapeutic messages, personalizing and adapting the content to their own lives. As one client complains about conflicts with a roommate, all others in the group (and those who are now reading these words) must ask themselves: How am I getting along with my spouse/friend/roommate? What things in this relationship am I willing to fight for, and which freedoms am I prepared to sacrifice? How much do I value my privacy? Do I want to live alone? How could we better settle our arguments?

Group work has the distinct advantage of permitting others to learn by observation. Clients are able to monitor the leader's behavior, imitating the actions that they admire: how to speak with confidence, how to create metaphoric language, how to take risks. The clients also scrutinize one another. When one member experiences success, the rest will live it vicariously. When a member is censured for monopolizing too much time, the others note the lesson as well.

The learning effects become contagious as an active participant is silently or not so silently cheered by the enthusiastic spectators. Each time a client opens up, takes a risk, or tries out a new behavior and doesn't die as a consequence, the other clients will feel more ready to test themselves.

## Stimulation Value

It is no surprise that the quantity and quality of ideas generated through group interaction are significantly more enriched than the results of solo brainstorming (Brilhart & Jochern, 1964; Meadow, Parnes, & Reese, 1959). Discovery of this phenomenon revolutionized industrial product design: Experts from compatible fields teamed to pool their problem-solving efforts.

The atmosphere of a therapeutic group is a virtual utopia of emotional and cognitive stimulation, with its emphasis on freedom of expression, honest feedback, interchange of novel ideas, acceptance of individual differences, prizing of creativity and spontaneity, experimentation without fear of failure, and focus on risk taking, sharing, and giving. In such an environment it is impossible to be bored or to repeat an experience in exactly the same way.

Group sessions provide an exciting and fertile atmosphere for change because of the collective energy available. The whole is greater than the sum of its parts. Giggles quickly become contagious. As new ideas are passed around, they grow with each input, contribution, refinement. You can feel the hearts beating in a group. You can smell the sweat and sense the nervous shuffling. You can hear the pounding in your brain as it tries so hard to understand. And the sights are a visual Disneyland—nonverbal behavior to monitor, facial expressions, territorial imperatives, positioning and status hierarchies, insight in action, gestures of defiance, respect, or affection. A group is alive with ideas and emotion and change. It is stimulation itself. It is a dozen people struggling to understand themselves and one another.

Therapeutic groups not only prevent burnout in the counselor, who must constantly stay on top of things, but also energize the clients through lively interactions, spontaneous humor, and abundance of stimulation. Many practitioners with hectic schedules often deliberately plan group sessions to help both their clientele and themselves. The groups are often so professionally rewarding that the leader—although carefully monitoring his or her own behavior to avoid self-indulgence or meeting his or her own needs in the session—nevertheless cannot help growing.

## Opportunities for Feedback

Where can you go for truth? Ask your mother or your best friend for an opinion on your new shoes or what you should change about yourself. They will lie, or at least hedge, to water down an unpleasant truth. Where can you go to find out what people really think of you?

A counseling group provides the opportunity for participants to receive straightforward, honest, and constructive reactions to their behaviors, both attractive and unattractive. After role playing or risk taking, a client gains feedback from astute observers that helps in making needed adjustments, identifying areas that could be upgraded, and providing reinforcement by acknowledging progress. When feedback is diplomatically confrontive, honest without being destructive, expressive but devoid of clichés, sensitive but not overly evasive, and concise by boiling down the essence of a person's behavior into a memorable image, it becomes one of the most powerful of therapeutic devices for promoting change.

In one introductory exercise used to open groups, for example, the leader encourages an exchange of first impressions among participants. Early in the therapeutic experience, the exercise helps them to give one another the gift of honest reactions. After members are instructed about the purposes of such an exercise—to encounter one another in a personal way, to collect information on possible areas of needed growth, to hear (perhaps for the first time) of the effect they have on others—they are then educated in the requirements of effective feedback. They are reminded to avoid stereotypes and clichés, to be brief rather than long-winded, and to be honest, helpful, and constructive by including both effective and ineffective behaviors. To give the exercise structure and direction, which are often necessary in initial sessions until members learn rules and roles, the leader asks the members to write down the name of the animal that each person in the group brings to mind. Using their observations of each person's gestures and appearances, their own intuition, and any other data available, trying to be creative in their thinking, clients send feedback to one another by disclosing the animals of which they are most reminded and the reasons why.

■ | VOICE FROM THE FIELD

I tell kids in my groups to avoid giving "yearbook" feedback. You know, the kind where they write in your yearbook: "You're so sweet. Don't ever change." That feels good for about two minutes, but then what have you got? There's nothing there you can learn from. The best kind of feedback is far more direct and honest. It might hurt for a little bit, but with a lot of support, it can change your whole life.

Just imagine being able to hear from others what they really think of you. Just think how amazing that would be to hear people tell the things they would usually never say out loud.

---

Angela, a shy, withdrawn girl, learns that some of the others see her as a turtle because "she loves to swim beneath the surface where no one can see" or a golden retriever "because she appears loyal, affectionate, and maternal" or an Opaline Gourami (the speaker is a fish expert) "because she's cautious when people are around but prances when alone; she has a beautiful display of colors and grace, yet she hides behind the plants even if she sees a tasty morsel to eat; she prefers to wait for things to come to her." Other members learn from the feedback on first impressions that they may resemble a Colorado River mule, because they are survivors, are self-sufficient, and have a flexible diet; or a Hobbit, because of their playfulness, innocence, perceptiveness, and love of adventure; or a queen bee, because they are good organizers but manipulative and overdemanding.

Any and all feedback in a group is aimed at providing experiences that are rarely available in the "outside world"—direct, honest, and sensitive statements describing exactly how one person feels and thinks about another.

## Support

The tarpon, among the world's greatest sport fishes, will fight for hours longer against the hook and line when accompanied by others of its school than when alone. It is as if it couldn't give in with its peers watching, urging, goading it to fight a little longer. Humans also need to give and receive support in groups. Our ancestors huddled together in their caves for security and division of labor. In the evolutionary scheme of things, the PTA, fraternity, and neighborhood club have inherited many of the social and protective functions of the bonds we originally formed as hunter-gatherers. Groups supply the nurturing elements of intimacy and psychological bonding—the cohesion that results from close proximity over time. A therapeutic group can develop into a surrogate family, without the rigid, authoritarian hierarchies of some natural families. Such an experience can even be sampled within the relative artificiality of your classroom. Although the physical environment, seating arrangement, competition, professional authority, and threat of grading are something less than ideal circumstances for promoting a sense of true cohesion, nevertheless a feeling of belongingness often develop among classmates. Students can draw support from one another, pool their emotional and cognitive energies to get through the hard times, and savor the enlightening experiences.

Yalom (1995) identified eleven curative factors that are believed to be crucial to the healing and growth process of groups. Many of them have already been alluded to—such things as instilling hope, developing social skills, creating cohesiveness, and facilitating catharsis of emotions. Support is certainly at the top of the list; however, Bemak and Epp (1996) more unabashedly claim that love should be considered the twelfth agent of healing in groups. More than mere support in groups, they believe that a kind of "group love" operates in high-functioning groups in which members genuinely and authentically care for one another and that this deep regard is indeed a healing force beyond anything else that transpires.

## Structured Practice

Within a group, not only can we receive feedback, but we can also experience the support and encouragement necessary to practice new behaviors. Often individuals undergo stress and frustration in their daily lives because they lack needed skills. Shyness prevents them from initiating new relationships, or frustration keeps them hostile and defensive, or low self-esteem triggers procrastination; each of these limitations can be viewed as a skill deficit, and the group becomes a place to develop and refine useful life skills. A man who is passive with his wife, for instance, can practice assertiveness skills. Group members provide feedback and help him to monitor the development of those skills. Laboratory experiences such as these help group members to put insights to use and to rehearse new behaviors in a nonthreatening setting.

The group, as a learning laboratory, can also be used for reality testing. Fears, anxieties, and inhibitions can be examined and explored, permitting the member to test out the validity of those feelings. Commonly a person will hold feelings in to avoid "hurting" someone else. This concern can be tested in the group by checking out others' reactions and practicing giving both constructive and critical feedback to determine the recipient's reaction. Often the person will learn that being protective and withholding honesty are more hurtful than disclosing it, and he or she can then work toward a personal awareness of what hurting means.

# BASIC ASSUMPTIONS ABOUT GROUPS

One human life is so complex in its origins, history, functioning, and consciousness as to defy complete understanding by all the social and physical scientists in the universe. Yet when this solitary life is combined with a group of other lives, the network of ideas and interactions that could be generated is staggering. A single action by an individual group member—rearranging his position on the chair, for example—could signify restlessness, agitation, back pain, hemorrhoids, a desire for attention, postural difficulties, a need for increased blood flow, or an itch. If that same person were to communicate with another in the group, with his eyes or gestures, not to mention the possible variations of his voice, the effects would ripple like waves through the minds of all those present. Each person would seek a personal interpretation of the action and would respond to the stimulus both internally and externally. And it is the leader's task to sift through the confusing assortment of often conflicting stimuli, to attend to those that have relevance to the present situation and goals, to make sense of and give meaning to the behavior, to predict likely consequences, and, finally, to act therapeutically in the best interests of those who are present.

The group leader must not only have mastered basic counseling technology but must also understand dynamics and assumptions as they are applied to group behavior. Initially, each client comes to the group with different expectations, interests, and goals. The most basic assumption about groups, therefore, is that there are often discrepancies among the participants' hopes and expectations and even between those of the leaders and the members. Coalitions are formed on the basis of these common interests and backgrounds and often on the basis of perceived similarities in attitudes, abilities, or attractiveness. The leader may be viewed as the "outsider," as a function of his or her expert role, or possibly as the only "insider," because the counselor alone really knows what is going on during the beginning sessions.

Assuming a diversity of expectations helps the group leader to plan for and permit the realization of individual goals that are compatible with the flexible structure. Individual members are thus helped to clarify their reasons for attending the group and encouraged to set specific goals that may be realistically attained during the time allotted.

> LEADER: Before I discuss some ideas regarding what options are available for you in this group and how we can spend our time, let's hear from some of you as to why you decided to come.
>
> ELKA: I didn't decide to come. My parents threatened to ground me for the semester unless I agreed to try this a few times. They think I'm too young to get married; I don't.
>
> NANDO: I heard that this was a good place to meet girls. I could always use a few new ladies in my life.
>
> BETH: I've got some problems at work—I don't know what to do. I was hoping to get some advice.
>
> FRED: Too much booze. Every day. I want to stop. Maybe y'all can help me.

Another assumption about therapeutic groups to which most (but not all) practitioners would subscribe is that the leader is not a participant of the group but a trained expert. Efforts are thus devoted to keeping the focus on the members, avoiding self-indulgent excesses, and generally staying in the role of paid professional who does not deliberately use group time for self-serving purposes.

CASSANDRA: Oh wise one, you always sit here so omnipotent like you know everything about anything. You are leading us, helping us. What are some of your problems? Why don't we help you?

LEADER: I do have lots of things I could work on in this group—my impatience, my overdriving ambition—and I know that you are all skilled enough to help me; but I don't feel comfortable using your time to work on my concerns. I'm being paid to help you. I can go to another group (and I do occasionally) where I get help. Thanks for your concern, Cassandra. But did I hear you resenting the control you feel I have? Is that something you would like to work on, since your lack of control has been an issue before?

For group work to be successful, or even to get off the ground, there must be an atmosphere of trust. Even more so than in individual sessions, the issue of confidentiality must be directly addressed so that it is clearly understood that all communication within the group is to be private and secure. Actually, there is no way confidentiality can ever be guaranteed or enforced in a group setting, for members are not legally bound to comply with any particular codes. Inadvertent breaches of trust can also occur, destroying the hard-won confidence. It is for these reasons that the leader openly, forcefully, and explicitly discusses the issue.

HECTOR: Why should I ever spill my guts here? I don't know you people. How can I believe anyone is trustworthy if I don't know them?

LEADER: Your point is a good one. There is a risk involved in being open, in this group or anywhere else. You should therefore pace yourself so that you disclose only what you feel ready to share. You will have to trust your own instincts on this. But remember, the degree to which you risk is related to how much you grow. Let's work on some situations that could test your confidential oath and discuss how they might be handled. What would you say, for instance, if your best friend asked what's going on in your group? What are you permitted to talk about outside the group? And what are some of your fears about what would occur if someone in here did tell others what you said?

In counseling groups, perhaps even more than in individual sessions, client discomfort is often associated with change. The very structure of a group environment, with its active audience, stimulates approval seeking, fear of failure, peer pressure, and other forces that do little to help the client feel at ease. This phenomenon isn't necessarily undesirable. A "healthy" amount of discomfort can motivate a person to get off dead center, to reduce dissonance, to make changes, and to restore equilibrium. As risk taking in a group accelerates, with members sharing their feelings, admitting inadequacies, and confronting themselves and one another, there are direct pressures from other members (which are usually held in check by the leader to protect individual rights) and subtle pressures from within to conform to the risky norm. Some begin to squirm as they watch others grow, leaving them behind. The more they hang back and remain passive, the more dissatisfied they become with their present ineffective functioning. The only way to reduce their discomfort is to leave the group (which sometimes happens if the leader doesn't carefully monitor readiness levels of each participant) or to make needed changes in themselves.

MONICA: This is the eighth session and I know I haven't said much, but I'm just not all that good at talking in front of groups.

STEPHEN: As long as you believe that crap, you don't have to do anything else. Just sit there and watch us sweat. I'm tired of you getting a free ride.

LEADER: [Interrupting Monica before she can defend herself]: Back off, Steve. Your point is well taken, even if you put it so harshly. Monica, before you answer him, what's going on inside your head?

MONICA: Just that maybe he's right. I wish I could get involved, but I'm too scared. And yet I hate coming here because I can't open up. I tried to stay home. But I can't do that either. Then I'd really feel like a chicken. I'm so confused; I just don't know what to do.

LEADER: How did you feel about what Steve said?

MONICA: I think he—

LEADER [POINTS TOWARD STEVE]: Talk to him.

MONICA: Ah, I don't know. . . . OK Steve, I think you're a bastard and you tried to hurt me. You didn't have to be so cruel about it. I heard what you said, but I didn't like the way you said it.

LEADER: Now we're off and running.

Much of the growth in groups occurs through observation, identification, modeling, imitation, and other social-learning processes that are often not found in individual sessions. There are opportunities to watch the leader in action, presumably an expert in social-interactive skills, a model of the fully functioning person. The leader disperses wisdom or settles disputes with Solomon-like grace. The leader articulates metaphors and speeches worthy of a Shakespearean soliloquy. The leader orchestrates behavior, structures situations, organizes, takes charge. The leader radiates warmth and kindness and enthusiasm. And, all the while, the others watch carefully, nodding to themselves when they see something they like, consciously selecting behaviors for their own repertoire, captive to the power and force of the leader's personality.

A client also learns while watching peers struggle with their concerns. Every presented problem is internalized by the attentive audience, adapted to their particular lives. Clients learn from one another's successes and failures.

ORLANDO: Last week, Gianina, when you were talking about how bored you were being a housewife, I was at first bored listening to you. I mean, what could I get out of your situation? My problem is that I'm too busy. I have too much work to do. Then I realized that, although our styles are different, we are both hiding from the same thing.

GIANINA: I don't understand. Your life is far from boring. I stayed a housewife, until last week anyway, because I was afraid to venture out.

ORLANDO: Exactly. And I keep myself so occupied so I don't have to deal with myself and confront how boring I feel I really am.

LEADER: Who else identified with Gianina's concerns last week?

Groups provide many opportunities for realistic rehearsal of new behaviors. Much of what constitutes the permanent acquisition of new learning involves not only the observation of desired behaviors but also the opportunity to practice skills under supervision. Clients spend a good portion of their time applying what they have learned in the laboratory. They can experiment and refine interaction skills and social behaviors. They can take risks or confront others and, afterwards, receive constructive feedback. Before they venture out into the world to wrestle with a problem, they can first use other group members to help rehearse their performance.

LEADER: Okay Jerry, who in the group most reminds you of your family members? Let's role play the disaster you expect to occur when you get home tonight. Maybe we can even give you some ideas on how to handle it.

JERRY: Well, Brenda for sure reminds me of my mother. No, Brenda—I mean you're both are so calm and relaxed.

LEADER: Don't apologize—just choose your characters.

JERRY: Okay. I guess Joe would be good to play my dad. But act real gruff. Grunt a lot and don't look at me when you talk. That's right. Also fidget more. Perfect. Patty, you can be my older sister. But you have to act confident but aloof. And, Louis, you're crazy enough to be my older brother. I guess that's it. Unless someone wants to be my dog.

LEADER: All right, now set the stage and program everyone the way they would normally act. Then you enter the scene and we'll see what happens. We will periodically stop the action, analyze what you did or didn't do, and give you some helpful suggestions. Perhaps we should even add a helper: Nancy will be your alter ego. Every time you are evasive or wishy-washy or back down, she will say aloud what you really want to say. Ready? Lights, camera, action!

The structure and ambience of therapeutic groups are well suited to working on interpersonal conflicts. The arrangement of chairs in a circle encourages direct communication among all as equals. If particular members make eye contact only with the leader while talking, that behavior is quickly extinguished. Constructive confrontations are stressed 'by encouraging the open and honest expression of feelings toward one another. Members are also helped to communicate and offer feedback sensitively and empathetically while they are taught to hear and interpret personal messages nondefensively.

# GROUP PROCESS STAGES

Each group goes through four or five distinct process stages that require a specific focus and agenda beyond the individual goals of each member (Corey & Corey, 2000; Gladding, 2003; Kottler, 2001). Even with minimal group training, you will find it instructive, if not amusing, to watch the underlying dynamics and stages of any group unfold, whether that takes place at a family dinner, party, committee meeting, or counseling group. It is important to keep in mind, however, that like in any developmental process, stages are often not

VOICE FROM THE FIELD

It sometimes seems so magical to me the way a group transforms itself. You walk in the first day and everyone is so cautious and nervous. You wonder to yourself how you're ever going to get these people to trust one another. The whole task seems overwhelming.

I think to myself how many times I've been through this before. I've run hundreds of groups and I can't think of a single one—okay, maybe only one or two—in which something amazing didn't happen.

It starts out so awkwardly. Everyone is careful and polite, or in some cases, really insensitive. I'm the leader, the one supposed to be running the show, but I often feel like it's out of my hands, too. The group process itself, especially if it's structured right, seems to act with a life of its own to build the kind of safety that everyone needs to get some work done. I watch this with wonder. I try to make it happen—I even think I'm the one who is making it happen. But that is delusional. The group members make it happen, if I've set things up in a way that trust becomes possible.

---

linear and as predictable as we might hope. Under conditions of stress or transition, a group, like an individual, may regress or experience oscillations in patterns (Rubenfeld, 2001).

**Forming Stage**   A group begins before its first session. Recruitment and screening take place in which members are often prepared for the group, informed of what to expect, and helped to get ready for the first meeting. Whether this orientation takes place during a pregroup meeting, individual consultations, or in an introductory letter, members still begin thinking and anticipating what to expect.

If a few group members know each other prior to the first meeting, then they are likely to have discussions sharing their perceptions and anticipatory feelings. The leader or leaders (when possible, coleading is certainly preferred), as well, spend considerable time talking about what they want to do, how they want to proceed, what problems they expect, and how they imagine various group members will get along.

The point to remember, whether in group work or any form of counseling, is that the treatment actually begins long before clients walk in the door. For most people, the decision to join a group involves a long struggle before action is finally taken. Lots of internal dialogue probably takes place, as well as conversations with loved ones. By the time clients actually show up for the first group meeting, they have already been doing quite a bit of work, some of it constructive, some of it more anxiety provoking. Keep this in mind before you make assumptions about where people are before you have checked them out.

**Initial Stage**   The beginning stage is the time when introductions are made, the purpose is determined, ground rules are established, and trust issues are initially explored. The beginning stage can be as short as a few minutes—

when the agenda is clear and trust is high—or as long as two or three sessions when more material regarding trust and comfort needs to be resolved.

The initial stage is about not only building trust but also establishing norms that are likely to be helpful throughout the tenure of the group. Participants have some ideas about what is expected, but many of these beliefs are misguided. They may engage in a lot of approval seeking and vie for attention. They may think that being a good group member means being "nice" all the time, but avoiding being honest or confrontive. At this stage it is important for group members to establish and enforce group norms that they believe are optimal to accomplishing desired goals. The leader must provide the right amount of structure at this stage so the group can accomplish process goals and move to the next stage.

**Transition Stage**    There are a number of critical incidents and predictable problems that come up in most groups—mostly signs of resistance or confusion (Conyne, Rapin, & Rand, 1997; Donigian & Malnati, 1999). Between the time when members are first getting to know one another and getting down to some serious work, there is a period of transition. You can recognize this stage by a number of signs: long silences, demands for leader structure, expressions of discomfort or anxiety, someone acting out as a distraction, prolonged conflict, or even attacks on the leader (Gladding, 2003).

If these critical incidents are processed in a constructive manner and members are helped to own, express, and deal with their fears, wonderful things often follow. The mood of the group changes from one in which people only pat one another on the back to one in which it is safer to disagree respectfully, to confront constructively, and to experiment with more freedom and flexibility that is necessary if real work is to take place.

**Working Stage**    In a healthy, high-functioning group it is safe to focus on deeper issues and to interact in new ways. During this stage, members work on specific issues, confront inconsistencies, explore issues, and share personal material. The leader must attend to the individual member on whom the group is focused as well as the overall interaction patterns and attitudes within the group. This is a most challenging assignment and one that often requires two leaders to do best, especially when you are first learning to do group work (Hazler, Stanard, Conkey, & Granello, 1997; Kottler, 1994b).

A number of signs and symptoms tell you that you are well into the working stage:

- When there is good movement from one member to another with almost everyone participating
- When there is less reliance on the leader(s) to direct and structure things
- When individuals are accomplishing their stated personal goals
- When cohesion, intimacy, and trust are operating at consistently high levels
- When game playing, conflicts, and acting out behaviors are labeled, confronted, and worked through successfully

◼ | VOICE FROM THE FIELD

It was awesome what I learned about groups as part of my training. And I'm not talking about job-related stuff, although that was certainly important. I'm talking about the dynamics of groups—you know, the way people behave predictably in certain situations.

I used to hate going to family get-togethers. At best they were boring and at worst I'd go home with a stomachache from all the tension. Dysfunctional family and all that. Then when I learned about group behavior and process, I became a student of the way my family—and all groups for that matter—act. I'd watch people at staff meetings. I especially loved watching my classes. It was amazing to me that the same stages and dynamics I was reading about I could actually see unfolding before my various eyes. You know, you look around the room and you see the same group member roles that are talked about in the books—the monopolizer, the ass kisser, the one who is distracting and off-the-wall. It's all there if you just pay attention to what's going on.

---

- • When self-disclosure, constructive risk taking, and sharing are high
- • When it appears as if people are making consistent progress in their sensitivity and responsiveness to one another

Of course, these particular behavioral signs are indicative not only of a group in the working stage but really of any group at any stage that is high functioning in terms of its process and productivity.

**Closing Stage.**   The final stage allows the group members to assess what they have learned, discuss plans for change, and explore their feelings about the experience. In this stage, members attempt to resolve unfinished issues within the group, evaluate the performance of the group, and say good-bye and deal with ending issues. This stage generally takes anywhere from one to several sessions. Its primary purpose is to help members to keep their momentum going after the group ends.

Counselors should be familiar with the stages and group process issues so they can structure sessions to facilitate movement through each stage. Although group process is important, the group counselor should remember that the one primary purpose of the group is individual work and growth so as not to allow process variables to dominate group time. In many groups members have a good time, do lots of process work with one another, but don't necessarily change the target behaviors that landed them in treatment in the first place. The smooth movement through each stage will maximize individual opportunity for growth within the group.

## High-Functioning Groups

Successful groups are those that make their way through the various stages in such a way that their needs are met and that distinct and consistent progress is made. Furthermore, it is important not only that the content objectives and desired goals are met but also that the process is relatively smooth and constructive. You have attended meetings in your life, or participated in certain groups, in which they may have been very efficient gatherings that quickly reached the declared goals. Yet you (and others) left the experience feeling badly about what happened. Perhaps people's rights were trampled, or individuals were not fully heard and respected, or the discussion felt unfinished.

On the other hand, you have attended groups in which the process was lovely. Everyone had a good time. Each person felt honored and understood. There was good will among all. The problem, however, was that very little work was completed and very few items on the agenda were worked through. In some cases, it may very well be the process that is far more important than the content or formal objectives. But in other situations, a balance must be reached between the two. High-functioning groups are often both process- and content-oriented. They can be both efficient in meeting stated goals, and yet still attend to the participants' experience in such a way that interactions are satisfying and constructive.

Several other indications are important in evaluating whether a group experience is high-functioning or not (Kottler, 2001):

1. Do members feel safe? Are people supported? Has trust been established to the point where people are willing to take constructive risks?
2. To what extent are differences respected and honored? Each group will include a great variety of cultural, value, gender, political, and personal beliefs. Yet there is often pressure to conform to the majority. Are people's different worldviews respected?
3. Have constructive norms been established and clear boundaries enforced? Good groups need rules around appropriate behavior (coming late, missing sessions, interrupting, etc.). People have to know what is expected and they have to count on the rules being enforced consistently.
4. How is conflict acknowledged and worked through? High-functioning groups do not avoid conflict but seek to deal with the underlying issues. Such disagreements can be helpful if dealt with in therapeutic ways.
5. How are resources shared? Is there reasonable distribution of contributions or are sessions dominated by only a few members? The best groups are those in which everyone feels a part of what is going on.
6. How are distractions, digressions, and acting out handled? It is a certainty that some members will say and do things that may not fit with what is going on. Chaos will ensue if these behaviors are not redirected. Good leaders know how to redirect the focus in such a way that things remain on task yet without humiliating the person(s) who need feedback.
7. Is there follow-up and follow-through? It is not nearly enough to have a high-functioning session unless it results in some sort of action. It is crucial to follow up on each participant to make sure they are doing what they say they will do, and what they need to do.

# CUES FOR INTERVENTION

Although a group leader's behavior involves a degree of intuition, artistry, and feeling for the situation, there are some fairly specific instances in which therapeutic intervention is almost always necessary. In individual sessions the counselor relies heavily on "gut wisdom" but also knows that, when a client becomes self-deprecating or self-deceptive or drifts from reality, an intervention is called for. Group situations contain a virtual overload of stimuli to attend to. The most difficult task, therefore, is to describe not just how and when to intervene but with whom. A leader's behavior can be at best distracting or at worst destructive if ill-timed or inappropriately directed. For these reasons, even the beginning student ought to become familiar with the minimally prescribed instances that signal therapeutic action (Kottler, 1994b).

## Abusive Behavior

Without exception or qualification, in the event that it can be determined that the physical safety or emotional welfare of any participant is in danger, the leader must intervene. Much of the research on casualties in group work supports the idea that the leader should take responsibility for protecting client safety (Lieberman, Yalom, & Miles, 1973). This can be done only by carefully monitoring each member for cues of internal distress, as well as by keeping a close eye on group interactions to ensure that verbal abuse is minimized.

Usually, interactions that are hostile in their intent are quickly dissipated, or at least brought into the open to be dealt with in a relatively controlled manner. When a member is unaware of or insensitive to the negative effects generated by a comment or outburst, the leader also steps in to repair any damage. However, the vast majority of therapeutic efforts are directed toward heading off potential abuse before it occurs. With some experience, a leader can detect the signs of imminent explosive behavior and can therefore intervene before a fight or screaming match breaks out, in much the way that a skilled classroom teacher always knows when trouble is about to erupt.

## Rambling and Digressions

For any number of reasons—to avoid meaningful dialogue, to resist treatment, to play games, or often simply because a client is verbally disorganized—the flow of conversation will stray from anything of therapeutic value. Perhaps someone will tell a long-winded story with no direct relevance. Or another might interrupt proceedings to prove some obscure point. Or there is a client (as inevitably there has been in every group I have ever known) who is just scatterbrained. His or her interjections can be maddening, interrupting a meaningful silence, badgering the leader with questions intended to win approval, or breaking into every interaction with the preface, "That reminds me of the time. . ."

Whether the group member's ramblings are mildly inconvenient or downright pathological, the leader will usually establish some norm for appropriate input. Initially, interventions are used subtly to play down digressive comments and reinforce those that are on target. Sometimes the interventions must be more direct. For Cindy, a client who is particularly prone to digressions, the leader may finally cue feedback to indicate when comments aren't appropriate: "Jacob, was it helpful to hear what Cindy just said when she interrupted you? Oh. It wasn't? You wished she would wait until you were through?" and then, "Cindy, what feedback did you just hear?"

Providing such focused input and reactions can be among the most powerful and useful things that can happen in a group. So often in our lives we do and say things that are off-putting to others, but we rarely hear about it in direct ways. We are left to guess how people respond to us rather than relying on honest data. Yet groups can be invaluable for providing honest feedback, especially to those who so desperately need it the most and don't even know it.

## Withdrawal and Passivity

Often the effects of verbal abuse, needless rambling, or other factors internal to the client will result in withdrawal in one or more members. This is a situation that is particularly difficult to deal with: The leader wants to safeguard the right to privacy yet does not want clients to slip into complete passivity. Furthermore, withdrawal is not obvious; it is recognized only by an absence of behavior. The leader must identify individual patterns for each client in order to read signs of withdrawal in averting one's eyes, scooting back one's chair, answering in monosyllables, or acting in some other uncharacteristic manner. The counselor may decide to draw the person into the group directly ("You're not saying much today. What's going on inside your head?"), consult with the person after the group in a private conference, or even wait and let other members bring up the issue.

## Lethargy and Boredom

One function of the group leader is to spice up the learning experience to maintain participants' interest. After only a few sessions, a routine sets in that can become predictable or boring. The leader uses humor, spontaneous actions, dramatic gestures, and a playful spirit to keep things stimulating. Whenever yawning becomes prevalent, or monotonous voices, or behavior in which clients appear only to be going through the motions (which happens frequently), the leader intervenes.

> It is up to each one of you to accept responsibility for your own growth in this group. Usually when you are confronted with a repetitive episode or when you feel lazy, you are content to daydream or doodle, biding your time until the ordeal is over. However, when you feel your mind drifting away in here, as many of you were doing just now, you are cheating yourself of a potentially valuable experience. It is too easy to write off the times you aren't intensely involved in what is

happening. You are in this group because you wish to learn to be more focused in the present, to enjoy each moment to its fullest. Why not begin now? Throughout the rest of this session, and those thereafter, when you catch yourself feeling restless or bored, force yourself to focus on what is going on. There is always so much to attend to, even if you find a particular discussion uninteresting. Watch the reactions of the others—how they are responding nonverbally to what they are hearing. Notice what I am doing or not doing and what my rationale might be. And closely scrutinize your own internal behavior. When you drift away, what are you hiding from? There is never a legitimate excuse for feeling bored in this group.

## Semantic Errors

Depending on theoretical preferences and linguistic sensitivity, every counselor has a list of favorite semantic errors to pounce on. Language is the principal evidence we have of a client's thought patterns; how a person speaks aloud and expresses ideas—the choice and arrangement of words—accurately indicate how that person thinks and feels about his or her situation. Group leaders will intervene when clients distort reality, exaggerate, or use illogical communications. A facilitator versed in the client-centered approach may correct participants by asking them to change "I think" to "I feel." Cognitive counselors would interrupt members when they express themselves with "I must" or "I should," asking them instead to substitute more accurate verbalizations such as "I may" or "I could." And a follower of neurolinguistic programming techniques would correct variations that are incomplete in their surface structure. For example, "They made me do it" is converted from a statement having ambiguous referents to a complete communication: "Several of my elementary school teachers [they] made me play without making any kind of a mess [it]."

The leader of a group has the responsibility to understand, to relate, to facilitate, and to structure the interaction of the group members in a way that maximizes the therapeutic potential of the experience for all participants. This is a challenging and, at times, overwhelming task that demands the total energy and concentration of the group leader, who must be trained and skilled in individual and group-focused counseling skills.

# SPECIALIZED SKILLS OF GROUP WORK

Working with groups requires the use of numerous techniques in addition to those used in individual counseling. Some practitioners are reluctant to lead counseling groups because of their anxiety over the responsibilities and techniques needed to function effectively. To some extent, inadequate preparation is the result of limited training in group leadership, and counselor educators have expressed concern over the teaching of group counseling skills and abilities (Dye, 1980). One of the main challenges has to do with the kinds of emotional material that is elicited, the performance anxiety, that come up as a result of learning group leadership experientially (Bemak & Epp, 2001; Christensen & Kline, 2001; Kottler, 2001).

Another area of difficulty has to do with the kinds of group leadership skills that must be mastered in order to work effectively in this setting. While many of these skills are similar to what you would do in individual sessions (reflective listening, confronting, interpreting, questioning, goal setting, giving feedback, and so on), other skills are somewhat unique to group practice. At the very least, generic therapeutic skills must be adapted considerably for group settings and the multiple participants involved. In fact, one of the interesting things that happens is that, over time, group member begin using the skills the same as they interact with others both in session and in their lives.

An overview of some common group leadership skills may be summarized as follows (Corey, 2000; Dyer & Vriend, 1975; Nolan, 1978):

*Active listening.* Just as you would in individual sessions, you must attend to verbal and nonverbal communications that arise in sessions and help other participants to do the same. This is what helps to build trust, facilitate deeper exploration, and encourage greater self-disclosure.

*Paraphrasing.* Again, not unlike what you would do with an individual client, you frequently let group members know that they have been heard and understood accurately. Whereas the previous skill focuses on affective dimensions, this skill attends to content of communication. If you are successful in modeling these behaviors, you will notice other group members begin to use them as well.

*Summarizing.* Periodically, throughout any session, you will want to help members to take stock of where they are. This also gives greater focus and direction to how things proceed.

*Questioning.* This involves drawing out additional material and data that is needed to understand a situation. Ideally, "open" questions are asked, or the kind that don't come across as interrogating. At times you will have to step in and stop members from using this skill too much as there may be an over-reliance on probing too much.

*Interpreting.* This is where you offer alternative explanations for what might be going on. The intent is to expand group members' perceptions and understanding.

*Confronting.* This skill is especially important in groups but must be handled in different ways so that people do not feel humiliated or censured. The best sorts of confrontations are those that come from other members, rather than the leader, so this is another skill you want to teach to others. Basically, you are challenging people to look at themselves and discrepancies in their behavior.

*Supporting.* This involves providing encouragement as it is needed. There are times when members begin struggling and may need help to work through the impasses. You want to communicate consistently that the atmosphere is safe in groups, that people will not be left to struggle on their own.

*Facilitating.* In order to promote open communication between members, it is your job to encourage people to talk to one another. One way you do this is by directing people to talk to one another instead of just to you.

*Initiating.* Groups need more structure and direction than individual sessions. You must intervene to increase or decrease the pace of what is going on, to introduce new directions, or to prevent a waste of time.

*Setting goals.* More so than in individual counseling, you must focus on helping each member work on personally declared goals. Otherwise, it is easy for people to get lost in the crowd.

*Giving feedback.* As with the other skills, it is preferable to get other members to do the work rather than you having to be the one to initiate things. This is where you help people to hear honest reactions as to how they are perceived.

*Suggesting.* You may have situations when you will offer advice, information, or directions for new behavior. Be careful not to do this too much or members will follow your lead and start telling people what to do.

*Protecting.* Remember your job is to keep members safe from harm. This skill involves protecting people against attacks and against unnecessary risks.

*Disclosing.* In order to encourage group members to reveal personal material you may model this behavior. Be careful not to be excessive or self-indulgent as this skill is often overused.

*Linking.* This skill involves making connections between group members—building further cohesion and shared intimacy.

*Blocking.* You must intervene during times when someone is being hurtful, disrespectful, or inappropriate.

## Special Training

The skills just described are absolutely critical to help groups proceed effectively and to deal with critical incidents that will inevitably arise (Donigian & Malnati, 1999). This would include situations when members gang up to attack the leader, when there is mass denial or a mutual conspiracy among members to avoid real issues, when a member abruptly decides to leave the group, when a member withdraws, or when any of the other cues for intervention mentioned in the previous section occur. In addition, group leaders need a thorough understanding of individual counseling methods and theory, a solid grounding in group dynamics and behavior, and good planning, organizational, and conflict-resolution skills (Jacobs, Masson, & Harvill,1998; Kline, 2003). In addition, perhaps more than any other treatment approach, group leadership requires an extraordinarily high degree of intuition and creativity in order to go with the flow and respond quickly to the ever-changing circumstances (Forester-Miller & Gressard, 1997; Gladding, 2003; Kottler & Markos, 1997). This means adapting the concepts and skills you have already learned to fit the specialized needs of various client populations and group contexts (Capuzzi, 2003; Capuzzi & Gross, 2002).

It is for all these reasons that you will receive specialized training in group leadership as part of your counselor education. Ideally, you will have the opportunity to study the various approaches to group dynamics and leadership, to experience a therapeutic group as a client in order to work on personal issues, and, finally, to receive supervised experience as a coleader of a group. After you have completed this sequence of training, you will likely find group leadership among the most invigorating, powerful, and satisfying professional experiences possible—not only for your clients but for yourself as well.

# SUMMARY

Counseling in groups represents a powerful and economical strategy for counselors to deliver services in a variety of settings. Group work is especially effective because it more closely simulates social interactions and interpersonal communication patterns than does individual counseling. At the same time, group work is more demanding of the counselor, who has a much more complex task in both structuring the effective development of the group and accepting the responsibility for the growth of multiple clients. Specialized training and supervision are essential so that counselors can learn to use group-focused skills effectively and include group work as a part of their professional activities.

# SELF-GUIDED EXPLORATIONS

1. Describe an experience you have had as a member of a group of some kind in which you felt some attachment (encounter group, study group, discussion group, counseling group, etc.). What factors are you aware of that operated in that group that made it especially helpful to you?
2. Think of a group in your life that you are currently part of. Describe the characteristic roles you play in this group (rescuer, placater, consensus-seeker, rebel, leader, etc.).
3. Look at your behavior in one of your classes right now. How do you imagine that you are perceived by your peers and instructor? Ask two or three other students for honest feedback regarding your interpersonal style. Ask them specifically for one thing you do that they especially appreciate and one thing that pushes them away. Discuss your reactions to the feedback, including how it coincides with your self-perceptions.
4. What are the group dynamics, stages, and processes that you observe unfolding in this class?
5. Imagine that you are leading some type of counseling group. What are some aspects of that prospect that frighten you the most? What are some of your personal strengths that you hope to bring to the group experience?

## For Homework:

Make plans to join some type of growth group as a participant. If that's not feasible for you at this time, then arrange to observe a group in action. If you should have difficulty obtaining permission to view groups (observers are ob-trusive), then find alternative opportunities to view group dynamics within human organizations, movies, television shows, families, or work settings.

Pay particular attention to leadership style—what you notice works best and least. If possible, talk to the group leaders afterwards to get their reactions and impressions of what took place. Write down what you learned from the experience.

## SUGGESTED READINGS

Corey, G. (2000). *Theory and practice of group counseling.* Pacific Grove, CA: Brooks/Cole.

Corey, M. S., & Corey, G. (2002). *Groups: Process and practice* (6th ed.). Pacific Grove, CA: Brooks/Cole.

Gazda, G. M., Ginter, E. J., & Horne, A. M. (2001). *Group counseling and group psychotherapy.* Boston: Allyn & Bacon.

Gladding, S. (2003). *Group work: A counseling specialty* (4th ed.). Englewood Cliffs, NJ: Merrill.

Jacobs, E. E., Masson, R. L., & Harvill, R. (2002). *Group counseling: Strategies and skills* (4th ed.). Pacific Grove, CA: Brooks/Cole.

Johnson, D. W., & Johnson, F. P. (2003). *Joining together: Group theory and group skills.* Boston: Allyn & Bacon.

Kline, W. B. (2003). *Interactive group counseling and therapy.* Upper Saddle River, NJ: Prentice Hall.

Kormanski, C. (1999). *The Team: Explorations in Group Processes.* Denver: Love.

Kottler, J. A. (2001). *Learning group leadership: An experiential approach.* Boston: Allyn & Bacon.

Shapiro, J. L., Peltz, L. S., & Bernadett-Shapiro, S. (1998). *Brief group treatment: Practical training for therapists and counselors.* Pacific Grove, CA: Brooks/Cole.

Yalom, I. (1995). *The theory and practice of group psychotherapy* (4th ed.). New York: Basic Books.

# 10

# MARITAL, FAMILY, AND SEX COUNSELING

## KEY CONCEPTS

Family system

Circular causality

Differentiation of self

Joining

Structural approach

Strategic approach

Symmetrical relationship

Complementary relationship

Boundaries

Hierarchy of power

Structural map

Identified client

Symptoms as solutions

Symptoms as metaphors

Genogram

Reframing

Externalizing

Forcing the spontaneous

Pretending

Emotional engagement

Sensate focus exercises

# MARITAL, FAMILY, AND SEX COUNSELING

It has been said that all counseling is, in fact, family counseling, because working with one person to change behavior cannot help affecting the feelings, attitudes, and behavior of others with whom the person lives. Whether the other family members are actually in attendance or not, they will most certainly be influenced by what happens in counseling sessions. For this reason, working with family members together is considered by many clinicians to be more humane, efficient, responsible, and realistic than individual counseling.

What was once an obscure specialty for radical social workers has become mainstream counseling for practitioners of all disciplines who seek to initiate changes through the involvement of those persons who wield a significant influence in the client's life. Since psychiatrists, psychologists, educators, counselors, and social workers have joined forces under the American Association for Marital and Family Therapy (AAMFT), an influential and relatively cohesive movement has developed. More recently, other organizations such as the International Association of Marriage and Family Counselors (IAMFC) have evolved as well, contributing specialized training standards, credentialing, and ethical codes for family practitioners.

## FAMILY VERSUS INDIVIDUAL COUNSELING

Family counseling bears some similarity to group counseling in that the systemic dynamics are as important as individual behavior. The field, however, has carved out a distinctly unique niche in its theory, research, practice, and distinct way of approaching a helping relationship (see Table 10.1). When compared to individual counseling, family work is different in a number of ways (Becvar & Becvar, 2003; Nichols & Schwartz, 2001):

1. Family practitioners view problems as located not within the individual but within the larger context of interactions between people.
2. Clinicians must generally be more active, directive, and controlling than they would be in individual sessions.
3. Rarely can the counselor afford the luxury of operating from one theoretical approach. Family practitioners tend to be very pragmatic and flexible.
4. Focus is directed toward organizational structures and natural developmental processes that are part of all family systems. This includes attention to family rules, norms, and coalitions.
5. A model of circular rather than linear causality is favored. This means that when determining the causes of events or behaviors, it is important to look at the bigger picture of how each person's actions become causes and effects of everyone else's behavior.
6. Developmental models are employed that describe the family life cycle, including predictable and natural transitions, crises, and conflicts.
7. Rather than a single notion of "family" structure, counselors recognize that multiple versions are common, depending on the dominant culture. More often than not, any clients will be members of a nontraditional structure: a blended family of stepparents and children, a single-parent household, a dual-career family, a cohabiting heterosexual or homosexual couple.

What should be clear is that family counseling involves additional training and specialization. Many of the skills and theories that you learned previously about doing individual counseling also fit when doing family counseling, just as they do with all group work. You would probably not be surprised to learn, for example, that all the disagreements among counselors about the best way to do counseling in general also apply to family specialists. Nevertheless, in spite of the disagreements about whether to do insight- or action-oriented family work; whether to stay in the present or the past; whether to focus on feelings, thoughts, or behavior; whether to concentrate on the presenting symptoms or underlying issues; whether to work with one or two members or the whole extended family, there is some consensus about some universal knowledge and skills to master.

Almost all family practitioners would agree, for example, that in order to attain a degree of competence in this type of work you must have specialized

TABLE 10.1 | DIFFERENCES BETWEEN INDIVIDUAL AND FAMILY COUNSELING

| Individual Counseling | Family Counseling |
|---|---|
| Asks "why" questions | Asks "what" questions |
| Linear cause-effect | Reciprocal causality |
| Subject-object dualism | Holistic |
| Either/or dichotomies | Dialectical |
| Value-free science | Subjective |
| Deterministic | Freedom of choice |
| Historical focus | Present-oriented |
| Individualistic | Relational |
| Reductionistic | Contextualistic |
| Absolutistic | Relativistic |

*Source:* Becvar, D. S. & Becvar, R. J. (2003). *Family therapy: A systemic integration* (5th ed.). Boston: Allyn & Bacon.

training in family systems dynamics, family theories, family interventions, and professional/ethical issues unique to this practice. Given the increasing popularity of this modality, it is likely you will have at least one and probably more courses dedicated to family counseling practices; if not, consult a basic textbook on the subject such as Carlson & Kjos (2001), Gladding (2001), Goldenberg & Goldenberg (2002), or Nichols & Schwartz (2001). You will also wish to supplement this basic education with additional training and supervision because family counseling has all the challenges of individual and group counseling, *plus* you have the added burden that everyone is related to one another and so comes with a history of interactions you have not been privy to. As if this doesn't seem daunting enough, consider that one or more family members are often working actively to sabotage any of your therapeutic efforts. It is for this reason you need a solid grounding in family theory, research, and practice.

## FAMILY COUNSELING THEORIES

Like everything else in this field, there is a tremendous diversity in the ways in which family counselors operate. Similar to the approaches we explored in the chapters on counseling theory, various counseling systems can be organized according to their basic perspectives (Gehart & Tuttle, 2003; Goldenberg & Goldenberg, 1999; Nichols & Schwartz, 2001). Thus, some approaches examine underlying family structures or patterns of communication, while others fo-

## VOICE FROM THE FIELD

One idea I've used over and over is the notion of developmental struggles, that every family, no matter how healthy, still will face certain challenges. When I see a couple, for instance, and they are agonizing because their adolescent is acting out, it is just so useful to explain how, developmentally, this is perfectly normal. I have favorite stories I tell about how important it is for adolescents to rebel. That's how they become individuals with their own values. They need to create disturbances in order to separate. At least that's true in white, middle-class homes. I know with other cultures, it's often a different story altogether.

cus more on dysfunctional thinking or behavior, and still others concentrate on the individual issues with which family members struggle.

As you would expect, some family counselors (Nathan Ackerman, James Framo) employ a psychoanalytic model. They deal with unresolved conflicts of the past, looking especially at family of origin issues. Also expected are some approaches (Virginia Satir, Carl Whitaker) that are humanistic in their orientation. They remain in the present as much as possible and examine issues of freedom and choices. Likewise, cognitive approaches to family counseling (Robert Liberman, Richard Stuart) that emphasize the same kinds of maladaptive behaviors that are present in individual counseling.

In addition to these familiar models that have been adapted to family settings, several unique theories were designed only for family work. Family systems theory (Murray Bowen) introduced the concepts of differentiation of self from the family. Structural family theory (Salvador Minuchin) looks at the ways that families become enmeshed and disengaged. Strategic approaches (Jay Haley, Cloe Madanes) look at alignments of power and communication in families. Psychodynamic family therapy explores family of origin issues as they shape current struggles (David Scharff), Milan theory (Mara Selvini-Palazzoli, Luigi Boscolo) introduced the paradoxes and games that families get caught in. Constructivist approaches (Michael White, Steve de Shazer) look at the ways that family narratives determine perceived reality. Finally, as you would expect, integrative models (Richard Schwartz, William Pinsoff) combine features of several other theories into a more encompassing framework.

The intent here is not to overwhelm you with a bunch of new names and concepts. At this point, I wouldn't worry too much about remembering anything other than the realization that family counseling is a very complicated field with a lot of interesting ideas that are helpful in unraveling the interactions that occur among people living together. As with each of the chapters in this book, which are intended to merely introduce you to the basic concepts, there will be plenty of time in later courses to master this material.

## VOICE FROM THE FIELD

Family counseling is hot stuff these days. I know counselors who even call themselves family counselors as their primary identity. In lots of ways, there are some very powerful things you can do with everyone together. But on the other hand, I've had some bad experiences too.

I remember one time I got the whole family in my office—the kids, the parents, even one of the grandparents—and it was total chaos. One kid was drawing on the wall. Another was punching her brother, who kept crying the whole time. The parents were screaming at one another. And grandma, she was gettin' in the act too. I just sat there with my mouth open, not knowing what to do.

Finally, I was able to regain some control—but not for long. I resolved, then and there, that if I was going to do this sort of work again, I was going to have to exert a lot more control on the proceedings. Now, whenever possible, I like to work with a cotherapist. Sometimes, though, that just isn't feasible and you've got to do it all yourself.

---

After studying the various family theories, you will be struck not only by how different they all seem, but also by the fact that they share some universal features. For beginners to the field in particular, it is useful at this point to understand that most family counselors agree on several areas:

1. Most family counselors rely on the same set of skills, such as "joining the family" or building rapport, assessing power hierarchies within the family system, restructuring coalitions among family members, reframing problems to make them more solvable, and engaging all members in resolving their difficulties.

2. All family counselors think in terms of social systems. Rather than viewing problems in terms of simple cause-effect relationships—that Mother causes Child to act out—they are seen in terms of circular causality: Chain reactions influence each family member, who in turn influences everyone else. For example, a mother becomes impatient because her daughter is slow getting dressed in the morning, making everyone late for work. The child feels pressured and resists the mother's efforts to control her. The father feels jealous because his wife is devoting so much attention to their child while ignoring him. He sabotages his wife's efforts to motivate the child. The mother feels angry at her husband for siding against her, withdrawing further. The child becomes even more obstinate, with more pressure applied by the increasingly exasperated mother. So who is causing the problem?

3. Family counselors, by and large, are more flexible, more active, and more structuring than practitioners of other treatment modalities. Because sessions can become so emotionally charged, things can rapidly get out of

hand if the counselor allows family members to become abusive, violent, or out of control. In addition, family practitioners focus more on the present than on the past, tend to be more didactic in their style, and are concerned primarily with patterns of communication.

Despite their similarities, each approach has distinctive features that permit the counselor to switch from one to the other according to the requirements of the situation. It is often desirable to begin structurally in order to diagnose, analyze, and test boundaries and rules, because this approach is more direct and comprehensible. They can move to strategic intervention once they have encountered resistance, defensiveness, or confusion. Then it may be effective to revert back to structural theory to pull together any loose ends. In this methodology, therefore, it is possible to think structurally and work strategically. By thinking structurally, the counselor is aware of various predictable patterns and styles that will commonly arise.

Of course, as with any form of counseling, whether in group, individual, or family contexts, success is often related to the quality of the alliance that has been developed with the participants. What has been emphasized previously applies equally well to family counseling: Any interventions and structural realignments take place only after a solid bond has been established where there is a sufficient degree of safety and trust.

## POWER IN RELATIONSHIPS

Relationships among family members can be *symmetrical* or *complementary*. The former, according to Haley (1976), has much competition, whereas the latter emphasizes reciprocal exchange as people maneuver for position and power. Minuchin (1974) introduces the notion of *boundaries* to describe how the various coalitions in family relationships tend to intersect. Sometimes, for example, the boundaries between parents and children are clearly defined and at other times an alignment may develop between mother and son, with a disengaged boundary between them and the father. Matters become considerably more complicated as the counselor joins the family system, creates different boundaries by manipulating the various coalitions, and finally restructures the system so that more constructive lines of affiliation develop.

Power within the family must also be carefully understood and balanced. Each family has a regimented hierarchy, within which each person has a specified amount of control and responsibility. Counseling often takes the form of reestablishing a single hierarchical organization in which the boundaries are more clearly delineated so that the parents are in charge and the children have less power.

Madanes (1983) records the case of a depressed man whose symptoms were treated by resolving the hierarchical incongruity in his marriage. The husband had previously been dominant in the relationship, but as the wife developed outside interests and a career as a therapist, his own life and business began to fail. The husband's depression became a source of power in the marriage because the wife, as a professional helper, could do nothing to bring re-

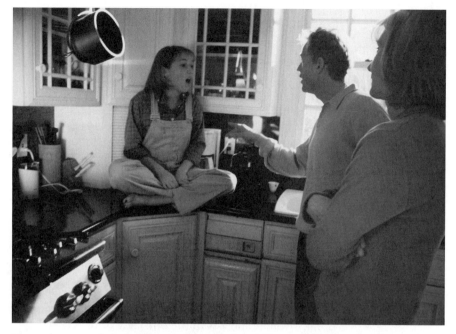

Counselors must help families to diffuse their conflicts and build on their resources to develop more constructive communication patterns. © Buccina Studios/Getty Images.

lief. The counselor's interventions focused on restoring a more balanced power hierarchy by reorganizing the way the couple dealt with each other. No longer useful as a form of one-upmanship, the depression vanished.

Balance of power between spouses can be viewed as a metaphor for other communications in the marriage. Consider a case in which the husband has all the power—in career, in decision making, in finances. The wife develops symptoms of depression. Husband tries to help but fails repeatedly. Husband becomes restricted in his own life by catering to wife. Wife indirectly controls husband and situation is reciprocal: Husband tells wife what to do about her life, then complains because she doesn't comply. Wife complains that husband is insensitive and can't or won't solve the problem. Both use power and helplessness, metaphors for submissiveness and rebellion.

Following is another example of the power struggles within a family. The counselor initially plots the family organization, then identifies the problems of each member, and finally develops a series of interventions.

FAMILY STRUCTURE

Mother is overinvolved with grandmother and daughter.

Grandmother and daughter have a friendly alliance.

Father and son have a weak and peripheral affiliation.

Father and mother are minimally involved.

FIGURE 10.1 | STRUCTURAL MAP OF FAMILY ORGANIZATION

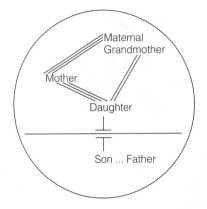

Father and son are both isolated from power in family.

Daughter and son are actively engaged in conflict.

Complete circle (Figure 10.1) represents a closed boundary separating the family from influences of the outside world.

FAMILY SYMPTOMOLOGY

*Son* is the identified client, who brought the family to counseling because of fighting at school and home.

*Father* is passive, withdrawn, uncommunicative, and depressed.

*Mother* is domineering, controlling, manipulative, and anxious.

*Father* and *mother* have marital problems; only son's acting out keeps them together.

*Grandmother* is lonely, isolated, and dependent on mother.

*Daughter* spends more time with *mother* and *grandmother* than with age mates; provokes her brother.

INITIAL THERAPEUTIC INTERVENTIONS

1. Solicit cooperation of mother, who is in control.
2. Build relationships with other family members and help them to tell their stories—and hear one another.
3. Rearrange coalitions with mother and father together against distracting influences of children and grandmother.
4. Invite father to take more power and control.
5. Strengthen bonds between mother and son, father and daughter, to equalize involvement.
6. Help grandmother to expand her social world. Help son to stop rescuing parents.
7. Open boundary isolating family from outside world.

VOICE FROM THE FIELD

Sometimes it's stunning how obvious the coalitions are in a family. I've designed my office in such a way that people have lots of choices in where they can sit. There's a couch along the back wall, another couch perpendicular to it, then several chairs scattered around. When a new family comes in for the first time, they arrange themselves in very revealing ways. Say, the mom and two kids sit on the couch, one on each side of her. The dad sits alone across the room. Now it may be mere coincidence but often this says a lot about who is aligned with whom. Here we have a father rather isolated and a mother enmeshed with her children. The first job I have, then, is to redirect the parents to sit together and the kids to sit together, sending a clear message about where the boundaries should be.

A child will often develop problems as a way to protect the parents from having to face their own difficulties. For example, the son in the family described here began to act out and became a common focus for the parents. In responding to the child's misbehavior, the parents were allowed to ignore their problem interaction pattern and the child felt powerful because he was keeping the family together. Although this intervention by the child kept the parents "together" in their interaction, it resulted in a serious family breakdown. As a counselor, you will often see families like this who present a "problem" child and view themselves as concerned parents who have no problems of their own. Counselors in a variety of settings observe this phenomenon, and it accounts for why even school counselors are now attempting more and more family counseling interventions (Davis, 2001; Evans & Carter, 1997; Ho, 2001).

## SYMPTOMS AS SOLUTIONS

Family systems analysis provides a larger context within which to view the problems of the identified client. Rather than approaching treatment with the usual intention of promoting individual insight and then helping the client to make specific changes, the family counselor often looks at the behavior of the disruptive family member as helpful or constructive in some regard. The disruptive behavior continues because it is unconsciously supported and maintained by others within the family system.

Haley (1980) suggests that counselors, particularly when working with severely disturbed adolescents, view the child's disruptive behavior as stabilizing the family structure. The child's behavior protects the parents from each other, forcing them to find solace in sharing their frustrations over the inability to control the unruly behavior. All family members, therefore, must be seen together to clarify the power and hierarchy structures. The family counselor's role is to help the parents regain control over themselves and the adolescent.

Haley finds it helpful when working with disruptive children to assume the following: (1) The client's symptoms are serving a protective function; (2) the client has the capacity to assume responsibility for disruptive behavior (and is not a victim of external forces); (3) the power hierarchy of the family is confused, with the "little" people controlling the "bigger" people; (4) the real problem is the family communication pattern, not the young person; and (5) once power is restored to the parents and the child is no longer permitted self-indulgence and failure—once the confusions, inconsistencies, and conflicts in family communications are cleared up—then the child can act more normally and responsibly without destabilizing the other family members.

When the child's destructive acting-out behavior is diagnosed as the solution to another, more important problem within the family, then interventions can be directed toward helping the parents to resolve their conflicts. Once the child's "help" is no longer needed, the child can then revert to more appropriate behavior to deal with his or her own internal conflicts.

This particular conception of symptoms as solutions certainly doesn't apply to all situations. In fact, those applying a more constructionist approach would try not to make very many assumptions about families and their problems until their own narratives are shared and understood. Some family therapies are more gender and culturally sensitive in their approach, looking at issues of power, sexual politics, and collaboration in very different ways (Hare-Mustin, 1978, 1994; Worden & Worden, 1998).

## CASE EXAMPLE OF FAMILY COUNSELING IN ACTION

The diagnosis and analysis of the interdynamics within a family, or even a couple's relationship, are often extremely complex. A 45-year-old salesman and his 40-year-old partner enter counseling to resolve a long-standing and increasingly frustrating problem between them. Although George can quite easily become erect during sexual foreplay, he quickly loses penile rigidity once he attempts to initiate intercourse with Joanne. The questions that come immediately to the mind of the counselor operating strategically within a family diagnostic structure are: "How is this particular problem of erectile dysfunction helping this couple?" "What solutions to another problem is the symptom offering?"

Naturally, some data collection and exploration are in order. The counselor learns in due course that George had nursed his cancer-ridden wife for a period of fifteen years, until her recent death, and suffers some residual guilt. Joanne, too, has had some life concerns. Her own romantic history is speckled by three failed marriages. Both Joanne and George are genuinely trying to create a loving, respecting relationship, and they care deeply for each other. Yet they are unable to proceed beyond their current impasse as long as their lovemaking is doomed to mutual frustration. Interestingly, however, George's "failure" occurs only with Joanne. In several attempts to test himself with prostitutes, he has found, to his relief, that he was easily able to consummate the sexual act.

What, then, do we know about this couple?

1. George's erectile problem is not organically caused, as evidenced by his awakening with morning erections and the occurrence of the problem only with Joanne.
2. George, as a salesman, has a high need for continual success to feel complete as a man. His area of greatest vulnerability is repeated failure at something—making a sale, for one thing, and, certainly, satisfying the woman he loves.
3. George still feels incredibly guilty about his failure to be a perfect nurse and husband to his dying wife. During the last three years of his wife's illness, he had a few sexual relationships, but only for physical relief.
4. The most difficult thing for Joanne to handle is the idea that she may not be attractive or sexy enough for George. Her anger and frustration are building as she realizes that an unknown prostitute can elicit sustained sexual arousal in George and she, his intimate friend, cannot do the same.
5. In their adult lives neither George nor Joanne has ever been able to sustain an intimate romantic involvement. Joanne forces relationships by pushing things too quickly; George has a desperate fear of losing control in relationships in which he would feel vulnerable.

Now the counselor can begin to help the couple put pieces of the puzzle together. What would be the likely consequence of solving this problem? The answer is: marriage.

Marriage is the one thing that both fear most. George still has unresolved guilt and feels the unconscious need to punish himself by not performing as he is capable. Joanne is desperately afraid that, once the relationship moves on to the next stage, it will certainly fall apart, as have all her other relationships. Yet as long as they remain at this current stage—admittedly locked in a frustrating dance—they can at least stay together. Their fears are temporarily displaced by focusing on the sexual problem.

Most of the traditional sex counseling techniques, of course, prove useless in eliminating a symptom that both partners unconsciously wish to continue. To remove much of the performance anxiety, the counselor tells them to do what they already can do—play in bed during foreplay—and not to worry about intercourse. They comply, and the inexplicable occurs: George can no longer become erect at all.

"It's as if this were the smartest penis in the world," the counselor explains to the couple. "It is so smart that, in spite of our best efforts to resolve this problem, your penis persists in figuring out ways to continue its stubborn unwillingness to cooperate. The lack of complete sexual fulfillment is actually helping both of you in the only way that could ever save your relationship in the long run. You are forced to slow down the pace of your relation ship. Because you can't relate sexually, you have to relate emotionally. You are spending hours together holding hands, hugging, talking. You are really developing intimacy before you can ruin the relationship by removing the sexual mystery.

"But that's not all. It is also permitting you, George, to pay for your guilt, or at least to work through your feelings. Yes, the problem provides you both with time to adjust to each other emotionally by restricting your sexual options."

George feels as if he has been saved! So he isn't a failure after all. Although he certainly doesn't believe that his penis has made decisions, he begins to recognize that he has, indeed, needed time to explore and develop a truly intimate relationship. He recognizes that subconsciously limiting his sexual activity is a way to force himself truly to know Joanne. She, too, feels relieved. Maybe it isn't her fault after all. She does agree that she feels closer to George than she has to any other man in her life. The reason is that the absence of sex has allowed them to become more alluring to each other. They feel more nurturing and caring than they could have with a normal sex life, because both have had so many other issues interfering with the development of intimacy along with active sex.

The counselor next instructs George and Joanne to appreciate each other by talking about all they have gained from each other. Now they can finally relax and enjoy each other without worrying about their inadequacies. The counselor then sends them away from the session with a reminder: "This problem will be resolved when both of you are ready. Meanwhile, just enjoy each other and continue to work together to achieve complete intimacy."

With the pressure lifted, they are able to appreciate each other and their relationship in spite of the sexual dysfunction, which persists for a few more weeks. The following sessions deal with the issues of guilt, sense of failure, and intimacy, until they are able to experience sexual intimacy without fear. After a follow-up several years later, George and Joanne were happily married and able to appreciate each other sexually, emotionally, and intellectually.

Although not all family counseling cases such as this end happily—nor is there even overwhelming evidence to indicate that this modality works significantly better than more traditional individual sessions—this type of systemic conceptualization is revolutionizing the way counselors plan their intervention strategies. Probably no movement within the field in the past decade has had more impact on the way counselors think about their work.

## INTERPRETING SYMPTOMS AS METAPHORS

Most communication has messages on two levels: *digital* and *analogical*. One part of communication is literal and content oriented, whereas another,

## VOICE FROM THE FIELD

Training in family therapy really changes you on many levels. Sure it's cool to learn all the techniques you can use with clients. But far more than that, it sensitizes you to look more closely at all your relationships, especially with those you live with. When you're first learning how to do a genogram [a diagram of family relationships], you do one of your own family, and this is absolutely mind-blowing. The same is true when you learn to read family dynamics: You apply it all to your own family. At least I do.

At first it's scary. I mean all this dysfunctional stuff has always been going on that I've been oblivious to. Then after awhile, this greater sensitivity helped me to be more understanding. The worst part, though, is that I can no longer get away with the games I used to play with my own parents since now I catch myself. It's just no fun any more.

---

deeper, communication expresses messages of a more subtle kind. For example, when a woman says to her spouse at the dinner table, "You eat so fast I don't know how you can even taste or enjoy your food," she is, in fact, making a literal comment about her husband's table manners. But in addition to this digital statement, she may also be communicating metaphorically about another aspect of their relationship that is rushed without enjoyment: their sex life.

Now, the counselor has the choice of interpreting the disguised meaning of the communication or responding on a similar symbolic level. Haley (1973), in writing about Milton Erickson's preferred strategy, relates that "whatever the patient says in metaphoric form, Erickson responds in kind. By parables, by interpersonal action, and by directives, he works within the metaphor to bring about change. He seems to feel that the depth and swiftness of that change can be prevented if the person suffers a translation of the communication" (p. 28). The couple in this example may be requested to go out and have a slow, drawn-out, leisurely meal. This message and its subsequent action permit the partners to practice their foreplay in an indirect, minimally threatening situation.

Because people communicate on these different levels, the family counselor must learn to recognize the ways in which children and adults express different issues through their behavior. Presenting complaints or identified symptoms are thus often interpreted as something quite different from their surface messages. This theoretical construct is common to many individual therapeutic approaches, such as psychoanalytic and Gestalt counseling. The main difference may be that the strategic family counselor is less interested in explaining or interpreting the metaphor and instead prefers to operate on the same level as the family members.

# DIAGNOSTIC QUESTIONS

One other unique contribution of the family systems perspective is the way it has encouraged practitioners to think diagnostically about client behavior. The narrative approach to counseling presented in Chapter 5, the strategic approach introduced in Chapter 6, and the systemic approach to diagnosis mentioned in Chapter 8 are all examples of different ways of asking questions. In some cases, the goal is to find out information not only about the symptomatic client's experience but also about how everyone in the family is affected and, in turn, affects the problem in their interactions. In other instances, especially in a narrative approach, the very act of asking questions is designed to promote changes in the ways that clients view their predicaments.

Operating strategically, the family counselor would be interested in sorting out the confusing connections among symptoms, metaphors, power hierarchies, and other relevant variables by asking some specific questions:

- What is the problem?
- When does the problem occur?
- Where does the problem occur?
- Where are various family members when the problem occurs?
- What is each member of the family doing when the problem occurs?
- What are the effects on each family member?
- What are the benefits to the client? (To other family members?)
- Who in the family has had a similar problem?
- Where is the power (money, decisions, time)?
- Who is being protected?

The *genogram* is another useful tool for gathering information about family relationships and structures. It consists of a comprehensive map of all the members of a family over several generations, including their coalitions, conflicts, and connections. It thus provides a blueprint for the counselor in understanding the cross-generational themes that repeat themselves over time, as well as the current interpersonal conflicts that are evident in the structural map (Figure 10.1) presented earlier.

For example, using symbols standardized by McGoldrick and Gerson (1985) in their book on family assessment, Erlanger (1990) plotted a four-generation genogram of Lucy, a 75-year-old client (see Figure 10.2). A review of this chart reveals several issues that Lucy may wish to explore: her father's suicide, her son's alcoholism, her relationships with her aging husband and mother. All of this is clear before any efforts are made to include existing conflicts among family members.

During the process of constructing a genogram, a number of issues will emerge, often in a nonthreatening way. You are simply taking a rather structured family history, learning as much as you can about patterns of relationships in the present and past. Such background information will be critical to you later when you are attempting to unravel dysfunctional interactions that may have their origins in previous generations.

FIGURE 10.2 | A FOUR-GENERATION GENOGRAM

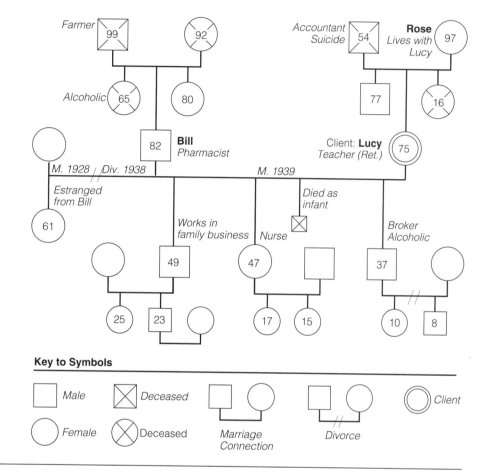

*Source:* Erlanger, M. A., (1990). Using the genogram with the older client. *Journal of Mental Health Counseling,* 12(3), 321–331.

# REFRAMING

Two types of diagnosis are useful in family counseling. The first variety includes applying those labels that help the counselor to grasp the processes and problems involved. We have already examined diagnosing client position, family hierarchy, communication style, and symptoms as solutions and metaphors in this context. But there is a second kind of diagnosis—the one communicated to the client. The counselor's initial task, therefore, is to define or reframe the present problem to the client or clients in such a way that it may be resolved.

Clients come into counseling sessions with preconceived notions of what is wrong with them and why:

- "My marriage is on the rocks because my wife wants to go back to school and start a career rather than taking care of the family."
- "My boy is having trouble in school because his teachers are too strict and don't appreciate his uniqueness."
- "I've never been able to hold a job because everyone in my family has always been lazy."

In the process of reframing, the counselor redefines the presenting complaint for the family, using both ingenuity and creativity to think on concrete and metaphorical levels. In the resulting working diagnosis, the counselor identifies issues that can, in fact, be responsive to change, so that the family will be more willing to work on them. There isn't much that can be done to help a client who is complaining about another person's behavior, unless, of course, the other person will come in for counseling and willingly change what the accuser dislikes. In initiating counseling for clients with the complaints quoted on the previous page, the most important task would be to reframe the client's perceived difficulties. The husband who wants compliance from his wife would be helped to view the problem more as a lack of communication: He hasn't conveyed his desires in such a way that his wife could understand (and accept) them. The problem of the boy having trouble in school would be reframed to say that, although he is clearly a talented comic, he is performing for the wrong audience. The person without a job would be helped to redefine his problem as a lack of skills and/or motivation rather than a lack of employable genes.

The value of reframing is exemplified in the case of a 35-year-old client who arrived for his session huffing and puffing, his face flushed, and his hand wrapped in a towel that was quickly turning red with blood. The flustered counselor, a tiny woman of 90 pounds, looked up at the 230-pound mechanic and responded, "Oh, I see you had some trouble. What happened?"

Still standing in the foyer, the man smiled with a glazed, stunned look and answered, "I locked my damn keys in the car and I got mad. And when I get mad I like to hit things. Anything. I can't help it. Boy, am I mad. Now, what's all this shit about you wanting to see me about my kid?"

The counselor went to her supervisor immediately following the session. She calmed down, at least enough to hear the more experienced clinician reframe the man's behavior: "What do you think about this guy? Blustering his way into a first session with his hand all bloody. This is funny. This is hysterical. This guy is no bully—this guy is a clown. Next time he comes in, treat him like a clown and see what happens. And, just in case you need me, I'll be close by."

During the next session the man responded with a burst of anger to the counselor's accurate confrontation about how he had been neglecting his son. He stamped the floor and rose with a menacing stare. The counselor, of course, was startled, but she regained her composure and looked at the humor in his behavior. She smiled, seemingly unaffected by his threatening behavior, thinking: "This guy really is funny."

The man anxiously demanded some explanation of the counselor's calm appearance. He was used to having people feel afraid of him. She told him compassionately how silly he really looked stamping around like a child; then, as an afterthought, she moved back a little and waited.

Yes, he agreed, he probably did look funny, but he does get what he wants by intimidating other people. He eventually admitted, though, that he hated himself for behaving so badly and appreciated the counselor seeing through the mask and allowing him to discuss his vulnerable feelings.

Although this was a risky strategy, it nevertheless demonstrated the power of reframing behavior, casting it in a different light. Not only is the client able to view his behavior as more manageable, but the counselor is also able to see the behavior in compassionate rather than threatening terms.

Another variation of reframing occurs in the narrative approach to family counseling. Called *externalizing,* the method is essentially the same; the counselor introduces another way of viewing the problem. In the narrative approach, however, this new diagnosis is offered in such a way as to make the symptoms located *outside* the family so everyone can work together as a team to defeat the problem (Monk, Winslade, Crocket, & Epston, 1997). This also prevents the family from blaming themselves or the identified client, because the enemy is now seen as being on the outside rather than the inside.

## DIRECTIVES

The idea of deliberately telling clients what they should do goes against the grain of almost all counseling systems. Counselors are, after all, supposed to be neutral, objective, detached, and not prone to giving advice. A rationale for the violation of this golden rule is that such interventions are often successful. Furthermore, family counselors, by the very nature of their work, are more active, structuring, and directive than they would ever consider being when working with individual clients. Put all members of a family together in a room—particularly those who are so conflicted they had to ask for help—and the situation often turns chaotic. Unless the counselor is prepared to jump in and take the initiative, the family counseling session could make matters considerably worse.

A number of directive options are available to the family counselor. They may be designed to be either obeyed or disobeyed, depending on which is more likely to work. They can be simply and straightforwardly presented or explained in such a complicated and confusing way that the client will rebelliously do the opposite. The best directives are those that involve everyone in the family, are precisely described, provide sufficient motivation to encourage completion of the task, and are simple enough that they can be reasonably accomplished.

In using directives, the counselor seeks to initiate changes in the family structure by getting people to act differently. The goal is to realign the hierarchy of power along more desirable paths—for instance, with the parents in charge rather than the children or grandparents, or with both spouses on an equal footing. The process of initiating all directives usually involves (1) redefining the problem in a less threatening form and describing it in a way that allows resolution, (2) motivating and preparing the client to follow (or not follow) the directive, and (3) presenting the directive clearly, simply, and realistically, ensuring that all participants understand what they are to do or not do.

According to Fisch, Weakland, and Segal (1982), all directives (and for that matter all therapeutic interventions) are designed to interrupt the current attempted solution to a family problem—that is, the symptoms of the identified client. Fisch et al. offer the following tactical maneuvers that require active counselor direction.

## Forcing the Spontaneous

Many psychosomatic complaints, performance problems, and thought disturbances occur spontaneously, in spite of a client's attempts to control them. Trying too hard to fall asleep, reach orgasm, or stop a tic only makes things worse. Asking the client to cease behavior that is not within conscious control is not reasonable. Instead, the client can be directed to continue the behavior at will. A person who can't sleep may be told to stay up or to get up after fifteen minutes and work on an important but nonstimulating task. The client is then able to make the first step toward resolution of the problem: If she or he can exhibit some control over the uncontrollable problem by exercising some choices around its occurrence, then the problem seems less ominous and not as wayward as the client originally believed. A paradoxical directive of this type allows the counselor to be successful, and the client perceives himself or herself as making progress. The client who complies with the suggestion is exhibiting control, and the client who doesn't abide by the directive to fail is then cured of the problem. This type of directive is safe for both the counselor and the client because it provides ample opportunity for positive outcome.

## Opposition through Compliance

In the physical world, when we attempt without success to solve a problem by a certain action, we will try something else—usually the opposite action. If we try to open a door by pushing it and it won't budge, we may try pulling it. If we attempt to loosen a screw by forcing it to the left and it doesn't move, we will try forcing it to the right. Yet when an attempted strategy doesn't work in emotional family struggles, with participants locked into no-win battles, a person will often try the same thing harder. If a wife fights for her independence in the marriage by repeatedly resisting her husband's orders and then discovers she is worse off, she will nevertheless struggle harder. If parents have attempted on numerous occasions to get their rebellious adolescent to comply

## VOICE FROM THE FIELD

The thing you gotta be careful of with directive counseling is that these brilliant ideas usually come from behind a one-way mirror. What I mean is that when you see demonstration videos at workshops or read about cases in books, the presenters inevitably include these amazingly creative solutions to problems. Of course, they often came up with these interventions as part of a team. Sitting behind the one-way mirror is one or even more colleagues watching the session, talking among each other about all the possibilities, then calling on the phone into the session when they'd like to make a suggestion. It's a fabulous idea, naturally, one that changes the whole course of treatment.

When you read about this, or see it on a video, you think to yourself, "Wow, I gotta try that!" Then you get back to your own practice where you don't have the luxury of having the most brilliant minds in the city watching and contributing to your sessions, and the stuff you come up with on your own isn't nearly as sterling as what the master therapists invented.

Don't get me wrong. I think using directives and all are powerful strategies. It's just that it's damn hard to come up with them at the time. That's why you always need to be connected to a great supervisor to consult with.

---

to house rules and they have found that the youngster is only getting worse, the parents will demand even more compliant behavior.

This second category of directives takes the form of suggesting to those without power that the only way they will get any control is to back down. By deliberately taking a "weak position" and "giving in," they finally break the vicious, repetitive cycle. Thus, benevolent sabotage begins to defuse the conflict: "I'm sorry I burned your toast. I don't know what's getting into me." The powerless client is able to feel more dignity and control because she or he backs down by choice. The key to using compliant tactics effectively is to avoid sarcasm or overt game playing. The client must attempt a "one-down" instead of the "one-up" position that didn't work. Once the opposition ceases, the cycle is often broken, and the other family members no longer derive satisfaction from their positions. It's no fun to dominate if the other person won't fight back. And it's no fun to rebel if the others won't force compliance.

## Pretending

A favorite ploy of Madanes in working with children is to direct the parents to encourage the symptom deliberately and to ask the child to pretend to have it. Much of the tension associated with the symptom is thereafter dissipated because everyone is "only pretending." Consider the case of a "28-year-old adolescent" who was still so dependent on his father that he carried around a paging device so that his father could reach him at any time, usually to scream at him for some mistake he had made in the family business. The young man was constantly late, missed appointments, and botched orders, and each time his father would furiously bawl him out. Neither man much enjoyed the pattern, but each felt powerless to stop it.

The counselor directed the son to bungle something deliberately at least three times a day. He was to pretend to make mistakes so that his father could no longer determine when the young man was truly irresponsible and when he was only faking. The son improved after discovering that because he could control when he made mistakes, and pretend to do so, he could certainly refrain from such errors whenever he chose.

A way to involve other family members is to encourage them to criticize the person's "performance." Another pattern is thus broken, because instead of trying to deter the symptoms, they are now trying to help the person do them even better. With the introduction of directives to pretend, the metaphorical symptoms are no longer allowed to be part of reality. The problem diminishes because it is no longer taken seriously.

## Slowing Down

Whenever anyone tries too hard to do something, the task becomes more difficult. The directive to slow down is often most effective during initial interviews, when clients are apprehensive about being asked to do something they won't be able to do. If the presenting problem is resolved too quickly, before the clients have had the opportunity to make new adjustments or discover other ways of relating to one another, it is possible that the family structure will break down.

During the first session with a woman complaining of a marriage that is falling apart, the counselor specifically directs her to stop trying to fix things: "Leave things just the way they are for now. This way your husband, too, will have the chance to get involved in solving the problem. I know he's saying that he won't come in for counseling. That is certainly the case as long as you keep nagging him, but let's see how things change once you slow down. The marriage isn't comfortable anyway, so by backing off you can hardly make things worse."

The therapeutic circumstances are now programmed for success no matter what the outcome. The client immediately feels released from her sole responsibility for fixing the marriage. She can loosen up and take a deep breath. She also focuses on herself rather than trying to change her husband. And, if things don't improve immediately, the client will be more patient and willing to keep working.

## COUPLES COUNSELING

Even if you never end up doing sessions with whole extended families present, you will inevitably do a significant amount of work with clients and their partners. This is especially true because problems in intimate relationships is the number one reason why people show up for counseling services (Johnson

## VOICE FROM THE FIELD

I know how important it is to see both people in a relationship when they are having problems but I still struggle with this a lot. I grew up in a home where my parents were fighting all the time. They screamed at one another. They slammed doors. They threatened to leave—and us kids sometimes hoped that one of them would—then we'd have some peace. But, of course, we were terrified our parents would break up.

What this means for me is that I have a hard time being in a room with people who are being mean and hurtful to one another. I know that sounds funny for someone in my line of work but I still have difficulty watching people yelling and screaming at one another. I have a low tolerance for that sort of thing and I don't put up with that behavior in my office.

To a certain extent, this compromises my effectiveness because sometimes couples need to express themselves passionately. That part is fine with me, but not if it means raising your voice. So I enforce strict limits. I make people behave themselves when they are with me no matter what they might do when they are by themselves.

If I had my choice, I would much rather see individuals than couples, just because I have more control over the situation. I am pretty confident that anyone who comes in to see me will leave better off than when they came in. But with couples, I want to save their marriages in a way that I never could with my parents who divorced. I am successful at this maybe half the time, and that isn't nearly good enough.

---

& Lebow, 2000). The consequence of *not* involving spouses or significant others in the process is that one person grows while the other gets left behind. It may not be necessary to involve both members of a couple in every case, or in every session, but you will still need to become reasonably comfortable with the nuances involved in doing counseling with more than one person present. This means, for example, being especially sensitive to not taking sides or to be perceived as showing favoritism that might compromise your credibility.

It also means knowing the basic research and practice related to the practice of couples counseling (see Berg-Cross, 2001; Brown & Brown, 2002; Carlson & Sperry, 2000). In one study of what predicts successful marriages, for example, Gottman (1999) identified several dimensions most associated with continued marital conflict: criticism, defensiveness, contempt, stonewalling, and belligerence. He also found that emotional engagement between partners is the best predictor of success, even if these feelings involve heated, angry exchanges. Although these findings have been challenged (Stanley, Bradbury, & Markman, 2000), they have nevertheless led us to mistrust what we might ordinarily assume about couples and what works best for them. Doing couples therapy is not simply a matter of applying what you already know to two people in the room.

Working with partners or cohabitants brings up a number of other issues—violence, money issues, sexual dysfunctions, child rearing, lifestyle compatibility, role definitions, health, jealousy, fidelity, career, and leisure choices. Anything you would hope to do with one person in the room is infinitely more complex when you are managing the interactions between two people who may already be locked into resentments and heated battles. This presents a series of new clinical challenges as well as ethical conflicts.

## ETHICAL ISSUES IN COUPLES AND FAMILY COUNSELING

If you have gotten the impression that marital and family counseling are powerful treatment methods that can often effect "cures" in a matter of weeks, that is indeed true. It is because these modalities are so potent, however, that they bring with them a number of moral dilemmas for the practitioner. A later chapter will focus on ethical and legal issues as they relate to the practice of counseling, but I nevertheless wish to mention briefly some of the conflicts you will face in your work as a marital and family counselor. Some of the following issues may already have occurred to you:

- Is it ethical to be deceitful and manipulative (using paradoxical techniques, for example) if it is for the client's own good?
- If your primary function is to treat family problems, what about the individual goals of each member, which may conflict with those of the others?
- How do you handle confidentiality issues if one family member or marital partner confides a secret (that he or she is having an affair, for example) but instructs you not to tell anyone else?
- Because family conflicts frequently involve value issues related to fidelity, sexuality, promiscuity, divorce, child rearing, and life priorities, how can you possibly keep your own values in check regarding how you believe people should behave?
- Because family counselors are often highly directive and dramatic in their interventions to break up dysfunctional patterns, aren't there greater risks for doing harm?

Last, but by no means least, is the area of family violence and the special ethical problems it raises. The abuse of children, spouses, and the elderly creates problems not only for the victims and perpetrators but also for the helping professionals caught in the middle who are trying to stabilize explosive situations (Green & Hansen, 1989; Huber, 1994). In their survey of ethical issues related to violence, Gross and Robinson (1987) describe several cases that highlight the conflicting loyalties counselors have (1) to state laws that mandate the reporting of abuse, (2) to the identified clients who are requesting help, and (3) to the victims (or potential victims) of the dangerous action.

Both the American Association for Marriage and Family Therapy (AAMFT) and the International Association of Marriage and Family Counselors (IAMFC) have developed ethical codes for this specialty. In addition to the universal ethical issues that all counselors face (confidentiality, conflicted loyalties, social responsibility, competence), these codes will help guide you to sort out dilemmas as they emerge, often in consultation with your supervisor.

# SEX COUNSELING

Sex counseling is the single most successful result of integrating many diverse theoretical structures into a unified technology of helping. With reported success rates of well into the 80–95 percent range for a variety of sexual dysfunctions, such as impotence, premature ejaculation, and orgasmic dysfunctions (in the absence of physical causes), sex counseling is one of the most well developed therapeutic specialties. First, the treatment is successful because it attacks sexual problems using insight methods as well as structured homework. Second, the treatment is relatively short term (usually three to ten sessions). And, third, the nature of the counseling strategy requires the practitioner to be flexible and pragmatic.

Helen Singer Kaplan (1974), in her classic book on the theory and techniques of sex therapy, readily admits that treating clients with sexual problems by insight methods alone is probably unethical, because the technology does exist to help people relatively quickly by more behavioral interventions. The sex counselor, therefore, not only uses much of the family counseling theory already discussed but also uses other insight theories with solid applications of behavior modification. Such techniques as relaxation training, sensate focus exercises, and cognitive restructuring are frequently employed.

Sex counseling is a specialized application emphasizing behavioral treatment to reduce symptoms. It is often a part of marital counseling, begun once basic communication problems are addressed. For sex counseling to be effective, the couple's commitment to the relationship and willingness to experience the therapy are essential prerequisites. The basic treatment plan usually takes a six-step form: clinical assessment, physical exam and medical history, exploration of relationship, sensate focus exercises, specialized techniques, and evaluation.

## Clinical Assessment Interview

With both partners present, or in separate intake interviews, the sex counselor does a detailed data-gathering interview to learn about family history, sexual attitudes in the childhood home, religious influences, early sex education, first sexual experiences, and current attitudes toward various sexual practices. The assessment includes consideration of previous sexual difficulties, as well as a detailed description of current problems and attempts to solve them.

Once a working relationship has been established, the counselor feels free to ask direct questions: "What do you think about during sex?" "How do you initiate sex?" "What would you like to do that you are not doing?"

## Physical Exam and Medical History

It is extremely important with sexual difficulties (as well as with any other psychological problem having a possible organic origin) that any physical causes be ruled out before attempting psychological interventions. It would be important to know about any drugs that the clients are taking; certain medications for high blood pressure, for instance, will affect sexual responsiveness. Chronic alcoholism also presents special problems, as do diseases such as diabetes. Hormone levels can be assessed to detect estrogen or testosterone deficiencies in the blood. A thorough medical history and exam are also valuable to rule out certain physical processes that can affect sexual performance.

Counselors who do any sort of sex counseling with couples have developed referral contacts with medical specialists who are trained to do these sorts of assessments. It is also important to work with physicians who have not only the requisite background but also the sensitivity to work with patients who often feel embarrassed and uncomfortable acknowledging their difficulties.

## Exploration of Relationship

If organic causes are eliminated, the next place to look for the sources of sexual problems is in the relationship between the couple. Sexual behavior is one way in which partners communicate with each other. Time (at least a few sessions) is generally spent working to improve the communication between partners, helping them to build trust and commitment for the work that lies ahead. In an open, accepting therapeutic atmosphere, clients are helped to dispel their fears of failure, often a contributing factor to sexual problems. They are asked to share their likes, dislikes, and fantasies with each other, all the while becoming more sexually intimate in a nonthreatening, verbal manner.

Often it isn't even necessary to begin the formal sex therapy program because it is the relationship that was the problem in the first place. That's why it's critical to make sure underlying relationship conflicts have been addressed before the more difficult sexual issues are dealt with.

## Sensate Focus Exercises

The counselor will next introduce the behavioral sequence in the treatment, essentially a prescribed series of progressive exercises that the couple will do at home. Initially, all pressure is removed by specifically prohibiting the couple from any further attempts at intercourse. They are absolutely forbidden to try, thereby removing the threat of failure. The sensate focus exercises involve selfishly, yet sensitively and nondemandingly, giving and receiving nongenital pleasure through touching. Very gradually, the couple add to their repertoire by (1) mutual back rubs for one week, (2) nongenital touching and mutual pleasure in other areas of the body, (3) light genital stimulation without orgasm, (4) genital touching to orgasm, (5) intercourse without orgasm (or erection), and (6) intercourse to orgasm.

The couple can progress slowly through these steps, doing no more than they are comfortable doing at any one time. Success is virtually guaranteed if the couple will follow the structure and resist the temptation to jump ahead to fulfilling the sexual act.

■ | VOICE FROM THE FIELD

Learning the techniques of sex counseling and education is the easy part. I mean, it's not brain surgery or anything. There are these structured programs that teach you about the techniques and all. The hard part, though, is confronting your own attitudes and values and beliefs related to sex that might get in the way of your work with people. That's why the training almost always includes experiential-type groups where you look at your own sexual issues and get used to talking about sex in an open, honest way.

One standard way that they often start the training is that they put the words penis and vagina on the board and have everyone in the room yell out all the names they can think of for those body parts. It's hysterical. People start out saying the standard ones but then they end up blurting out their own pet names for their private parts. While everyone is laughing, they don't realize that what the exercise is supposed to do is desensitize you to sexual terms so that you can talk about them to couples without shame.

If couples you're working with sense that you feel the least discomfort talking about sex—I mean any aspect of it—they won't deal with their stuff. They are looking to you for guidance and the best way to offer it is to be really calm and matter-of-fact about the subject.

## Specialized Techniques

The sex counselor will use a variety of educational and therapeutic options to facilitate better communication, awareness, and sexual responsiveness. Specialized approaches are also taken for particular clients, depending on their age, sexual orientation, and presenting problems (Kleinplatz, 2001). Films and books may be used for demonstration purposes. Vibrators are often recommended for nonorgasmic women. There are also several specific procedures, such as the "squeeze technique," that are used for premature ejaculation. Certain sexual positions are often suggested for various problems, and focused fantasy exercises help combat distracting thoughts.

## Evaluation

Throughout the duration of treatment, the counselor works with the couple to combat the usual resistances. The recognition that, when the symptoms go away, the couple will have to find another way to communicate is a problem that should be addressed early in the counseling. Once sexual functioning is restored, the counselor helps the spouses to integrate what they have learned and continue their marital growth and enrichment.

In addition to applying these sequential steps in the treatment of specific dysfunctions, sex counselors are also called on to be of assistance to those suffering from sexually transmitted diseases, such as HIV and herpes, and to individuals troubled by chronic disease, aging, chemical dependency, sexual assault, abortion, and physical disabilities. In any and all of these situations, counselors must not only be highly trained in the technology of sex treatments, but they also must have thoroughly worked through their own inhibitions, discomforts, and values related to the subject. Organizations such as the American Association of Sex Educators, Counselors, and Therapists (AASECT) and the Scientific Society for the Study of Sex (SSSS) and training centers such as the Institute for Sex Research (Kinsey Institute) and the Masters and Johnson Institute provide training experiences for those interested in specializing in these areas. You may also wish to consult basic primers (Kleinplatz, 2001; Leiblum & Rosen, 2000) that introduce you to the methodology.

## SUMMARY

In this chapter you have learned about the basic theory and techniques of marital, family, and sex counseling. Most counselors are faced with many clients who experience adjustment problems in these areas. Professionals who work with children and adolescents in particular need knowledge and expertise in family counseling. The major focus of these techniques is to clarify the system of relationships occurring in marital and family interactions and to identify opportunities to interrupt dysfunctional patterns. In working with family systems, counselors attempt to help clients restructure relationships toward developmentally healthy goals and to reduce the impact of destructive systems of relationships. Counselors must skillfully blend specific marital, family, and sex techniques within the framework of individual and group counseling skills.

## SELF-GUIDED EXPLORATIONS

1. What are some experiences from your family of origin that have influenced you to become a counselor?
2. Using the following notations, create a genogram or structural map of your family relationships. Clearly highlight the coalitions, boundaries, conflicts, and patterns of communication.

   ☐ Male family member      ══ Strong relationship
   ○ Female family member      ------ Weak relationship
   ◎☐ You      ≡ Dependent relationship
        ∿∿ Conflicted relationship

3. The concept of *reframing* is central to the practice of family counseling. In this process, you attempt to recast the way a problem is viewed so that it is easier to resolve. For example, a mother keeps pestering her son about doing chores that he consistently avoids. The more she nags him, the more obstinate the boy becomes. Once the counselor reframes the mother's behavior as a way of showing love and caring, the boy stops feeling so resentful toward the mother's intrusions. Think of a problem or conflict in your life that could be reframed in more constructive terms.

4. What are some sexual issues that a couple might present that would be uncomfortable for you to deal with? Imagine that a client walked in presenting that very issue. How would you help this person?

## For Homework:

Arrange to interview several "normal" families. Explore their family dynamics, coalitions, cross-generational issues, decision-making style, and other factors that you have learned are important in healthy family functioning. Be sure to look at strengths of the family and individual members, as well as any problem areas.

## SUGGESTED READINGS

Becvar, D. S., & Becvar, R. J. (2003). *Family therapy: A systemic integration* (5th ed.). Boston: Allyn & Bacon.

Berg-Cross, L. (2001). *Couples therapy* (2nd ed.). New York: Haworth.

Brown, J. H., & Brown, C. S. (2002). *Marital therapy: Concepts and skills for effective practice.* Pacific Grove, CA: Brooks/Cole.

Carlson, J., & Kjos, D. (2001). *Theories and strategies of family therapy.* Boston: Allyn & Bacon.

Carlson, J., Sperry, L., & Lewis, J. (2003). *Family therapy techniques.* New York: Brunner/Routledge.

Gehart, D. R., Tuttle, A. R. (2003). *Theory-based treatment planning for marriage and family therapists.* Pacific Grove, CA: Brooks/Cole.

Gladding, S. T. (2002). *Family therapy: History, theory, and practice.* Upper Saddle River, NJ: Prentice-Hall.

Gladding, S., Remley, T. P., & Huber, C. H. (2000). *Ethical, legal, and professional issues in the practice of marriage and family therapy.* Upper Saddle River, NJ: Prentice-Hall.

Goldenberg, I., & Goldenberg, H. (2002). *Counseling today's families* (4th ed.). Pacific Grove, CA: Brooks/Cole.

Gottman, J. M. (1999). *The marriage clinic: A scientifically based marital therapy.* New York: W. W. Norton

Kleinplatz, P. J. (Ed.)(2001). *New directions in sex therapy: Innovations and alternatives.* New York: Brunner/Routledge.

Leiblum, S. R., & Rosen, R. C. (eds.) (2000). *Principles and practices of sex therapy* (3rd ed.). New York: Guilford.

McGoldrick, M. (1997). *You can go home again: Reconnecting with your family.* New York: W. W. Norton.

Nichols, M. P., & Schwartz, R. C. (2001). *Family therapy: Concepts and methods* (5th ed.). Boston: Allyn & Bacon.

Young, M., & Long, L. (1998). *Counseling and therapy for couples.* Pacific Grove, CA: Brooks/Cole.

# I I CHAPTER CAREER COUNSELING

KEY CONCEPTS

Vocational choice

Work functions

Meaningful work

Career information systems

Employability skills

Life coaching

Career identities

Holland personality types

Social learning theory

Career education

# CAREER·COUNSELING

# 11

Historically, career development has been the principal domain of counselors. It is through the process and techniques of vocational guidance that the counseling profession was introduced and implemented in numerous settings. In recent years, however, there has been a gradual yet perceptible shift in emphasis from vocational issues to personal/emotional issues (Dorn, 1986) and the systemic context for career development (Patton & McMahon, 1999). Career decisions are no longer looked at in isolation but in a much broader developmental, relational context (Phillips, Christopher-Sisk, & Gravino, 2001) and also a more culturally responsive focus (Flores & Heppner, 2002). This means that when someone comes in to deal with some career-related issue, you will also likely end up exploring family, cultural, gender, and related issues that are part of the bigger picture.

You would only have to consider the complexities of your own career transition right now (Yes, you are in the throes of a major life transition) in order to appreciate what must be done in order to work through this developmental stage to a satisfactory conclusion. You are studying to be a counselor and, as such, there are many side effects, ripple effects, and consequences as a result of this choice. Certain financial resources are sacrificed to pursue this dream, monies that could be spent elsewhere. Your family and friends are also included as part of this journey, whether they wish to be or not. As you learn and grow and make changes in the ways you think and behave, the effects have far-reaching impact on all your other

## VOICE FROM THE FIELD

I think if they ever really told us what the impact of going back to school would be on our families, friends, stress levels, and economic situations, many of us never would have continued. At first, it didn't seem to be such a big deal. I'll just take a counseling class or two. It's only a few nights a week. No big deal.

But it's not just the time commitment that is so disruptive—or even the extra financial burden. When you get into this field, you not only learn things, but you also change your basic values and attitudes. So much of what we do is about learning and growth.

It's all very exciting, too. The problem, though, is that sometimes people get left behind.

I come home from school all excited about the things I'm learning. I'm working hard to be more open, to express myself more often. But if my friends and family are still stuck in the same old routines, then it can drive a wedge in our relationships. Even worse, I've heard from lots of classmates how their families are really threatened by them going back to school. I can really see that, too. Any career change like this creates a whole lot more problems, just as it solves others.

---

relationships. It would thus be impossible to talk to you only about your ultimate career aspirations without delving into your relationships, your family, your financial situation, your personal values, and what gives your life meaning. That is one reason why career counseling cannot take place without considering the personal, familial, and cultural context for a person's choices and lifestyle (Jackson & Scharman, 2002).

Keep this in mind as you study this field because, traditionally at least, many of the theories of vocational choice have tended to be rather limited and microcosmic in their view of human experience. They also have reflected a period of North American culture in which a person training for a stable life career was the norm, manufacturing and industry were primary employers, and discrimination against women and minorities was accepted. A number of changes have taken place as both scholars and practitioners are making efforts to adapt traditional theories and develop new ones that are much more reflective of diverse cultural populations and gender differences for both men and women (Flores & Heppner, 2002; Sharf, 2002; Zunker, 2002).

In spite of the changes taking place in the field, there is still a myth among many counselors that "real" counseling is personal/emotional and that vocational/career counseling is somehow a second-class cousin that requires fewer skills and is more "routine." This attitude is not only false but dangerous. As you will see in this chapter, much of your self-esteem and many of your needs are met by career activities. To achieve a modicum of personal fulfillment, you must participate in effective life/career planning. Individuals who experience vocational chaos (such as unemployment, underemployment, and job dissatisfaction) report high stress, relationship difficulties, and low self-esteem. It is likely that you have experienced these conditions as well at some point in your life, if not this very minute. You can therefore relate to the feelings of uncertainty, anxiety, and fear often associated with these changes.

# THE FUNCTIONS OF WORK

"Rich man, poor man, beggar man, thief. Doctor, lawyer, Indian chief." From our first day at school, we became eligible for that eternal question from well-meaning relatives—that question that still plagues (and will always nag) us: "What do you want to be when you grow up?" As if we had to grow up to be something—or as if we wanted to be something we are not—or as if we had to grow up. But even Peter Pan lost that fight.

Work is supposedly what we have prepared, educated, and trained ourselves to do. Long ago we shed our existence as hunter-gatherers whose only job was to find enough to eat. Now we are specialized. Everyone, and I mean *everyone,* is engaged in some purposeful, productive activity. Some receive financial remuneration for their efforts—they sell their time and talent. Others work for internal rewards or receive other forms of compensation by way of a cooperative division of labor. But labor we all do. Even the children are working—mastering new skills, taking in new knowledge. They may sometimes work in places called playgrounds, but we are not for a moment deceived that these little people are not laboring away at their age-related developmental tasks. They are working their bodies, testing their minds, and learning about cooperation, competition, and a million other things they will later find useful after they "grow up" and work in a "real" job.

Work is more than a source of income. For most people, vocation is very much tied into their sense of identity, self-image, and sense of worth. Jobs are a measure of status, a major object of devotion of one's time and energy. They are a testing ground for skills and information that have been accumulated over a lifetime. They are the source of many friendships.

People who are satisfied in their work are those who are often most content with their lives. Lonely, depressed, anxious, problem-ridden people—those who seek a counselor's help—are often those who are not content with their life's work, whether that role is one of homemaker, student, or corporate executive. Career frustration, job stress, and discontent with one's decisions and current vocational development are thus major preoccupations for many people and therefore a significant part of a counselor's work.

If you think back to a time when you were not engaged in meaningful work, when you felt unappreciated or understimulated, when you were frustrated or bored on the job, you are well aware of how this dissatisfaction affects every other aspect of your life. You are also probably aware of how bleak and hopeless the future can sometimes seem, how alone you feel in your struggles, and how confused you can be about which direction to take. If only there had been a counselor available to help you sort out your desires and goals, offer support and encouragement, and structure plans to make needed changes, it might have made a difference.

# ROLES OF COUNSELING

If work is what you have to do and play is what you want to do, then a major goal of counseling is to teach people never to work a day in their lives. Some people are able to adopt an attitude that helps them to enjoy their jobs, to have fun, and to feel fulfilled. When the alarm clock rings, they jump out of bed, eager to begin their day. Yet others, working in an exactly equivalent position, feel only dread, boredom, and disgust with what they do for a living. Take the case of the Pickens brothers described by Terkel (1972) in his book *Working*. Both boys have paper routes. They both get up at the same time and basically do the same things. Yet note how the difference in their attitudes about their jobs affects their perceptions. One boy plays; the other works.

CLIFF: It's fun throwing papers. Sometimes you get it on the roof. But I never did that. You throw the paper off your bicycle and it lands someplace in the bushes. It'll hit part of the wall and it'll go booooongg! That's pretty fun, because I like to see it go booooongg!

TERRY: I don't see where people get all this bull about the kid who's gonna be President and being a newsboy made a President out of him. It taught him how to handle his money and this bull. You know what it did? It taught him how to hate the people in his route. And the printers. And dogs. (Terkel, 1972, p. 161)

These different attitudes about the same exact job are indicative of the choices people make in how they treat their work. Some people are immensely satisfied; some are burned out. Counselors spend a lot of their time helping people, whether children or adults, to think and feel differently about what they are doing. Attitude is all important in any activity, and certainly in one that can become as routine as going to work. The ultimate goal of almost every person, and therefore every counselor who is giving assistance, is to wake up with energy and excitement, with enthusiasm and anticipation for the day's events that lie ahead.

Counselors help people with career indecision on a number of fronts. Developmental problems such as career immaturity are resolved by exploring the client's interests and career alternatives and applying decision-making strategies. Situational problems such as job stress are worked on within the context of a supportive, problem-solving relationship to develop alternative responses. And chronic problems such as psychological dysfunctions are resolved in longer term counseling to initiate more extensive personality changes. In each case, counselors strive to develop more positive attitudes, as well as to accomplish the following objectives.

## Facilitating Self-Awareness

The first step is to help clients discover what they really want and need—to become aware of what they value most. Many people who require career development assistance aren't exactly sure what is most important to them, or if they do know, they certainly haven't matched their priorities with their current work.

Clients may be asked, for example, to rank-order the following work values according to personal preference:

- long vacations
- opportunities for advancement
- big money
- security
- variety of tasks
- friendly coworkers
- creative opportunities
- physically active

- flexible hours
- lots of responsibility
- status
- independence
- minimum of pressure
- benevolent boss
- power
- chance to help people

The self-awareness or self-exploration process includes much more than clarifying one's values, including several aspects of self-exploration (Atkinson & Murrell, 1988):

1. *Concrete exploration* includes activities that allow the client to become more directly involved in career exploration activities. These activities might include using computer-based career guidance systems to clarify values, needs, and interests; writing a detailed vocational history; and describing in writing pivotal experiences and life decisions (Boer, 2001).
2. *Reflective exploration* might include activities to clarify the personal importance of life decisions, events, and transitions and to evaluate personal needs, wants, desires, goals, interests, and dreams in terms of their relative importance. During this phase of self-evaluation, it is useful to weigh the relative value of input from family, associates, friends, and other significant individuals regarding personal strengths, weaknesses, and skills.
3. *Actual exploration* might include activities such as résumé writing, videotaped practice interviews with feedback sessions, and informational interviews with individuals employed in possible career choices. The purpose of these activities is to increase self-awareness and to accurately assess strengths, weaknesses, aptitudes, skills, and lifestyle issues.

## Becoming Familiar with the World of Work

Whatever structure is used—a Career Day, guest speaker, reading and research, on-line computer dialogue, experimentation, on-site visit to a workplace, or even the use of stories with embedded work values—the stated task

## VOICE FROM THE FIELD

It's been years since I learned about the DOT [Dictionary of Occupational Titles]. I don't really use it that much in my current job because I use computer-assisted testing like the Strong [Strong Interest Inventory]. But I remember being fascinated with the idea that there's this huge book, or really two books, that has every job in it. Ever since then, I've been playing this game trying to think of jobs that aren't in the DOT. You should try it!

I was in this restaurant not too long ago. It has a Roman theme and so they have these scantily clad women and men walking around catering to customers. Each table has an assigned "wine goddess"—yeah, I know, not very politically correct but still fun—whose only job is to keep your wine goblet filled to the brim. Maybe I'd had a little too much to drink but I couldn't help but giggle when it occurred to me that I'd discovered another occupation not in the DOT—wine goddess. It just kind of gets you thinking all the time about what people do for work.

---

is to help people become more aware not only of themselves but also of career options that are possible (Heitzman, Schmidt, & Hurley, 1986). A person might ask herself, "Given the parameters of a profession that allows me to work with people, use my verbal fluency, and structure my own time, what jobs are likely candidates?" or, "Which careers would involve being outside, using my creative energies, and moving around a lot?"

There are more than thirty thousand different occupations, each divided into one of nine categories, in the *Dictionary of Occupational Titles* (such as service, technical, processing, and clerical professions). Often entire families of careers can be explored, depending on a client's interest. A few may be examined in greater detail, eventually narrowing down the choices to realistic possibilities.

Because of the sheer numbers of available jobs and the complexity of matching aptitudes, interests, values, and required educational level to accurate career information, the use of computer career information systems has become widespread. These systems allow users to access job information based on education, values, interests, and other user variables, greatly simplifying the task of becoming familiar with the world of work. Although these career information systems are useful, they cannot replace a trained counselor who can assist the client to understand, interpret, and apply the information.

## Teaching Decision-Making Skills

Because career development is an ongoing life process, it is hardly functional to focus only on finding a first job for a client. More and more often, people are making radical changes in what they do for work, sometimes enjoying two, three, four, or even more distinctly different careers during their lifetimes. People make decisions to try different careers for a number of reasons—early retirement, boredom, desire for growth, new interests, or in the case of women and minorities who have been closed out of certain sectors, new opportunities. In particular, many individuals at midlife are faced with the need to make career decisions; some do so for personal growth, whereas many others face forced career change because of structural factors in the workplace (Perosa & Perosa, 1987). Many companies have been taken over, with duplicate positions being eliminated. Budgetary issues have forced other firms into a reduction in workforce; some companies have eliminated entire departments in an attempt to sharpen their focus and reduce overhead. In each of these cases, many high-performing individuals find themselves needing to make often unanticipated career decisions.

People must learn to make quality decisions about when and how they should initiate career changes. As we get older, more established, and more secure, taking new risks becomes increasingly difficult, especially because career decision making affects family dynamics.

The counselor can help by teaching people how to make intelligent decisions. The process often involves learning to collect and assess useful information, generating alternative courses of action and predicting their probable consequences, narrowing the field to a plan of action, taking risks, and dealing with the aftershock of change. The counselor is the one who helps organize this process.

## Teaching Employability Skills

There are other even more practical skills that can help people find and maintain satisfaction in their careers. Clients are helped to develop personal marketing strategies to sell themselves and their potential during interviews. They are also encouraged to work on overcoming inertia, resisting procrastination, relieving job-related stress, building an interpersonal support system, and avoiding feelings of frustration and failure.

In other words, the goal of all career-counseling efforts ought to be to provide life skills for making and implementing decisions. How these decisions ought to be made and, in fact, how people even develop vocationally are topics of considerable debate.

## Life Coaching

Nowadays, some counselors are taking on a far more creative and flexible role in order to facilitate career development throughout the lifespan. The new specialty of "life coaching" has a number of differences from traditional counseling:

| Counseling | Coaching |
| --- | --- |
| Past and present oriented | Future oriented |
| Identifies problems | Identifies skill deficits |
| Therapeutic role | Consultant role |
| Focus on thoughts and feelings | Focus on goals and dreams |
| Builds on strengths | Builds on weaknesses |
| Licensed professionals | Unlicensed and unregulated |

Rather than having clients come to the office to talk about their career-related concerns, a life coach would most likely visit the person in the workplace or home. The coach functions less like a therapist and much more like a personal trainer, consultant, and a mentor. Very specific goals are identified. Action plans are set in motion. But rather than waiting on the sidelines for the weekly report, the coach follows up progress via the telephone, Internet, and personal visits. This specialty is still so new that it is not only unregulated but also somewhat controversial. Nevertheless, personal coaching is drawing attention to alternative ways that counselors may help people to make better career decisions and follow through on their declared goals.

## THEORIES OF CAREER DEVELOPMENT

Here is just what you didn't need at this point—*more* theories. You've been introduced already to general theories of counseling, theories of development and learning, theories of group counseling and family counseling, theories of assessment and treatment. Now come more theories of career development. Before you are exposed to new names, new concepts, and new theories, remember that all of this is just designed to provide you the tools you need to help people navigate the complex, turbulent waters of work. Don't overconcern yourself with memorizing names and terms at this point; focus instead on the very interesting ways that have been devised to explain how and why people end up doing the kinds of work they do.

Just as there are a number of theories that attempt to explain learning processes, personality styles, cognitive development, abnormal behavior, social functioning, and models of motivation and change, so too are there varied approaches to vocational development with which counselors are required to familiarize themselves.

Pertinent questions may come immediately to mind:

- How do people make career choices?
- Which variables are most influential in making career decisions? What parts do genetics, the environment, and cognitive and emotional responses play in career development?
- What makes some people happy and others so miserable in their work?

- How does work fit within the larger context of life satisfaction?
- What roles ought counseling to play in the shaping of career development?

Clearly these questions need answering—if not for our own peace of mind, then to better enable us to help clients select fulfilling occupations and learn the skills for remaining satisfied and productive. As we review each of the major theories of career development, try to approach the subject with the same critical eye you applied to glean useful concepts from other counseling models. Look for concepts that make sense and help explain this complex process of development. Note the value and applicability of their ideas to your own career choices and confusions.

## Theodore Caplow's Theory

The first and certainly the simplest theory we will attend to is one based on the notion that career choices are the result of random events, accidents, or errors of being at the right/wrong place at the right/wrong time. Although not exactly using an astrological model, the sociologist Caplow (1954) believed that birth order and the accidents of inheritance (parentage, race, nationality, gender, and background) strongly influence your chosen occupation.

When people are asked how they ended up in their current profession, their responses are often muddled. Answers such as these are not uncommon:

- "I don't remember. I always wanted to be an electrician. My dad is one. And his father was too."
- "My cousin got me this job, and it seemed kind of easy to stay with it."
- "I didn't really intend to go into psychology, but there were no girls in business administration. So, at orientation, I walked out the door and psychology happened to be across the hall."
- "I didn't have much choice. In our town there were only two options for a girl—waitressing and working in the mill."
- "I was just walking down the street when I saw this sign that said, 'Help Wanted.'"

Many of our life's decisions are affected by quirks of fate and the "roll of the die." If we were to subscribe to a theory of random movement, however, there wouldn't be much point in having counselors to provide guidance and encourage self-responsibility.

## Donald Super's Theory

For Super (1957), a person's self-concept is all important in determining vocational development, a process that he views as ongoing and orderly through successive stages. An occupation is the individual expression of one's interests and abilities at a particular time. As a person's preferences and skills evolve, so does his or her career, reflecting the changing self-concept.

Super introduced his theory in a series of ten propositions (1953) about the nature of developing career identities:

1. People differ in their abilities, interests, and personalities.
2. They are qualified, by virtue of these circumstances, for a number of occupations.
3. Each of these occupations requires a characteristic pattern of abilities, interests, and personality traits, with tolerances wide enough to allow both variety of occupations for each individual and variety of individuals in each occupation.
4. Vocational preferences, competencies, situations, and self-concepts change with time and experience, making choice and adjustment a continuous process.
5. This process may be summed up in a series of life stages, characterized as those of growth, exploration, establishment, maintenance, and decline.
6. The nature of the career pattern (that is, the occupational level attained and the sequence, frequency, and duration of trial and stable jobs) is detected by the individual's parental socioeconomic level, mental ability, and personality characteristics, as well as by the opportunities to which he or she is exposed.
7. Development through the life stages can be guided partly by facilitating the process of maturation of abilities and interests and partly by aiding in reality testing and in the development of the self-concept.
8. The process of vocational development is essentially that of developing and implementing a self-concept; it is a compromise process in which the self-concept is a product of the interaction of inherited aptitudes, neural and endocrine makeup, opportunity to play various roles, and evaluation of the extent to which the results of role playing meet with approval of superiors and peers.
9. The process of compromise between individual and social factors and between self-concept and reality is one of role playing, whether the role is played in fantasy, in the counseling interview, or in real-life activities such as school classes, clubs, part-time work, and entry jobs.
10. Work satisfaction and life satisfaction depend on the extent to which the individual finds adequate outlets for abilities, interests, personality traits, and values; they also depend on establishment in a work situation and a satisfying way of life.

Super recognized that people differ in their personalities and unique strengths and therefore choose occupations that will permit them to use their competencies. The pattern of development begins during adolescence with the *exploratory stage,* in which a person uses fantasy, play, and role experimentation to help clarify the emerging self-concept, and moves tentatively onward in the early 20s to a first job. The *establishment stage,* through experimenting and trying out various options, helps the person to discover an occupation well suited to satisfy personal needs. The self-concept adjusts to fit the stabilized career choice. Stability may or may not last into the *maintenance stage;* during the 1950s, when Super was writing, there were far more opportunities and less mobility and economic pressure, and it was more the norm to continue evolving in a single career. In today's times of high unemployment, greater flexibility, and changing situations, the maintenance phase may involve a return to earlier developmental tasks in the search for personal and professional satisfaction. The *decline stage* is characterized, naturally, by dealing with reduced energy and trying to maintain one's position until retirement.

More recently, Super (1990) saw counselors as aiding an individual's progressive development across the whole life span, helping to facilitate the maturation of ability, improving the self-concept, encouraging reality testing, expanding interest, and negotiating a compromise between fantasy and reality and between the various roles that are played throughout life.

## John Holland's Theory

Whereas Super focused on self-concept, Holland (1973) believes that career choices are expressions of the total personality. Satisfaction thus depends on the compatibility of a person's work situation and personality style.

Holland rested his theory on four major assumptions:

1. Individuals can be categorized into six different personality types—realistic, investigative, artistic, social, enterprising, or conventional—depending on interests, preferences, and skills.
2. Environment can also be classified into the same six types and tends to be dominated by compatible personalities.
3. People search for environments in which their personality type can be comfortably expressed; artistic people search for artistic environments, whereas social people look for social environments. They wish to exercise their skills and abilities, express their attitudes and values, and participate in agreeable problems and roles.
4. The behavior of an individual is determined by the interaction between personality type and environmental characteristics. If personality type and work environment are known, the outcomes of vocational choice, achievement, and job changes can be predicted.

The six different personality types that Holland described predispose people to do well in certain careers that capitalize on their strengths. Certainly these personality types do not describe everyone, but they do provide a structure for understanding why some people do better than others in particular jobs. The following is a more detailed description of each type.

1. *Realistic.* This person is logical, objective, and forthright. Preference is given to dimensions such as physical prowess, aggression, and domination. A realistic type prefers activities in which to manipulate objects, tools, machines, and other tangible things. This person is likely to be emotionally

stable but less sociable and inclined to select technical, agricultural, or trade occupations. He or she is practical and tends to have underdeveloped verbal and social skills but highly developed motor skills. The realistic person chooses careers such as laborer, farmer, carpenter, engineer, or machine operator. The realistic environment allows realistic people to perform preferred activities and be rewarded for technical abilities.

2. *Investigative.* By relying on intelligence and cognitive skills, this personality type is a problem solver. Socially aloof and introverted, the investigative individual prefers intellectual tasks that require academic proficiencies. He or she also tends to be analytical, critical, intellectual, methodical, precise, rational, and reserved. This person exhibits traits of creativity, independence, and self-confidence but is often not realistic or practical. Career choices for this type include scientist, scholar, research worker, and theoretician.

3. *Artistic.* This is a sensitive, impulsive, creative, emotional, independent, and nonconforming individual who values cultural activities and aesthetic qualities. This person may develop competencies in art, drama, music, writing, and language and avoid structured situations. Not surprisingly, a creative type chooses careers such as actor, writer, musician, and artist.

4. *Social.* This person is highly skilled at dealing with other people. She or he is usually accepting, responsible, cheerful, nurturing, and caring. If you have noticed a similarity between this type and yourself or your classmates, it is because this category is most often descriptive of those who choose helping professions. Take note, however, because this type often evades intellectual or physical tasks, preferring to use strengths in interpersonal manipulations.

5. *Enterprising.* This person uses highly refined verbal skills for leadership and sales professions such as marketing, business, and politics. He or she is enthusiastic, energetic, dominating, persuasive, extroverted, and aggressive. Much concern is devoted to attaining status, power, and leadership roles. Some examples of enterprising vocations are business executives, salespeople, politicians, and promotional workers.

6. *Conventional.* This type of person prefers activities that are routine, structured, and practical. A conventional type is self-controlled, orderly, inhibited, and efficient. Examples of conventional vocations include bankers, bookkeepers, office workers, and clerks.

To a large extent, Holland believes that there is a real relationship between personality and educational/vocational decision making. He further believes that interest inventories are really personality measures. Members of a vocational group have similar personalities, and each vocation tends to attract and retain people with similar personalities.

Because people in a vocational group have similar personalities, they respond to situations in like ways and therefore tend to create characteristic environments. Vocational satisfaction, stability, and achievement depend on the

## VOICE FROM THE FIELD

I know that many students don't much like their careers class. I probably never learned to hate it because I started doing it before I had ever had a vocational theory course. I came into it as a "career" by accident, learned about it by modeling other counselors and by doing it, and liked it because I was never subjected to being bored by it by a tired university professor who'd rather be teaching something else. I mean, wouldn't everyone rather teach anything but voc? I figured out on my own what was important in vocational counseling, and later had that validated by many of the theories when I finally began to read them. Also, by learning about it "from the trenches" I saw what was actually done in the real world, not what books said was done. In my experience, more than any other type of counseling, there is a big gap between what is done in career counseling and what books say is done.

congruence between an individual's personality and the environment in which he or she works (Holland, 1996).

## Robert Hoppock's Theory

Hoppock (1976) stressed the function of the job in satisfying personal needs, but his theory has attained wide popularity also because of his efforts to integrate ideas from a number of other theories. Vocational development begins with the first awareness that a job can help meet one's needs and continues as the person is better able to anticipate how potentially satisfying a particular career could be as compared with others. Once a person becomes aware of other jobs that could satisfy personal needs, then occupational choices are subject to change. The degree of job satisfaction can be determined by assessing the difference between what a person wants from a job (emotionally, financially, and so forth) and what she or he actually has attained.

Hoppock describes his composite theory in ten basic postulates:

1. Everyone has needs: basic physical needs and higher order psychological needs such as self-esteem, respect, and self-actualization. People vary in the pattern of their need structures, and the individual reaction to needs influences occupational choice.
2. People tend to gravitate toward occupations that serve their perceived needs. A person who has a strong need for power and status will be influenced to seek occupations that have them. Few people are controlled by a single need; most have a variety of needs that act in concert to influence occupational choice.
3. A person does not necessarily have a clear intellectual awareness of needs for them to affect choices. Individuals with self-understanding and insight

may understand the forces that influence them, and others may simply experience pleasure or satisfaction in certain occupational areas.

4. Life experiences help to develop a pattern of individual occupational preference and, as such, suggest a developmental perspective on vocational choice. Contact with occupations occurs both experientially and vicariously, supporting the need for both work or occupational experiences and occupational information, especially during the years of formative development.

5. Given the great diversity of occupational choices, the individual must develop effective decision-making skills based on solid self-awareness and a rich informational base. A trial-and-error process of occupational experimentation is usually not appropriate. The number of occupations and the extensive training many of them require preclude that approach.

6. Self-understanding is the basis on which occupational choice rests; thus it is a primary goal for career counseling.

7. Understanding the self is only half of the occupational choice process; one must also have accurate and thorough information about available occupations. A person cannot choose a career without the knowledge that it exists. Likewise, accurate information dispels stereotypes and myths about the activities involved in various types of work.

8. When a person's needs are met by a job, then he or she experiences job satisfaction. Money is not the only need satisfied by a job; other higher order needs are just as crucial to satisfaction as basic security needs. For a worker to perform effectively and with the motivation to deliver quality, the ratio must be positive. Industrial and assembly workers are often good examples of this principle: Although they may be well paid, many do not have higher order needs satisfied; as a result, their performance on the job is low, the quality is erratic, and absenteeism is a problem.

9. Individuals can delay need satisfaction if they perceive their job as having the potential to satisfy their needs in the future. Opportunities for advancement and career mobility are, therefore, important if a firm wishes to maximize satisfaction.

10. If the balance between needs and satisfaction is unfavorable, then a worker will change jobs if another position appears to offer the potential to meet needs more fully.

In using Hoppock's theory of occupational choice, the counselor's role is to: (1) stimulate the client's self-awareness of interests and needs, including the clarification of values; (2) promote insight into that which gives life personal meaning; (3) provide accurate and complete occupational information; and (4) help match the client's perceived strengths and weaknesses with occupations likely to provide maximum need satisfaction. Hoppock's theory has a number of implications for counselors:

• The counselor should always remember that the needs of the client may differ from the needs of the counselor.

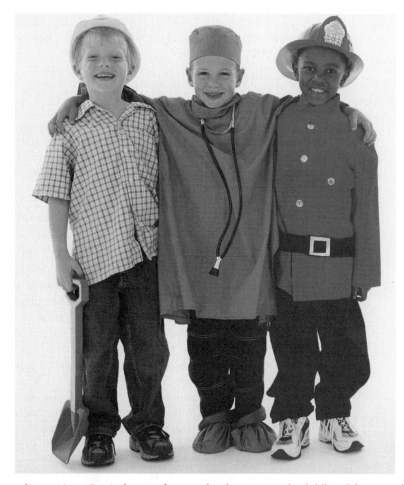

According to Anne Roe's theory of career development, early childhood fantasies form a strong motive for later employment choices. © BananaStock/Bananastock, Ltd./PictureQuest.

- The counselor should operate within the framework of the client's needs.
- The counselor should provide every possible opportunity for the client to identify and to express his or her own needs.
- The counselor should be alert to notice and to remember the needs that the client reveals.
- The counselor should help the client gather information about occupations that may meet his or her needs.
- The counselor should help the client to anticipate how well any contemplated occupation will meet the client's needs.
- The counselor should stay with the client through the process of placement in order to provide the further counseling that will be needed if the desired job is not available.

- The counselor should follow up with the client some months after place-ment in order to see how well the job is meeting the needs that the client thought it would meet.

## Anne Roe's Theory

On the basis of her intensive investigations of scientists' early childhoods, Roe (1957) created a theory that emphasizes need satisfaction in career choices. Persons from child-centered, rejecting, or accepting homes are predisposed to compensate for (or duplicate) in their jobs experiences that they missed (or en-joyed) in their childhood homes.

Roe suggested that the emotional climate of the home is one of three types: (1) emotional concentration on the child, (2) avoidance of the child, or (3) acceptance of the child. Emotional concentration on the child has two ex-tremes: overprotecting and overdemanding. Overprotecting parents limit ex-ploration by the child and encourage dependency. Overdemanding parents set very high standards for the child and rigidly enforce conformity.

The avoidance type is divided into those ranging from rejecting to neglect-ing. A rejecting parent resents the child, expresses a cold and indifferent atti-tude, and works to keep the child from intruding into his or her life. A neglecting parent is less hostile toward the child but provides no affection or attention and only the bare minimum of physical care.

An accepting pattern is divided into casual acceptance and loving accep-tance. Casually accepting parents are affectionate and loving but in a mild way and only if they are not otherwise occupied. They tend to be easygoing. Lovingly accepting parents provide much warmth, affection, praise, and at-tention. They encourage the child and help in an appropriate way.

These six subdivisions produce, according to Roe, two types of voca-tional behavior. The categories of loving, overprotective, and overdemanding tend to produce a major vocational orientation toward persons. The remain-ing categories—casual, neglecting, and rejecting—produce a major voca-tional orientation away from persons. The theory has generated considerable research, which has overall failed to bear it out. This may be in part because of misunderstandings and misinterpretations about what Roe intended (Brown, Lum, & Voyle, 1997). In any case, any theory that is more than forty years old is going to have some problems being applied to contempo-rary life without adaptations. She is still responsible for calling attention to the ways that jobs fulfill needs that were not met in early childhood.

## John Krumboltz' Theory

Krumboltz (1978) developed a social learning theory that attempts to synthe-size the factors that influence career decision making. First, Krumboltz ac-knowledges the impact of genetic endowment—how race, gender, cultural and

## VOICE FROM THE FIELD

Why do I like vocational counseling? It's challenging. It appeals to the detective or investigator in me, sorting through data and theories to try to help someone get clarity about decisions they want to make. It's personal counseling, in the most personal sense. What's more personal than the work one invests one's life in? If work isn't going well, it impacts the person's life, not just their work. If it is going well, the same is true.

Probably on a personal level, it appeals to me because the goal is relatively concrete—clarifying, deciding, narrowing choices. I also like functioning in the role of an expert. A vocational counselor needs to be a bit of a frustrated research librarian because he or she needs to know a lot of information about the world of work. I like that, too.

---

physical characteristics, native intelligence, and abilities limit some choices and expand others. Not everyone can choose to be a professional basketball player, brain surgeon, or ballet dancer, regardless of motivation or interest. Second, environmental factors play a part in career development. The economic climate, occupational opportunities available, labor laws, union rules, technological developments, family resources, educational systems, and other variables outside the individual's control influence occupational decision making. Third, previous learning experiences (in behavioristic terminology, *conditioned stimuli* and *reinforcers*) shape the person's attitudes and interests toward various professions. Some children are reinforced by their parents for reading, others for their physical or mechanical skills.

A final factor to be considered, according to Krumboltz, is a person's "task approach skills," which are his or her performance standards, work habits, unique perceptions, and abilities to alter problem-solving strategies flexibly according to the demands of the situation.

Krumboltz summarizes the responsibilities of a counselor in the career development process as helping people to: learn a logical sequence of career decision-making skills; arrange a series of exploration experiences that will provide needed information; and make informed choices about the consequences of what has been learned.

Subsequent development of this theory has led to several other practical applications that can be used in counseling (Mitchell & Krumboltz, 1996; Zunker, 2002):

1. Career decisions should be based not only on present interests and abilities but also on others that can be developed.
2. Structured learning experiences can be customized for clients so that they can expand the range of their choices and opportunities.

3. Efforts should be undertaken to prepare people for a changing world in which new skills and abilities will need to be developed.
4. Career counseling should be integrated into all counseling efforts rather than just restricted to occupational choices.
5. Cognitive restructuring methods should be employed to help people to think differently about their choices and situations.

## Other Models

As confusing as it might be to digest all these new theories, you are probably not the least surprised to learn that this is just the tip of the iceberg. There are actually at least a dozen other approaches to career development that space limitations (thankfully?) make impossible to cover in any depth.

Eli Ginzberg (1972), for example, described career development as a continual, lifelong process of decision making in which the person is trying to reconcile goals and preparations with the reality of limited opportunity. Like Super and Ginzberg, Tiedeman and O'Hara (1963) are developmentalists who suggest that career development is a process of identifying with work through the interaction between personality and society. They suggest the importance of decision making in the process of defining the relationship between personality and career. They have, however, been more precise than most other theorists in plotting the changes people experience in their evolving sense of identity.

One other development in the field that is likely to increase will be the continued evolution of career theories that deal with special populations that do not fit those derived from white, middle-class, male norms. Thus career theories related to women and multicultural groups will continue to proliferate as North America continues to become more diverse in its composition (Zunker, 2002). Finally, the constructivist approach that was described in earlier chapters has also been applied to career development in such a way that people's views of their options are examined within their cultural history and beliefs (Cochran, 1997; Savickas, 1997; Sharf, 2002).

## CAREER EDUCATION

Direct counseling service is only one way that counselors provide help to people; as with other specialty areas, practitioners are also called on to function in the roles of consultants and teachers. Career education, career development, and vocational assistance are lifelong processes that often require supportive services at various developmental levels. It is an ongoing process that has crucial significance in elementary, secondary, and postsecondary schools. In addition to professionals who work in school, college, and university settings, rehabilitation counselors are also involved in career education programs, most of which have several components:

1. *Every learning experience has career implications.* Career education must be accepted as an institutional responsibility rather than a function of the counseling and guidance staff.
2. *Skill training is necessary for entry into an occupation.* Educational experiences should have a work-related skills component attached to them. Counselors should be ready to work with clients and other professionals to structure appropriate skill-related activities.
3. *Cognitive and experiential ways must be provided for students to understand work-oriented values.* The counselor must help the student to gain self-understanding, knowledge of alternatives, awareness of values, and decision-making skills in both cognitive and experiential ways.
4. *Opportunities must be provided for observing work environments.* Individuals must have the opportunity to develop experiences and knowledge about the world of work. Counselors can coordinate with students, employers, and educational institutions to create these opportunities.
5. *The interrelationships among home, family, community, and societal values should be identified.* The impact of these values on career decisions and preferences needs to be clarified.

Each of these general components requires the assistance of counselors who provide information as needed, consult with other personnel, and structure activities and experiences designed to facilitate career awareness, self-understanding, and occupational information. Counselors who work in career education and career guidance settings must also be prepared to implement and use the services and information available through computer-assisted media.

1. Counselors must develop skills in computer-assisted management with regard to records and career assessment results, and they must attend to student confidentiality issues inherent in these systems.
2. Career guidance professionals must thoroughly understand the strengths and weaknesses of the various computerized career information and career guidance systems available to students.
3. Career education professionals must understand the need to integrate computerized career guidance and assessment systems as supplements to career education and career counseling.
4. Counselors must structure technological systems to enhance rather than to direct student choice.
5. DVDs, telecommunications, and Internet systems must be identified and infused into the career education process.
6. Counselors must maintain quality control of computer-assisted systems through ongoing dialogue with clients so that they are able to integrate the learning that is taking place.

## Abilities

Individuals must have an understanding of their abilities in order to identify potential areas for job exploration and career development. People must recognize the need to develop basic academic skills and to maximize potential abilities to participate fully in the career development process. In an era of rapidly changing technology and job obsolescence, the task of identifying abilities will extend well into the adult years. Most adults will confront periods of unemployment in their lives and that practically everyone will experience work adjustment problems at some time or another. A thorough understanding of abilities, including needs for remediation, will be helpful to both students and adults as they participate in the career development process.

## Interests

A knowledge of interests (and the personality tendencies they suggest) will be helpful to individuals as they attempt to match aptitudes with available occupations. Interests are often the key to occupational satisfaction; people whose interests are not represented in their occupational choice can suffer much unrest and dissatisfaction. It is also important for the counselor to emphasize that abilities and interests are not always neatly related and that interest alone is not a sufficient condition for job satisfaction in positions requiring abilities that the client lacks.

## Values

Values are an important factor affecting career development. Occupations that reflect values similar to those held by clients can lead to greater job satisfaction, especially with regard to motivation and job performance. The ill-defined or poorly defined values of many clients can interfere with effective decision making. Counselors must help clients to clarify their values and relate them to abilities and interests. Clients who are aware of the relationship among values, interests, and aptitudes can be described as vocationally mature and more likely than others to experience job satisfaction and career advancement.

# CAREER DECISION MAKING

In some ways, career development—and certainly career choices—can be viewed as a decision-making process. Clients who are unable to integrate knowledge about the self with occupational information will make sporadic progress in career choice. Helping clients to develop refined decision-making skills is an essential dimension of occupational assistance.

Some clients will come to career counseling aware of the skills involved in decision making. For others, knowledge may be absent or fragmentary, requiring the counselor to assess the client's level of decision-making skills and provide appropriate information. Most decision-making models contain several specific steps:

1. *Defining the problem.* The counselor helps clients explore various aspects of a stated vocational issue. Specific counseling skills are used to elicit information, establish priorities, and crystallize salient points. It is essential that sufficient time be spent on this step because it will set the tone for future progress. Problem identification may need to be done at several stages in the process.

2. *Finding and using information.* Once the vocationally related problem is identified, the counselor assists the client in gathering useful information. Sources might include testing; occupational, vocational, and educational information; and a computer-assisted job search. The counselor must also help the client to use the information in an appropriate manner by interpreting tests, clarifying misunderstandings, and generating conclusions.

3. *Creating alternatives.* In this step, the counselor and client combine forces to identify as many alternatives as possible. Those that are clearly inappropriate are excluded, and the remaining alternatives are examined in the light of information on aptitudes, interests, values, and availability.

4. *Developing plans.* In this stage, plans that may be either tentative or firm, depending on the client's needs, are developed. The planning stage should be detailed and sequenced and should have contingencies built into it. This is a crucial step in decision making because it translates the information into action-oriented steps.

5. *Implementing plans.* Implementing and following through on plans are primarily the responsibilities of the client, although the counselor should be available for consultation and support. Sometimes clients experience difficulty at this stage, and the counselor should intervene to determine whether there are flaws in the plan or whether personal counseling is needed.

6. *Evaluating plans.* Evaluation helps the client to determine the effectiveness of the decision-making process and to feed results into a new problem formulation. Counselors should emphasize to clients that they are ultimately implementing a process as much as a specific decision. Vocational decision making is a lifelong undertaking that requires continual refinement and development.

Counselors must be familiar with the decision-making process both generally and specifically as it is applied to career decision making so they can identify particular problems in style for clients who are experiencing difficulty. Career counseling, however, must focus not only on decision making but also on techniques to correct embedded or underlying difficulties beyond skills in making decisions. For example, a family systems approach may be appropriate for individuals whose pattern of enmeshment interferes with career decision making; for others who exhibit irrational beliefs and attitudes, cognitive restructuring may be indicated. Career counselors must be flexible and insightful as they diagnose the multiple variables affecting career decision making and be versatile in designing treatment approaches for specific problems.

The process of career education and vocational choice is highly complex. Counselors can help clients to perform this crucial lifework in a systematic and objective fashion, providing information and assistance at critical points. The ultimate goal of career education is to assist individuals to optimize their resources and to make vocational choices that are likely to lead to job satisfaction and career development.

# TRENDS AND ISSUES IN CAREER COUNSELING

The world of work is rapidly changing and evolving, requiring major adjustments on the part of the labor force and vocational counselors. There is little doubt that the fundamental nature of society has changed from an industrial base to an information base. Whereas once upon a time the economy was driven by the manufacture of tangible goods, more and more the marketplace is dominated by service-oriented jobs. We are living in the information age, with the impact of technology felt in every sector of the world of work, simultaneously creating labor shortages (in the case of computer specialists) and surpluses (in the case of assembly and manufacturing workers). Given recent developments in computer technology and the shift from industrial to service, professional, and technical work, two classes of workers are emerging: (1) skilled and specialized service, professional, and technical workers who form an elite and highly employable class and (2) an underclass of workers without employable skills. These forces are likely to create technical problems and labor shortages in addition to the human problems created by dislocations. Vocational counselors must be ready to respond to these issues, particularly those involving retraining and the use of technologically dense systems.

## Changes in the Workplace

The ways we function in our jobs change almost every year. If we look only at the task of word processing, an activity that most of us engaged in a decade ago on a typewriter, we can appreciate how quickly we are forced to adapt. Every six months we now receive notices that our software is outdated and if we really hope to keep up with everyone else, we have to learn another new version of a language. Relearning supposedly better ways to "process words" is so time consuming that by the time we have mastered the new system, it is already obsolete.

Similarly, as the pace of change accelerates, many workers are likely to experience unemployment and job elimination because they were unable to adapt quickly enough. Career guidance professionals will have major responsibility for helping workers who become occupationally obsolete to cope with the stress of transition and dislocation and to develop marketable skills through retraining and retooling.

As women increasingly enter the workplace, counselors must be aware of issues pertaining to sexual harassment, salary inequities, dual-career families, and the needs for child care. Estimates of sexual harassment, for example, have found the prevalence to be widespread (40–90 percent), resulting in damage at both the individual and the institutional levels (Barak, 1994). Career counselors must develop educational programs for women to assist them to respond to these and many other issues to gain equity and opportunity in the workplace.

Additionally, career counselors must recognize that the majority of the new workers entering the labor market will be women and immigrants. These groups are overrepresented in areas experiencing the least amount of growth and are less prepared educationally for the fastest-growing segments of the labor market. This change illustrates the challenges for career counselors who must develop programs to improve the educational and employability levels of these new job seekers. Innovative procedures must be developed in response to the career development needs of women, minorities, and immigrants.

## Work and Leisure

As productivity increases through the application of technology to work, efficiency is likely to increase, meaning that people will be able to work fewer hours (even if they are not yet choosing to do so). In fact, productive work may become a relatively scarce resource. To compensate for decreased demands of work, individuals must increase their skills and abilities to use leisure in a manner that will be personally fulfilling.

Work and leisure must be seen not as antithetical but as psychologically related aspects of a career. Career counselors must recognize the importance of leisure as they assist clients to engage in life/career planning that will include creative and fulfilling ways in which to use their time. Leisure can be used effectively once the misperception of leisure as nonproductive is eliminated. Some of the productive uses of leisure might include alternative ways of seeking fulfillment, techniques for managing discretionary time, and resources for reducing stress and maximizing consciousness. Leisure, then, must be seen by the vocational counselor as a companion concern to work.

## Use of Technology

Technology is likely to affect career and vocational counseling more than any other specialty within the counseling and guidance field. As mentioned earlier, there has been an increase in the use of computer-based interactive career guidance systems that allow users to integrate occupational and educational information with interests and values in order to improve career decision making. These systems are likely to continue to be used, with refinements that depict information more realistically. The availability of this technology requires that the career counselor be technologically literate and computer "smart" to assist clients effectively in career decision-making activities.

As computers become more widely used, simulation and virtual reality are likely to emerge as important career development strategies. Simulated work experiences will allow clients to gain concrete experience and to develop relevant career skills optimally in a "no-lose" environment. With computer networking, increasingly sophisticated software, and DVDs and CD-ROM simulations, clients will be able to sample interactively an ever greater and more diverse range of jobs, activities, and career guidance resources. These future technological developments will require a career counselor who has the skill and ability to use them in career education and vocational guidance.

# SUMMARY

In this chapter we have examined the value and diversity of career counseling. The importance of this specialty will increase with the impact of technology on our society. The counselor's role in a high-tech society is to help individuals assimilate the effects of technology, thereby allowing them to develop to their fullest potential.

# SELF-GUIDED EXPLORATIONS

1. List some of the most helpful things that people have said to you in your life regarding work and careers.
2. What are some of the things people have said to you about work and careers that have not been very helpful?
3. The circumstance in which you presently find yourself—taking a counseling class—is the result of a number of forces and factors that have affected you in particular ways. Describe as many influences as you can identify that have shaped your conscious and unconscious choices to be where you are now.
4. Describe your fantasy of what you will be doing five, ten, and twenty years in the future.
5. Rank-order the factors that would be most important to you in a job.

| | |
|---|---|
| _____ Variety of tasks | _____ Minimum of pressure |
| _____ Supportive co-workers | _____ Excellent supervision |
| _____ Subsidies for further education | _____ Promotional opportunities |
| _____ Good salary and benefits | _____ Lots of responsibility |
| _____ Opportunities for creativity | _____ Attractive office |
| _____ Job security | _____ Freedom of movement |

How have these rankings helped you decide what you will focus on when you look for a job after you graduate?

## For Homework:

Talk to several different people of various ages and socioeconomic backgrounds to find out what it is about their work that they find most and least satisfying. List the principal factors that you discovered are most significant.

## SUGGESTED READINGS

Gysbers, N. C., Heppner, M. J., & Johnston, J. A. (1998). *Career counseling: Process, issues, and techniques.* Boston: Allyn & Bacon.

Herring, R. D. (1998). *Career counseling in the schools: Multicultural and developmental perspectives.* Alexandria, VA: American Counseling Association.

Isaacson, L. E., & Brown, D. (1999). *Career information, career counseling, and career development* (7th ed.). Boston: Allyn & Bacon.

Luzzo, D. A. (2002). *Career counseling.* Boston: Houghton Mifflin.

Niles, S. G., Goodman, J., & Pope, M. (2001). *Career counseling casebook: A resource for students, practitioners, and counselor educators.* Washington, DC: National Career Development Association.

Patton, W., & McMahon, M. (1999). *Career development and systems theory: A new relationship.* Pacific Grove, CA: Brooks/Cole.

Sharf, R. S. (2002). *Applying career development theory to counseling* (3rd ed.). Pacific Grove, CA: Brooks/Cole.

Terkel, S. (1979). *Working.* New York: Avon.

U.S. Department of Labor. *Dictionary of occupational titles* (latest ed.). Washington, DC: U.S. Department of Labor.

Zunker, V. G. (2002). *Career counseling: Applied concepts of life planning* (6th ed.). Pacific Grove, CA: Brooks/Cole.

# 12 $\overset{\text{CHAPTER}}{}$ ADDICTIONS COUNSELING

KEY CONCEPTS

Addiction

Drug culture

Prevention programs

Medical model

12-step programs

Therapeutic model

Abstinence

# ADDICTIONS COUNSELING

# CHAPTER 12

Almost everyone has some kind of addiction—if not to drugs or alcohol, then to gambling, cigarettes, risky behavior, exercise, television, computer games, the Internet, adult videos, work, shopping, and so on. The key question here is not whether you are addicted but if that attachment interferes with the satisfaction and productivity of life.

There is probably no presenting complaint that will be brought to you as a counselor that is more common than some form of addiction—and quite likely none that you will find more frustrating to treat. The incidence of addiction to drugs and alcohol is staggering, estimated to cost the nation billions of dollars alone in economic loss, not to mention the debilitating effects on physical, social, and family life (Shute, 1997). In the United States alone more than 700,000 people receive alcohol treatment for chronic abuse (National Institute on Alcohol Abuse and Alcoholism, 2001). And this number doesn't include the other 25 million people who are chemically dependent but not seeking treatment (Biancoviso, Fuertes, & Bishop-Towle, 2001).

When you add to substance abuse problems the many other addictions common to contemporary life (computers, video games, excessive exercise, eating disorders, workaholism, etc.), you can appreciate the magnitude of the problem. Increasingly, for example, more and more people are becoming hooked on the Internet, spending more time in front of a computer screen than they do face to face with human beings (Fearing, 1996). As with any other addiction—from excess television viewing to abusive levels of daily exercise—these problems are often chronic, intractable, and even life-threatening.

# SYMPTOMS OF ADDICTION

An addiction is defined as a persistent, chronic, and intense focus on a single behavior pattern that feels (or is) out of control. Whether in the case of a drug or an activity, there are a number of symptoms in evidence (van Wormer & Davis, 2003):

1. Persistent and frequent thinking about the activity throughout the day.
2. Significant interference with enjoying other important aspects of life.
3. Inability to control, cut back, or stop the behavior, even after being aware of debilitating effects.
4. Restlessness or irritability when attempts are made to cut back the behavior.
5. Feelings of anxiety or agitation if behavior is stopped for a period of time
6. Use of the addiction to escape or avoid other responsibilities.
7. Dishonesty or exaggerations when reporting the incidence of behavior, minimizing the problem to self and others.
8. Engaging in high-risk behavior that jeopardizes emotional or physical safety.
9. Intense mood swings associated with the activity, ranging from euphoria to shame, guilt, and depression.

It is no wonder that addiction counseling is one of the fastest growing specialties in the field, spawning its own professional associations (International Association for Addictions and Offender Counselors, National Association of Alcoholism and Drug Abuse Counselors), its own certification bodies, and journals. In addition, self-help groups proliferate around the world to provide needed support systems—not only the familiar Alcoholics Anonymous, but also hundreds of other groups devoted to one addiction or another.

Among the various addictions that you will encounter as a counselor, surely treating alcohol and drug abuse will be among the most challenging. This will be the case not only because of the physically addictive properties of mind-altering substances but also because our culture is so steeped in drug-related behavior. In fact, three of the most common substance addictions in our society actually have their own institutions devoted to supporting the behavior: coffee houses, bars, and cigarette breaks.

# DRUG USE AND DRUG ABUSE

Everyone without a drug habit, raise your hand. Now, let those who are smugly confident that they hold nothing in common with your basic drug addict (and so are holding their hands quite high) consider the following:

1. A drug can be any substance ingested into the body that produces an altered state of consciousness or change in body chemistry.
2. Andrew Weil (1972, 1998) a noted pharmacologist, has a theory that all humans have an innate drive to alter their consciousness. From spinning in circles as children to eating spicy foods as adults, the goal is to experience sensory overload. For some people, it is stimulants like coffee, am-

FIGURE 12.1 | CONTINUUM OF DRUG BEHAVIOR

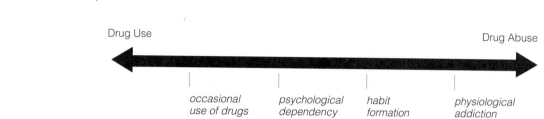

phetamines, or even chocolate that light their fire; for others, they prefer to medicate themselves with "downers" like alcohol or Xanax.

3. Drug use not only is common among human beings but also is found among other creatures. When animals in Africa are subjected to crowding, poaching, and other stressful conditions, they resort to intoxicants. Elephants will munch fermented fruit. Grasshoppers will literally get high (given their jumping prowess) after eating marijuana. Peruvian llamas are fond of cocoa leaves. Rats, when given choices between plain water and alcohol, prefer the booze, especially at bedtime.

4. The difference between drug use and drug abuse is a matter of degree (see Figure 12.1). Once a need for drugs has been established, in order to maintain effective functioning, addiction and physiological dependence prevail. The most widely used (and probably abused) drugs are those that happen to be legal. Coffee, cigarettes, chocolate, and cola beverages all contain sufficient quantities of amphetamines to create full-fledged addictions.

5. Almost every person alive has some oral addiction, and the world is filled with regional choices. Whereas alcohol has permeated every known culture (except that of the Eskimo, who live in a climate too cold to grow anything), more exotic drugs are found in every region. Cocaine originated in the Andes of Peru and Bolivia, coffee and hashish in southern Arabia, peyote in Mexico, opium in India and Mesopotamia, and, of course, tea in China.

It may now be evident that most people ingest drugs in some form, whether as food additive, beverage, medication, or intoxicant. Although the biological mechanism underlying drug use is not clearly established, one theory suggests that drugs have psychomotor stimulant properties that activate positive reinforcement mechanisms within the brain. This results in pleasurable sensations that are more powerful than those occurring naturally (Wise, 1988).

There are many factors that determine whether a person can safely and responsibly use drugs (such as an occasional cup of coffee or glass of beer) or will abuse addictive substances (heroin, for example) or become psychologically dependent (as is common with marijuana). Counselors are often required to work with these various forms of drug use and to make a determination with the client as to which behaviors are self-destructive and out of control.

## VOICE FROM THE FIELD

There's nothing my counselor could have done to help me when I was using. [Laughs.] There's nothing anyone could have done. And a whole bunch of people tried, I gotta tell you. [Laughs again, but he's not smiling.] I was in detox I don't know how many times. I was in and out of I don't know how many places. I saw more people like you than you could imagine. They all did their best, I know. Shit, I felt sorry for 'em all. That's why I played their games and all. I knew what they wanted—what they wanted me to tell 'em. So that's what I did.

So what did it take? Hey, good question. I guess that's why I want to be a counselor now to figure it out. I don't think anyone really knows. I think with me it was just that I was hitting bottom. Nothing left to lose. I had no money left to score. Couldn't risk gettin' caught again stealing stuff. My friends were sick of me, my good friends anyway; I always had buddies I could get high with. Who knows? Maybe some of the counselors did help me. Kind of a delayed reaction. [Laughs.] I do know, though, that when I got ready to get clean, that was it! I've never looked back since.

---

The subject of drug use and abuse merits its own chapter in an introductory counseling textbook for a number of reasons. First, most people, and especially clients who tend to be externally controlled, regularly use drugs in some form. Often alcohol, marijuana, coffee, tobacco, or excessive food is a troubled person's effort at self-medication for distressing symptoms. The externally oriented addict denies responsibility for problems, blames others for experienced misery, and feels that, because someone else has created the emotional pain, an externally available substance will fix things. The unfortunate part is that such a person is perfectly correct. Drugs do provide immediate relief. They dull pain and are great distracters. While using drugs at moderately abusive levels (whatever that means), people can still function through their day in a purple but painless haze. (See also Table 12.1 illustrating reasons for drug use and abuse.)

The second reason for studying a specialty such as drug counseling is that traditional therapeutic interventions tend not to work very well. Insight into the reasons underlying self-destructive behavior in the form of addiction is not sufficient to alter the behavior. Clients with chronic addiction problems are so immune and resistant to change that sometimes highly dramatic and creative interventions must be found. Finally, many such individuals may have the same expectations for their counseling sessions as they have for their drugs: instant, magical relief.

Many people engage in mood-altering behavior to create a sense of euphoria or well-being or to block out unpleasant events. Counselors must recognize that drug taking is a behavior and follows patterns that can be understood and modified to the same extent as any other. The behavior will persist if it minimizes discomfort or maximizes pleasure and satisfaction. Nothing will decrease the hold of drugs unless there is an adequate substitute

| TABLE 12.1 | REASONS FOR DRUG USE AND DRUG ABUSE |
|---|---|

| Why People Use Drugs | Why People Abuse Drugs |
|---|---|
| Euphoria | Biochemical predisposition |
| Availability | Physical addiction |
| Cultural exposure | Maintenance of intoxication |
| Pain suppressant | External control |
| Boredom | Habituation |
| Rebellion | Social reinforcement |
| Entertainment and curiosity | Poor self-image |
| Enhancement of reality | Addictive personality |
| Peer pressure | Escape |
| Stress reduction | Impulsivity |
| Social lubricant | Instant gratification |
| Self-medication | Few perceived options |

for the feelings drugs provide. Counselors need to assess and observe a client's behavior to determine whether the client is displaying symptoms of abuse and reliance on mood-altering substances.

## OUR DRUG CULTURE

People are constantly encouraged to purchase drugs to feel better and to buy products that help with weight loss. The implicit—if not explicit—message is that comfort and ease are of maximum importance. There is little glorification for the hard work or discipline involved in maintaining a healthy body. Advertising has clearly had some impact on drug use in our society. Ads on television and in other media promise to make you feel happier, younger, sexier, more attractive, and less tense. They persuade people to buy over-the-counter drugs as a means of relief from suffering and to create a desirable personal image. Advertisements clearly imply not only that the use of these drugs will create wonderful results but also that the drugs are harmless.

Although legislators try to keep current in providing protection for the consumer, our society continues to approve and even encourage use of substances such as caffeine, alcohol, and tobacco. Although the latter is becoming less than fashionable these days in North America, its use is increasing in other parts of the world. The acceptance of alcohol as an appropriate drug by all citizens over a certain arbitrary age encourages the development of a milieu in which drug use is considered normal.

## VOICE FROM THE FIELD

I've never understood how people in our field can have such disdain for addicts. Sometimes, you hear them made fun of and all. You see, there's basically two kinds of drug counselors: those who are recovering addicts themselves but who don't have much formal training, and people like me who have a degree but no direct experience as an addict. Sometimes, it feels like war in that each group thinks they have more credibility. Obviously, though, both points of view are valid. But I don't think you need to have been a drug addict and lost everything in your life in order to know what it feels like to be out of control. I think almost everyone knows that feeling. I think all of us, at one time or another, have had a problem with impulse control or whatever.

I'm pretty disciplined about a lot of things in my life. I eat right and exercise regularly. I never got into the drug scene and I don't drink very often. But still, I don't know what I'd do without my lattes and all. You can laugh, but I'm serious. I just don't think I could give up coffee for anything. Maybe that doesn't sound like a big deal, but it does give me an idea of how hard it would be to quit. And I use this to understand clients better. That's why I don't judge them so much.

---

Almost all drugs are available to adolescents, not only on the street but also on the school grounds. It is not uncommon to find adolescents sniffing glue, gasoline, or lighter fluid; using heroin; or taking barbiturates or amphetamines during school hours. Marijuana use is so prevalent among adolescents that it is often considered normal by school officials. There is also frequent use of drugs like MDMA (Ecstasy) and PCP, an anesthetic employed in veterinary medicine that, when used in excess, produces a toxic psychosis often associated with violent and self-destructive behavior.

Depending on the setting in which you practice, and the specific population that you work with, you must educate yourself about the various substance abuse problems that will be most common. This will alert you to watch for physical signs (fatigue, sleep disturbances, confusion), emotional symptoms like mood fluctuations, unprovoked hostility, and uncooperativeness, interpersonal signs such as hanging out with deviant groups, and those symptoms related to impaired work or school performance (Windle, 2001).

## EFFECTS OF DRUG ABUSE

There are many negative physical effects that result from drug abuse. These symptoms are in addition to the relationship casualties that usually occur as the abuser alienates friends, family members, and coworkers.

1. Death has to be at the top of the list. Reports of drug overdoses occur in the newspapers so routinely that they are no longer news. Suicide is certainly a distinct possibility for a person in an altered state of conscious-

ness, and it is not unknown for people to die from convulsions while withdrawing from barbiturates.

2. Through neglect, disinterest, and distraction, the diet of a drug abuser often suffers. Many drugs tend to stifle the appetite; other drugs (narcotics, alcohol) lead the user toward malnourishment.

3. Disturbances of sleep are common results of introducing artificial stimulants or depressants into the bloodstream. Certainly anyone who has had a few cups of coffee before bedtime or who has fallen asleep while still feeling the effects of alcohol knows that the quality of sleep is impaired. The loss or disruption of sleep presents added dangers for the drug abuser, whose perceptions and reactions are already less than optimal.

4. Many other physical symptoms can develop as a result of long-term drug use. Naturally, after foreign substances are ingested, the body reacts. Some problems are the result of the ways in which the drugs are introduced into the body. For example, nasal damage results from repeated snorting of cocaine, lung damage has been reported in marijuana smokers, and skin disorders occur in those who inject heroin. A variety of musculoskeletal, respiratory, gastrointestinal, and central nervous system disorders are also possible—even likely—after long-term drug or alcohol abuse. In addition, almost every system of the body is affected: Neurons are destroyed, neurotransmitters are sidetracked, genetic material is altered, and disease is more likely.

## ADOLESCENT DRUG USE

Many counselors interpret the drug abuser's behavior within the context of family dynamics. The family is sometimes stabilized in its distraction by and attention toward the abuser's behavior. The family has its scapegoat. And the abuser has feelings of control, at least over making others feel powerless. Everyone continues helplessly along, unable to break the destructive patterns that bind the family members together.

The significance of such early use of drugs relates to the development of crucial social and personal skills in adolescence. This is a difficult time, and drugs are an available way to ease pain and discomfort. Unfortunately, they also increase antisocial behavior, block completion of normal developmental tasks, and sometimes lead to the development of a deviant lifestyle. Frequent drug abusers often appear as withdrawn, alienated, and generally unhappy.

The frequency and intensity of adolescent drug use are of concern to the counselor. Early identification, treatment, and support are crucial to reducing the negative effects of drug and alcohol use in the next generation. Adolescent drug users present a troubled profile to counselors. They are unable to invest in or derive pleasure from personal relationships, work, or school or to direct energy to future goals.

Working with adolescents on drug abuse and alcohol use is sensitive and complex. In addition to providing individual treatment, counselors should include family counseling that focuses on reducing current levels of denial, shame, resentment, guilt, anger, and insecurity. In some cases, innovative programs that use a "boot camp" or a prison model are designed to frighten at-risk teenagers into making radical changes in their lifestyles (Alter, 1995). Although these programs have some serious ethical problems because of their dramatic—if not sometimes even abusive—formats, there is no arguing that they appear to have a higher success rate than more traditional models (Gladding, 1997c).

# PREVENTION

Although treatment of substance abuse receives considerable attention, it is through prevention efforts that counselors can have the best potential to affect alcohol and substance abuse problems. Prevention programs are especially important in schools because substance abuse often begins with school-age experimentation. Early and frequent prevention activities can provide needed knowledge and skills for children to learn alternatives to substance use and abuse. Because students find counselors to be creditable resources, we have an opportunity to broaden and expand their involvement with primary prevention in the school.

In designing prevention programs, counselors need to differentiate between two subgroups of adolescent drug and alcohol users: those who are primarily experimenters and those who use alcohol and drugs as a symptom of underlying personal and social maladjustment (Shedler & Block, 1990). The experimenter group is an appropriate focus for prevention efforts because the underlying personality pattern is normative, allowing prevention efforts to concentrate on reducing and eliminating destructive patterns of substance use. The second group requires treatment around the underlying syndromes rather than a focus on the patterns of drug and alcohol use.

Prevention programs can focus on alcohol and drug education, social resistance, and social-skills training. Focus should be directed toward understanding the reasons why people use drugs, especially variables like self-confidence, self-control, and impulsivity. Prevention programs designed to help build skills can be an important aspect of what counselors do.

Effective prevention programs have the following characteristics:

- They go beyond simple information sharing and publicity about substance abuse.
- They include parent and family involvement.
- They are long-term commitments, not Band-Aid approaches.
- They are integrated into a holistic concept of healthful living.
- They are closely connected with positive school climates.

Involvement with prevention activities provides the counselor with multiple opportunities to influence the substance abuse problem at the earliest stage before it becomes a negative factor interfering in the lives of adolescents and adults.

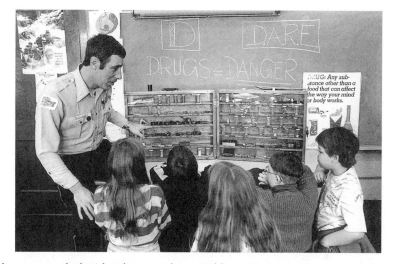

The best way to deal with substance abuse problems is a prevention program that equips children with the necessary attitudes and skills that will immunize them against future addictions. © Jean-claude Lejeune.

## ABUSE IN SPECIAL POPULATIONS

The major similarity among most special population groups with regard to drug and alcohol abuse is the willingness of society to overlook or accept the behavior. This tendency results in part from sympathy and denial. Because the lives of special populations are often viewed as lower in quality, many people view any form of pleasure as acceptable. Recognizing the serious problems of special populations means having to work with them to improve the quality of life; denial of problems reduces the responsibility to work toward change. The attitude of society and even of immediate family members is an important factor in treatment because it means that there will often be little support for behavior change. Two special populations that you are especially likely to encounter as a counselor are the elderly and the disabled.

### The Elderly

Drug abuse by the elderly may be intentional but often is not; most of the time it results from using prescribed medications. Older patients frequently visit several different doctors, each of whom prescribes a variety of medications. The elderly therefore form the largest group of consumers of legal drugs. Some estimates even show that half of all elderly patients who seek medical services are experiencing some drug-related problem (Blake, 1990). Furthermore, the elderly have a decreased ability to metabolize medications and are more susceptible to their actions, interactions, and side effects (Beechem, 2002). It is especially important for counselors to be aware of the potential for prescription drug/alcohol interaction effects in this population.

## VOICE FROM THE FIELD

I remember this one time I was seeing this little old lady in counseling. I wasn't even sure why she was coming in. I think she just wanted somebody to talk to because nobody ever seemed to pay much attention to her. I didn't know why because I found her to be delightful. She had lots of stories to tell and I felt honored to hear them.

Anyway, one day she brought in this oversized bag and set it next to her on the couch. I kept looking at it, wondering what was inside, but she didn't say a word. She just kept talking about whatever was going on in her life. Then when it came time to leave, she handed the bag to me and asked if I would hold it for her. I asked her what was inside and she just smiled at me with the innocent little ole lady look and then walked out.

After she left I looked inside the bag and found about two dozen different prescription bottles. I'm not exaggerating either! I looked at them more closely and saw she had scripts for just about everything: high blood pressure, sleeping pills, antidepressants, tranquilizers, and a bunch of other things—I couldn't imagine what they were for. And they were from about five different doctors, too. I have no idea how she could even get out of bed in the morning, she was so overloaded with chemicals in her body. I figured out later she brought them to me because she really trusted me and wanted me to help her cut down.

---

Although both prescription and nonprescription drugs are abused by the elderly, alcohol presents by far the most serious drug problem for this population. About one-third of elderly alcoholics have developed an alcohol problem later in life, usually as a reaction to stress. The remaining two-thirds appear to be long-standing alcohol abusers who drank heavily into old age. Because both types of elderly alcoholics tend to drink in response to stress, favorable responses to treatment, especially in the company of contemporaries, have been reported.

In the elderly, a number of characteristics have been identified that tend to trigger drug and alcohol abuse. Depression and its effects increase substantially with aging. Persons over 65 years of age account for 25 percent of all suicides. The health habits of elderly abusers are often poor; they do not eat regularly or properly, and their sleep is frequently disturbed. They tend to rely on medication for a sense of well-being. Behaviorally, they may stay at home, feel lonely and abandoned, and focus on the past; they have little interest in activities, remaining isolated and uninvolved. Drinking helps to pass the time.

Developmentally, elderly abusers are often needy, lonely adults who are angry and feel a sense of despair about their lives and selves. They are depressed and often feel powerless and unwanted, a state of mind that is temporarily blunted by drugs and alcohol. They sense—rightly at times—an attitude of indifference toward them because they are perceived as old and worthless. As a result, much professional care of the elderly abuser focuses on management and custodial issues. Little emphasis is placed on identification, treatment, and rehabilitation.

Doweiko (1996) suggests the following alcohol treatment considerations for the elderly:

1. A primary prevention program to warn of the dangers of using alcohol as a coping mechanism.
2. An outreach activity to identify those who might be overlooked.
3. Detoxification services by qualified personnel.
4. Structured living environments, so the elderly can receive treatment without the temptation of continued alcohol use.
5. Primary treatment programs for both inpatient and outpatient care.
6. Aftercare programs to assist in the transition from primary care to independent living.
7. Long-term residential care for those suffering from complications.
8. Access to counseling and social support services.

## The Disabled

Approximately 36 million people in the United States are physically or mentally disabled, a population particularly vulnerable to alcoholism, drug abuse, and related problems. Although the magnitude of the problem has not been clearly established, estimates range as high as 60 percent for patients with spinal cord injury. The National Institute of Alcohol Abuse and Alcoholism estimates a similarly high rate of alcohol problems for the disabled. Drug and alcohol abuse in the disabled is a significant problem that is generally ignored by the helping professions (Helwig & Holicky, 1994).

There are several explanations for the high risk of alcohol and drug abuse in the disabled population:

1. There is easy access to prescription medication, especially for pain and severe spasms. Physicians often prescribe drugs because of their own feelings of pity and guilt and a notion that this is the least they can do, given the tragedy of the situation.
2. The drug-abuse path is taken as a result of the frustration and anxiety of being disabled and being thrust into a nonproductive and dependent role.
3. The disabled are a marginalized group in our society; therefore, the lure of a substance that produces highs and numbness is an attractive alternative.
4. Abuse is often the result of medical intervention and the rehabilitation process.
5. Many disabled individuals have poorly developed social skills and are socially isolated.

A major problem in treating drug abuse and alcoholism in disabled populations relates to diagnosis. Counselors are often unaware of the problem, and treatment is often delayed until the symptoms become chronic. A growing advocacy movement has focused attention on the multidisabled alcoholic and encouraged programmatic responses at the community level. Although awareness of the problems of this population is improving, there is still a need for increased attention to the treatment of the disabled drug and alcohol user. Many people are unacquainted with the symptoms of alcoholism and drug abuse and unfamiliar with the treatability of the problems, and some administrators and clinicians are reluctant to become involved. In addition, services to the disabled are often provided by multiple agencies and individuals. There is a need for improved interdisciplinary and interprofessional collaboration to more accurately assess and treat substance-abuse disorders in this population.

Alcohol and polydrug use is widespread among the disabled due to lack of access to prevention and treatment services, architectural barriers, lack of training and sensitivity to the specific problems and needs of the disabled, and attitudinal barriers that negate the desired effect of these services by reinforcing the client's poor self-image. Substance abuse is an easy way to avoid the difficult and painful work necessary to develop social skills and overcome social isolation.

To varying degrees, the blind, deaf, paralyzed, and orthopedically impaired communities have reacted similarly in that they discourage the identification and treatment of alcohol or drug problems. They live in close association with one another and share a common identity and fear of being labeled by what a few deviant members might do. They already have shared the burden of the stigma of their disability. People who are constantly reminded of their disability rather than their ability find the addition of an alcohol- or drug-abuse problem an unwanted burden. Treatment for this population is therefore difficult and dependent on early identification, support, and reduction of the threat of stigma.

# PRINCIPLES FOR COUNSELING THE CHEMICALLY DEPENDENT

## Medical Model

In the medical model favored by many hospital, mental health, and clinic settings, substance abuse and alcoholism are classified as diseases similar to diabetes or cancer. It is presumed that the patient has some genetic predisposition to chemical abuse that may be exacerbated by family conflicts or other life pressures. The abuser is helped through a detoxification program that may include forced abstinence, intensive psychotherapy, family support groups, and possibly medications to help with withdrawal symptoms. Antabuse and naltrexone, as well as some antidepressants (Prozac) for example, are prescribed drugs that help alcoholics stay sober and prevent relapses. They are, however, effective only if the person agrees to take the preventive drugs on a regular basis and can live with the side effects. As such, their usefulness is limited. Medications are more likely to be helpful depending on how long the person has been drinking excessively and whether therapy or counseling are used as supportive adjuncts (Swift, 1999).

Because the medical model approach absolves the client of responsibility for his or her condition, the counselor works intensively on issues related to self-control and compliance to the prescribed program. Efforts are also directed towards helping clients understand the full implications of recovering from a chronic "disease."

The medical model operates on both an inpatient and outpatient basis. There is some evidence that, for the vast majority of individuals, outpatient treatment is equal in effectiveness to inpatient treatment at a fraction of the personal and monetary cost (Miller & Hester, 1986; Miller, Meyers, & Tonigan, 1999). Most programs will include the following elements (Beutler & Hardwood, 2000; Lewis, Dana, & Blevins, 2002):

- Detoxification
- Orientation to a treatment-structured regime, including substance abstinence
- Education about effects and consequences of continued abuse
- Motivational training and morale building
- Aversion therapy and behavioral self-control training to initiate change in drinking behavior
- Social-skills training
- Strong peer pressure/support
- Individual counseling
- Group counseling or self-help group
- Family counseling
- Relapse prevention strategies
- Follow-up by the treatment team

## AA/NA Model

The Alcoholics Anonymous/Narcotics Anonymous (AA/NA) model is somewhat compatible with the medical approach in that the abuser is labeled as helplessly addicted forever unless complete withdrawal is initiated. Through powerful peer support groups, the client is helped to make radical lifestyle changes, to abstain from all drugs and alcohol, and to admit that as an addict the only salvation is through rigorous adherence to the AA or NA program. As long as the abuser attends regular meetings (often several per week) and follows the prescribed steps, continued recovery is possible. Although 12-step programs are consistently reported by participants to be critical components of their recovery, there is little empirical evidence to support their long-term effectiveness without supplemental treatment (Tonigan, Toscova, & Miller, 1999). AA/NA programs are thus probably best conceived as a form of support rather than of treatment (Lewis, Dana, & Blevins, 2002).

Counselors need to be familiar with local AA/NA resources and to make referrals in a manner likely to result in client attendance at a meeting. It is also extremely important that the work you do in counseling complements rather than opposes the 12-step programs. Riordan and Walsh (1994) suggest several guidelines for making referrals to AA:

1. *Who to refer?* Most clients, except those with significant pathology, are appropriate referrals.

2. *Making the referral.* An AA referral should be based on a complete assessment and a recognition that outpatient treatment is indicated. Support should be offered so the client does not feel rejected.

3. *Timing the referral.* A referral should be made as soon as practically possible. Often a referral at a point of reduced denial is useful; for example, following a binge or other adverse consequence.

4. *Be aware of labeling.* Many clients are offended by the label of *alcoholic*. Consider neutral ways to refer to the problem without glossing over real issues. Also consider that while abstinence is often preferred (and a requirement of AA/NA), some clients can manage with controlled use.

5. *Personalize the referral.* It is helpful to have materials available and give written instructions to the meeting; the client might even make the first contact from the counselor's office. Establish a follow-up session after the initial referral to process the experience.

6. *Prepare the client.* Help the client to understand what to expect and explain the difference between a religious and spiritual program. Emphasize the anonymity of the meeting. Encourage the client not to make a decision on involvement on the first one or two meetings. Be aware of the variety of meetings, times, and locations. Each meeting has a distinctly different "culture" and composition. Warn clients that they may need to visit a half dozen or more different meetings to find one that feels right.

7. *Attend meetings.* It is useful for counselors to attend "open" meetings to get a more complete understanding of the AA experience.

One problem associated with AA and NA programs is the emphasis placed on external control—often a conflict with the values of therapeutic counseling. Participants may learn to substitute one form of dependency for another: Whereas they may no longer abuse drugs or alcohol, they nevertheless must go to meetings in order to maintain the cure. It is for this reason that individual counseling can be even more helpful in conjunction with AA and NA programs, giving focus to issues of autonomy, independence, and self-control.

Occasionally, some clients will not be well suited for AA because they don't care for the religious emphasis or are unwilling to engage in complete abstinence. Fortunately, alternative programs are available. In the case of those who want the benefits of a more secular support group, a number of other groups exist such as Secular Organization for Sobriety and Rational Recovery. For those who are interested in reducing their drinking but not stopping altogether, they may find assistance at Moderation Management or Drinkwise.

## Therapeutic Model

In the therapeutic model, the various approaches to counseling are applied to the specific problems of substance abuse or addiction. Whereas there isn't much evidence to support the effectiveness of traditional therapies with alcohol and drug problems, there are practitioners who nevertheless attempt such strategies with mixed results. According to the various theories, the counselor

◼ | **VOICE FROM THE FIELD**

It's a funny thing, this whole substance abuse counseling business. You've got to be very careful what you do, and how you do it. I'm not talking about with clients but within the community. A lot of what we do in counseling is in direct opposition to what they do in NA or AA. Here we're trying to work with people to take responsibility for their behavior, and AA groups often teach them to turn over the control to a Higher Power. They can't help the way they are and so should turn themselves over to God. For some people, this is an outstanding plan. They take like ducks to water with the 12-step program. But other people just drop out, and they get really confused with the messages they get in counseling versus those they get at AA.

---

may work on delving into repressed conflicts underlying the drug symptoms or perhaps concentrate on issues related to self-control. Any of the theoretical models presented in Chapters 5 and 6 could conceivably be applied to substance abuse programs. Regardless of the therapeutic model, however, several suggestions have been made for working with alcohol/drug abusers in particular or addictions in general:

1. Recovery from addictions is unlikely without some support system as an adjunct to counseling.
2. Group counseling modalities are often helpful in providing support, positive modeling, motivation, intimacy, and constructive confrontation for substance abusers.
3. Family counseling strategies help the counselor to recruit more power and support, to collect more information about the problem, and to resolve conflicts that are sabotaging recovery. The concept of family can also be expanded to include a wider network of friends, associates, and concerned others who wish to be involved. Among some indigenous groups, there is a wide network of extended kin, related by blood and affiliation, who are all involved in providing family support (the New Zealand Maori, for example, call this *whanau*; the Hawaiian *ohana* is similar in concept).
4. The counselor should explore the motivation to use alcohol by examining the availability of nonchemical incentives.
5. Alcohol and drug abuse is often a form of self-medication in which the client attempts to cope with debilitating depression or anxiety. Attempts should be made to identify and treat the underlying pain that is being anesthetized.
6. Time can be spent productively helping clients to grieve the time they've wasted, even the childhood they've lost. Help addicts resolve their feelings of shame and anger, leave the past behind, and move forward.

7. Physical exercise programs that involve daily structured commitments are often helpful in creating more positive addictions. Activities such as biking, running, swimming, and aerobics have been found to reduce tension, increase productivity, improve confidence, and provide an alternative to drugs.

8. The counselor should watch for manipulation, deceit, and lying, which are not uncommon among those who are used to saying anything to get what they want. Developing trust is a major issue in the counseling of addictions, especially in sufficient doses to make vigorous confrontation possible.

9. Rules and limits are often needed to structure acceptable and inappropriate behavior within the sessions. For example, the counselor may refuse to work with the client unless she or he can agree to maintain sobriety for at least eight hours prior to any session.

10. Because drug and alcohol abuse is often associated with low self-esteem, considerable work should be spent helping the client to improve confidence and self-worth.

11. Work on identity issues, because addicts often use "totalizing descriptions" of their own essence: I am an addict. A narrative counseling approach would locate the problem—the addiction—outside the individual ("The addiction is seducing you") but would also make certain that the clients did not confuse their behavior with who they are as human beings.

12. Varieties of adventure and constructive risk taking other than the drug-induced kind should be substituted. As the person finds more fulfillment in a career, course of study, hobby, intimate relationship, social network, travel experience, or any other passionate project, the need to use drugs for excitement or boredom decreases.

13. If the client cannot or will not practice complete abstinence, offer a compromise program of moderation. A number of self-help organizations such as Moderation Management and Drinkwise are having limited success with people who would otherwise drop out of treatment altogether.

14. Make sure to consider the factors and consequences of addiction as they affect a client's financial status, career, relationships, and stress levels.

15. Consider gender and cultural differences as a context for the addiction or substance abuse. Alcohol abuse, for instance, may have different meaning for some women who have histories of sexual or physical abuse (van der Walde, Urgenson, Weltz, & Hanna, 2002).

16. Regardless of the treatment model employed, systematic follow-up of cases is critical, ideally for up to two years after sessions have ended.

Regardless of the specific program that the counselor adopts for those clients who are struggling with the temptations of drug and alcohol use, this specialty has become a big part of the mandate of professional helpers. The demand for qualified experts in this field will only continue to grow at the pace with which children, adolescents, and adults abuse chemical substances.

## VOICE FROM THE FIELD

I was pretty discouraged when I first began my job in a treatment center. From reading the research on drug addictions, I saw that 98 percent of teens who go through treatment fail. Yet the place where I worked claimed to have a 75–80 percent success rate. But that's only as they leave the center. When they do follow-up three months later, they find that most of them relapse.

Still, there are several things you can do that increase the chances that counseling will be helpful. I learned the hard way. First, you have to be honest with them and you have to talk to them at their level; if you sound any way like a counselor, they will shut you out.

You have to stand up for them. They interpret loyalty as caring. For instance, when a lampshade was broken, the program director refused to let up on them until he found out who did it. I stood up for the kids and he backed down. That really made a difference in my relationship with them.

Treatment is all about setting limits. Strength gets their attention. Then, you have to follow through on what you said you were going to do. The limits should be balanced with showing that you care for them—really care. If they don't think they matter to you, you don't have a chance to help them.

## SUMMARY

Addictions present some special challenges for the counselor because (1) the problems are so widespread; (2) the effects of the drugs are intrinsically rewarding and resistant to extinction; (3) there may be pressure from peers to continue the abuse; (4) the abuser tends to be externally controlled and thus unresponsive to efforts toward self-control; (5) abusers tend toward irresponsibility—they may miss or break appointments—and so may be uncooperative clients; (6) physiologically addictive effects complicate change efforts made on a psychological level; (7) abusers are ambivalent in their motivation because the drugs do work—in spite of side effects—to temporarily reduce symptoms of boredom, anxiety, or depression; (8) there is some evidence that genetic factors may predispose some people to addiction in spite of their best intentions; and (9) addicts have learned, as a matter of survival, to be manipulative, deceitful con artists—qualities not generally considered optimal for a productive therapeutic encounters.

Because of these many factors contributing to an addict's situation, the counselor should develop a multifaceted treatment program to combat resistance on physiological, psychological, family, and cultural levels. Traditional insight-oriented counseling interventions are largely useless without additional therapeutic measures. Even with the best resources available, prognoses for chronic drug and alcohol abusers are guarded.

In general, when working with any kind of addict, the counselor is well advised to use every possible resource available in the client's world and in the repertoire of therapeutic options. Particular attention should be paid to factors such as family influences, peer pressures, underlying internal conflicts, and tendencies toward escapism and immediate gratification of needs. The counselor normally needs to spend more time than usual on trust dimensions of the therapeutic relationship and to define clearly what constitutes responsible behavior, both within and outside the counseling sessions.

## SELF-GUIDED EXPLORATIONS

1. Relive a time in your life when you "self-medicated" yourself for some sort of stress. This could have included the use of substances (alcohol, illicit or prescription drugs, coffee, cigarettes, etc.) or some other activity designed to provide escape (sleep, isolation, exercise, food, etc.). Describe the positive and negative impacts that experience had on your life. How did you decide to stop or cut down?
2. Describe a close friend or relative whose life was significantly changed as a result of drug/alcohol abuse. What impact did this behavior have on you and others who were close to him or her? What finally made a difference in helping him or her to stop?
3. Two different positions argue that: (1) addiction is a genetic predetermination and disease that we can do little about except to abstain from all temptations; (2) addiction is a choice based on our refusal to accept responsibility for our behavior. Create a dialogue between two proponents of these positions, each one trying to convince the other of their respective accuracy. Which position are you most sympathetic to? Defend your position with some evidence.

## For Homework:

Attend several different open meetings of Alcoholics Anonymous, Narcotics Anonymous, or some other self-help support group devoted to addictions. Consider ways that this research will help you to integrate your own counseling efforts with the work being done in these groups.

## SUGGESTED READINGS

Beechem, M. (2002). *Elderly alcoholism: Intervention strategies.* Springfield, IL: Charles C. Thomas.

Buelow, G. D., & Buelow, S. A. (1998). *Psychotherapy in chemical dependence treatment: A practical and integrative approach.* Pacific Grove, CA: Brooks/Cole.

Doweiko, H. E. (2001). *Concepts of chemical dependency* (5th ed.). Pacific Grove, CA: Brooks/Cole.

Harrison, T. C., & Fisher, G. L. (2000). *Substance abuse: Information for school counselors, social workers, therapists, and counselors.* Boston: Allyn & Bacon.

Lewis, J. A., Dana, R. Q., & Blevins, G. A. (2002). *Substance abuse counseling* (3rd ed.). Pacific Grove, CA: Brooks/Cole.

McCollum, E. E., & Trepper, T. S. (2001). *Family solutions for substance abuse: Clinical and counseling approaches.* New York: Haworth.

Peele, S. (1998). *The meaning of addiction: An unconventional view.* San Francisco: Jossey-Bass.

Senay, E. C. (1998). *Substance abuse disorders in clinical practice.* New York: W. W. Norton.

Thomas, D. L. (1999). *Introduction to addictive behavior* (2nd ed.). New York: Guilford.

van Wormer, K., & Davis, D. R. (2003). *Addiction treatment: A strengths perspective.* Pacific Grove, CA: Brooks/Cole.

Weil, A. (1998). *From chocolate to morphine.* Boston: Houghton Mifflin.

# 13 CHAPTER COUNSELING DIVERSE CLIENTS

# COUNSELING
# DIVERSE CLIENTS

# CHAPTER 13

Working with diverse populations requires the skills needed for all therapeutic counseling, plus knowledge about and sensitivity to the needs of particular groups. The same counseling skills are used with women as with men; the same theories of change apply to the physically handicapped as to the athlete. Depression or anxiety does not feel qualitatively different to a Latino, African-American, or white person. Group dynamics operate in similar ways in groups of children, middle-aged adults, and older adults. Gay men and lesbian women feel loneliness, frustration, or anger just as do heterosexuals. The delinquent, disabled, or drug-addicted clients all respond to empathy, confrontation, and other therapeutic strategies, depending on the counselor's finesse and sensitivity.

Yet in spite of these similarities, every client you will ever see requires you to adapt what you do—and how you do it—to a unique cultural context. Each person's ethnicity, religious and spiritual orientation, gender, sexual orientation, life stage, and primary cultural identities will challenge you to be sensitive and flexible in the ways that you work. To complicate matters further, often the differences you will see within particular identified groups will be so diverse that generalizations are next to useless. Nevertheless, your job is to (1) examine and explore your own cultural identity, (2) educate yourself as completely as you can about the cultural context for each client's experience, (3) learn about the effects of oppression on minority and disadvantaged groups, (4) acknowledge and confront your biases and prejudices with regard to particular groups, and (5) adapt all your

## VOICE FROM THE FIELD

I think it's the atmosphere of political correctness that makes it difficult to talk about the real issues in this field. I mean, we are all required to undergo cultural sensitivity training or whatever. Every journal is filled with articles on the subject. But I wonder how much really changes.

For lots of white counselors like me, we've just learned to pretend we aren't as racist as we really are. We don't say things out loud that we really think. We pretend that we're all liberal, enlightened souls, but that's a load of bull. I'm not saying things aren't better than they were, but the truth is that the people I help the most are just like me. They look like me. They believe in the same things. The real challenge is to help the ones most not like me. That's really hard because I'm not working in areas that I feel most comfortable and familiar.

---

counseling knowledge and skills in such a way that you can help diverse clientele. This is a tall order, indeed, but one that is absolutely necessary in order for you to function effectively and ethically.

## MULTIPLE CONCEPTIONS OF CULTURE

Traditionally, chapters, books, and discussions about multiculturalism referred to a person's ethnicity or race. Yet "culture" involves a set of multiple identities for most individuals (Robinson & Howard-Hamilton, 2000). Each person is not only strongly influenced by their ethnic/racial background but also the culture of their gender, religion, socioeconomic class, geographical location, first language, sexual orientation, political affiliation, profession, and similar identities. In fact, to some clients you will see, their choice of social group (Alcoholics Anonymous, Shriners, gang affiliation), leisure activity (coin collector, softball player, snowboarder), or even factors related to their appearance (tattoos, clothing) may be the most defining characteristic of their cultural identity. Table 13.1 provides examples of cultural groups as they are defined by their norms, rituals, characteristics, traditions, and shared beliefs.

A client walks in the door and speaks with a particular accent, or has a particular skin color, or exhibits features of some identifiable group. You may immediately assume that being African American, Native American, Latino, or Vietnamese is the person's dominant cultural identity (and so make further assumptions about the best way to structure the sessions) but you may be sorely mistaken. It is extremely important that you approach this whole subject of multiculturalism with a truly open mind and heart so you are best positioned to truly learn about any given client's experiences and multiple cultural identities.

Initial sessions may very well be devoted to asking questions such as the following:

| TABLE 13.1 | SOME EXAMPLES OF CULTURAL GROUPS |
|---|---|

Race (African American, American Indian, Chinese)

Country of origin (Mexico, Cuba, Chile)

Language (Gaelic, Spanish)

Political affiliation (Republican, Communist, Green Party)

Gender

Sexual orientation

Living situation (widowed, divorced with children)

Club (fraternity, Harley Davidson, rave)

Hobby (gun collecting, fantasy baseball, cooking)

Physical characteristics (blonde, tattoos, obese)

Physically challenged (hearing impaired, dwarfism, wheelchair bound)

Afflicted (HIV, multiple sclerosis)

Profession (athlete, police, counselor)

Religion (Mormon, Jewish, Southern Baptist)

Church/temple affiliation

Age (baby boomer, Gen-X, newly retired)

Alumni (Harvard, Marines, Peace Corp)

Geography (New Yorker, Southern Californian, Texan)

Victimization (Holocaust survivor, incest survivor)

---

- What would be helpful for me to know about you in terms of your cultural background?
- What are some of the groups with which you most closely identify?
- What is it that I need to know in order to understand where you come from and what is most important to you?

Your challenge is to learn as much as you can about the unique cultural background, history, and traditions of each client you see. This is not an additional burden on your job but rather a privilege of the profession that comes with the territory. Every client who walks in affords you the opportunity to learn about a variety of cultural identities that previously may have been beyond your experience. A skydiver comes in complaining of chronic anxiety. A Haitian immigrant is depressed because she misses her family back home. An Orthodox rabbi has just been diagnosed with inoperable cancer. On the way to helping them work on their issues you become an expert in their lifestyles. You learn all about their worlds, their languages, their beliefs and values. And all throughout this process you become more knowledgeable and wise.

## VOICE FROM THE FIELD

I can't tell you how often I've gotten myself in trouble by assuming that a client is a particular way based on what I think is the person's cultural background. I see someone who is black and I would think, okay, this is someone who has likely experienced oppression and discrimination because of his skin color. Then I find out he is also gay, and that cultural identity is far more important to him than being black. Then, there was another time in which I was working with a corporate executive who was also black and I again assumed that this must be important to him. Yet every time I tried to bring up racial stuff in sessions, he kept saying that this wasn't a big thing to him where he worked; it was his corporate culture that most strongly identified himself. At first, I didn't believe him; I couldn't believe him because my own race is so important to me. But over time, I've learned to be very careful to watch and listen and learn from clients rather than to assume that they hold particular values because of the way they look or speak.

## BEING CULTURALLY SENSITIVE

In one sense, the idea of multiculturalism runs contrary to some of the themes from the American idea of the great melting pot. Many people adamantly hold to the belief that people are essentially similar and any emphasis placed on the differences between "us" and "them" borders on discrimination. One major injustice inherent in that belief is the notion that if we are all the same, then what works for me obviously must also work for you. A counselor who operates from this belief system will undoubtedly play out the dynamics of domination and hegemony that the minority client has learned to distrust or abhor. This subtle bias in action looks harmless enough, but it may have dire consequences. Consider the interaction between a white, male school counselor and his Japanese American client:

> COUNSELOR: I heard about the death of your brother. I'm really concerned about our last few sessions because it seems that I've been doing most of the talking. I can imagine that you are feeling really sad right now, but you seem so disconnected. How can I help you explore your feelings? You know it's okay to cry in my office.

> CLIENT: [Looking down at the floor]: I don't know.

The counselor obviously holds to the notion of Western values that successful intervention requires the client to have a cathartic emotional process. However, for the Japanese American client, the expression of intense emotion and the exploration of his problem outside the family unit run contrary to his cultural values. Understanding clients from their unique cultural perspective has been the impetus that has driven the multicultural movement. Moreover, the definition of culture has evolved to describe more than racial and ethnic

## VOICE FROM THE FIELD

There are some clients I see who I think I should pay rather than the other way around. Their stories are so, so interesting. Their life experiences just blow me away—the things they have seen and done. There was this one guy who, when he was a teenager, was recruited to fight in Palestine. He kept this to himself his whole life. Didn't even tell his wife and children. Yet it was such a formative part of his life. I ended up learning a whole lot about that part of the world during that time period in history. I not only heard this client's stories but I ended up reading books so I could better understand his world. I've had other clients who are prostitutes, or stock brokers, or actors, or litigators, and with each one of them, I end up learning so much about their inner worlds. Oh, the books I could write on what I've learned.

---

barriers to now include social class, gender, age, sexual orientation, and physical capabilities.

Make no mistake, multiculturalism is hot stuff—perhaps the single most powerful movement in the profession in the past decade. No longer is it acceptable to have only one course on multicultural issues; the subject is ideally infused into *all* courses and textbooks because it is considered so critical to understanding each client's world and planning for respectful, appropriate interventions.

Pedersen (1991) writes of multiculturalism as the "fourth" force in counseling, complementing the traditional three forces of psychodynamic, behavioral, and humanistic as explanations for human behavior. The multicultural perspective emphasizes the value of diversity and the recognition that all people—and therefore all counseling relationships—are shaped and influenced by cultural patterns of thinking and acting. Therefore, the daunting task of working with a diverse population of clients is a complex endeavor. The counselor needs to have an awareness of the client's cultural worldview, while concurrently relating to the client as a unique individual. Furthermore, effective counselors approach this relationship with an understanding of counterproductive personal and cultural barriers that they may also present.

Clients are both alike and different. It is only through a connected humanness that counselors can positively assist clients. The need to blend a clear understanding and respect for myriad cultural patterns with a recognition of the universal human qualities that connect individuals is a core requisite for counseling diverse clients.

Culturally sensitive counselors have been identified as having several qualities (Baruth & Manning, 2003; Lum, 2003; Robinson & Howard-Hamilton, 2000):

1. They embrace the concept of cultural pluralism and are extremely committed to learning all they can about racial/ethnic groups different from their own.

2. They are aware of how their own ethnicity and cultural backgrounds influence their practice.
3. They realize the extent to which they are not only enriched but also limited by their own ethnic and cultural heritage, a circumstance that can be remedied only through greater openness to new experiences.
4. They have developed a perspective in which each person is seen as a unique individual with values that have been influenced by the cultural context of the environment in which he or she was raised.
5. They are extremely flexible and eclectic in the ways they work with people, depending on where the client comes from and what he or she needs. Furthermore, this flexibility is manifested not only in the kinds of alliances that are created and interventions chosen but also in the ways they live their lives.
6. They recognize the influence of cultural background on a client's concepts of *power, growth, time, solution,* and other terms that are part of the counseling vernacular.
7. They are free of prejudices and biases that tend to stereotype people and that alienate them by communicating an ignorant or patronizing attitude.
8. They are aware of and sensitive to the client's worldview and work to clarify it and understand it in assessment, diagnosis, and treatment selection.

When you put all this together, what you've got is a template for relating more effectively and sensitively to all your clients. As a society, we have reached a point where these qualities are not only part of a culturally skilled and competent counselor, but anyone who seeks to help others. Table 13.2 summarizes ten points to keep in mind when working with your clients.

## INFLUENCE OF BIASES

Are you biased? Of course you are! Think about it. How do you define happiness? How would you describe a psychologically healthy person? Your answers to most questions about human behavior, religion, philosophy, or health are rooted in your worldview. Is it your job to convince the indigenous client that his depression is not caused by demonic spirits but rather by his irrational belief system? Do you think that if you confronted the client about his ideas he would come back for a second session?

Even if you don't believe people who are different from you are substandard, such individuals may very well have sufficient injustice in their lives to sense such feelings from you that maybe even you are not aware of. So, although your desire to treat all people as equals is laudable, you may still unconsciously and unintentionally be harboring a number of biases and prejudices that can easily be picked up by others who have training themselves to be more than a little cautious, especially by people who look like you.

Members of diverse populations know they have some unique issues, and a counselor who fails to acknowledge them will likely be perceived as ineffective. Furthermore, biases and prejudices move in both directions. Picture your-

**TABLE 13.2** | DOING A CULTURALLY SENSITIVE INTERVIEW

1. Help the client to tell his or her story.
2. Monitor your assumptions about this person based on your first impressions and past experiences with others who may *appear* similar.
3. Use open-ended questions and probes to elicit information related to multiple cultural identities.
4. Flesh out the context and background through reflective listening skills.
5. Ask the client to teach you what you need to know and understand in order to be helpful.
6. Communicate your intense interest and convey what you've heard and understood.
7. Make sure that your communication style is sensitive, respectful, and appropriate to the particular values of your client.
8. Match your language and behaviors to those of your client.
9. Watch your biases and internal judgments as they arise during the conversation.
10. Deal with issues of marginalization, power, and oppression (if indicated and appropriate).

---

self as a white male counselor in professional practice. You've analyzed your biases and beliefs. You are especially aware that as a member of the majority culture, your beliefs reflect the ideas of those in power and have not exactly been sympathetic to those who have experienced oppression.

Imagine, for example, that thus far in your efforts to establish a practice you have only three clients and the bills are piling up. Your four o'clock appointment shows up and you are excited about this new referral, an African American 40-year-old lesbian. You run through your list of dos and don'ts as a multiculturally sensitive counselor before you invite her in and open the session with a warm greeting. She immediately sits down and wonders how this straight, uppity white boy can possibly understand her world, let alone help her! You have about ten minutes (if you're lucky) to prove yourself.

Biases, stereotypes, and prejudices are indicative of the cognitive processes that we use to understand the world (Hayes, 1996). In essence, we seek to categorize others in an attempt to understand ourselves. By observing what we are not, we can define who we are. Problems with biases and prejudices arise when we are intolerable to the differences between people. When we adamantly adhere to the notion that our way is the "right" way while others are wrong, corrupt, or naive, we exhibit a rigidity that can only be destructive to interpersonal relationships with those unlike us.

In one sense, biases and prejudices are the most natural thing in the world. Throughout history, human beings have been notoriously intolerant of others who are not of their "tribe," killing one another with abandon:

Assyrians versus Babylonians, Romans versus Carthaginians, Moors versus Spaniards, Boers versus English, Iroquois versus Algonquins, Paiutes versus Utes, Croats versus Serbs, Turks versus Armenians, Japanese versus Koreans, Peruvians versus Ecuadorians, Hutu versus Tutsi, Khmer Rouge versus Cambodians, Irish Catholics versus Protestants, Union versus Confederacy, Bloods versus Crips, Arabs versus Jews, Romans versus Christians, Montagues versus Capulets, Hatfields versus McCoys (Kottler, 1997b, p. 26).

Horowitz (1985) found that within forty years after the Holocaust, there had been twenty-five documented cases of genocide in which one group or another has tried to do its best to wipe out others of a different religion or skin color or geographical region. In the last twenty years since this survey, surely that number has doubled still again. It would seem that there is even a human tendency to expend our energy doing everything we can to protect resources on behalf of others who are members of our "tribe," who share our gene pool, and do everything we can to prevent others "not like us" from enjoying the benefits of limited resources (Wright, 1994).

So, it's senseless to deny that you feel biases toward one group of people or another. Notice who you gravitate toward at a party and who you naturally move away from. Such attraction/repulsion may not be based on skin color or physical features, but often you will find yourself preferring to be around others who share your basic values, socioeconomic class, or even professional affiliation.

Any one person or group of people who differ from societal norms almost inevitably face covert and overt forms of discrimination. Differences can be as obvious as physical characteristics or more subtle, such as education level, religious affiliation, or marital status. Discrimination can be as obvious as preventing African Americans or women from voting or owning property. Covert discrimination occurs more subtly but is just as harmful. An individual may not get a job because of sexual orientation, ethnicity, or gender. A child may not be picked to answer a question in school because he is lower class or black. There are countless ways in which people from diverse populations are quietly and discreetly discriminated against.

Some biases and prejudices result from the awareness that "bad" things can happen to all of us; the discomfort we experience at seeing a disabled or mentally ill person is often related to our own fears. Rigidity of thinking, fear of the unknown, avoidance of risks, and many other self-defeating behaviors likewise contribute to an individual's inflexibility.

There is also a danger that counselors who work with large numbers of people will class them in groups rather than seeing them as individuals: "I was seeing this Jewish housewife yesterday . . ." or "What do you do to get around the resistance in Asian families . . ." or "I've got this deaf guy on my schedule . . .". But that's my point. Their generalizations are likely to breed misconceptions.

How would you describe the following people: a Latina, a high school dropout, an African American teen, a truck driver, a priest? When you think of these people, what images do you see in your head? What experiences have you had with people that carry these labels?

If a member of a culture different than your own was to walk into your office, you might make a snap judgment about that person. This is not only a natural phenomenon but a useful one as well. Our survival, at least in the past, was based on making instantaneous and accurate judgments about who

## VOICE FROM THE FIELD

I'm sick of do-gooders who think they are being helpful but don't have a clue about what is going on with the people they are trying to help. There were some architects who got together to volunteer their time to design economic public housing for the inner city. They built these low-slung modern-looking buildings not at all like the usual concrete towers that are in most cities. They had courtyards. They were decorated in bright colors. Very attractive. The problem was that nobody would live in them. They were built according to the aesthetic tastes of the architects, many of whom were minority people but from a very different socioeconomic class. Their worldviews never considered that the so-called public spaces, the courtyards, allowed gangs to patrol freely. And the walls of the buildings might have been quite nice to look at, but they were too thin to stop bullets from penetrating. They never stopped to consider what the people really wanted who were going to be living in the housing project.

---

was safe and who was dangerous. We carry within us this legacy in which we are constantly making assessments and predictions about people based on our prior experiences with others who *appear* similar.

The problem, of course, comes when—in light of new, more complete information—you don't alter your initial judgments; you retain your prejudices and refuse to see individuals as who they really are rather than as a member of a group.

It is not uncommon for people to believe that although they are prejudiced against a certain group of people, they never let that belief interfere with their work. It is unlikely that anyone who has strong biases or prejudices is completely able to conceal those feelings from others. In counseling, for example, diagnostic biases abound (Snowden & Cheung, 1990). Many examples demonstrate greater frequency of certain diagnoses among specific groups (Jones & Gray, 1986). Diagnosticians are often seen to have a bias against lower class patients. A diagnosis of severe psychosis is more likely to be bestowed on a lower-class patient than on a middle-class patient, given similar manifestations of pathological symptoms.

Counselors, regardless of their sex, rated female clients with unusual career goals as being more in need of counseling than those with conforming career goals (Sinacore-Guinn, 1995). This finding raises an important issue: Bias is not necessarily directed toward someone who is different from us—the opposite sex, in this case—but can also be directed toward people who are like us. The societal expectations, norms, and socialization processes operate systematically to define appropriate roles for women, African Americans, senior citizens, and disabled persons. Prejudices and biases can be and are formed against any conceivably definable group of people: WASPS, veterans, Ku Klux Klansmen, homosexuals, hunters, blue-collar workers, executives, middle-class suburban housewives, and BMW owners are all groups of people for whom certain stereotypes have been established in our society. There are, of course, many more.

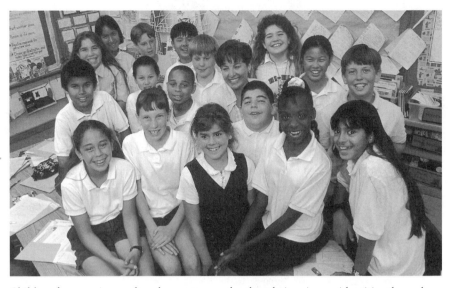

Children from various cultural groups may develop their primary identities through different influences, including their neighborhoods, families, schools, clubs, friends, and media. © Will Hart/PhotoEdit.

## IDENTITY ISSUES

How would you describe your own cultural identity? Are you a woman, a man, Latino, white, African American, gay, Southerner, or Methodist? Or are you a gay Hispanic man, an African American woman? If you are white, what does that mean to you? Are your European roots especially important to you? What would a counselor need to know and understand about your cultural identity in order to be helpful to you?

Or would you describe your cultural identity as something completely different? Think back to how you developed your sense of yourself and your culture. Does the definition of your culture differ from how others would see you? In fact, I would dare to guess that your cultural identity could be comprised of many cultures. Current researchers have been investigating that multiculturalism has been delineated into mutually independent categories and that a cultural identity is much more complex than association with a single group (Das, 1996; Phinney, 1996; Ramsey, 1996). To further complicate the issue, there has been much discussion about the applicability of the male Eurocentric treatment models to members of diverse populations (Hayes, 1996; Zayas, Torres, Malcolm, & DesRosiers, 1996). Gilligan (1982) and Nelson (1996) have argued eloquently that women's identity must be considered from a relational rather than an autonomous viewpoint. What, then, is the process for identity development of a disabled Hispanic girl?

Developing a positive identity is a universal human challenge often compounded by membership in a minority group or groups. Pervasive numbers of "isms" (ageism, sexism, racism) in society can act as barriers to positive identity development. Many individuals feel alienated and different when they do not live up to expectations because of cultural differences. Counselors must be aware of alternative models for identity that are culturally broad and inclusive to help clients build a positive sense of personal identity.

Facilitating identity development is a critical issue for counselors working with diverse clients. The presence of a clear and directed identity is essential to foster growth and development. Counselors must be aware of the limitations of traditional developmental theory for many clients and be able to work with alternative patterns if they fit more appropriately.

# PREFERRED CLIENTS

In a classic study of professional biases, psychiatrists, social workers, and clinical psychologists were surveyed to find out their preferred client types. What emerged was the YAVIS profile (Schofield, 1964). The YAVIS client is young, attractive, verbal, intelligent, and successful. All groups of clinicians in the survey preferred female clients between the ages of 20 and 40. Social workers and psychiatrists preferred married females, whereas psychologists did not differentiate. Psychologists and psychiatrists had rigid levels of acceptable education and preferred high school graduates with some college experience—but not "too much" education. For example, graduate-school experience was considered to create a difficult client. Nonpreferred clients included the very young (under 15) and those over 50, widowed or divorced clients, uneducated people, and those in agriculture, fishery, forestry, and semiskilled or unskilled types of jobs.

Although the evidence indicates that counselors and other professionals have definite preferences, the YAVIS population represents but a small proportion of the types of clients that most of you will work with in counseling settings. Part of the reason for preferring particular clients is that those clients make counselors feel more successful about their work. Clients who improve quickly allow counselors to feel powerful and competent.

Although it's easier to help someone who has the same background that you do, it's likely that many of your clients will come from cultures and value orientations that are quite different from your experience. The challenge for you will be to acknowledge your own cultural beliefs and, at the same time, reach beyond your own narrow world to embrace those who are different.

The idea I am about to introduce is provocative and may spark some defensiveness: it is my belief that *everyone* is a racist and *everyone* has biases and prejudices towards others. What I mean is that you prefer to hang out with folks who are "like me" and avoid people who are "not like me." These are people who are part of your "tribe," your identified peer group. This may not be based on skin color, or religious preference, but it is certainly based on shared interests, values, and preferences. Just consider the immediate impressions you might have, and prejudgments you might make, about someone de-

## VOICE FROM THE FIELD

Sure I have a preferred client: someone who is well educated and articulate—someone in touch with feelings. Probably a woman, since she's more likely to talk about feelings. I like clients who are a bit feisty, who stir things up, who challenge me, but who, when it comes right down to it, they're women of action. There's nothing worse than someone who talks and talks but never changes anything.

Who don't I like to work with? Well, in my experience, older men can be a pain in the butt. They just didn't grow up during a time when counseling was acceptable. They don't know how to be good clients. They want me to tell them what to do.

Because God is important to me, I have a hard time working with anyone who doesn't feel the same way. It's not that I can't help that person, it's just that my feelings come through. I know it.

---

scribed to you as: "Republican," or "a rodeo cowboy," or a "Seventh Day Adventist," or a "transsexual." It is difficult, if not impossible, to avoid forming some initial expectation. Furthermore, such impressions are in many ways highly functional.

Confronting your prejudices and biases is an important component of your counselor training (Kiselica, 1998; Sandhu & Aspy, 1997). You can do great damage to clients who may already be feeling somewhat vulnerable and insecure. If they sense and feel your critical judgments of them (and these are very hard to hide), it may further erode their already fragile self-esteem.

## COUNSELING AND GENDER

About three-quarters of the clients you will see are going to be women. This is not because females are inclined to have more problems than men but because they are often designated as the "identified clients" in their families, the ones who seek help on behalf of others. Furthermore, the whole enterprise of counseling is much more congruent with the values of women: Clients are expected to be self-disclosing, to share feelings openly, to be vulnerable, and admit to weaknesses. These are tasks not often associated with male socialization.

Though women are not definable as a minority group, they have been subjected to similar marginalization, discrimination, and prejudice that minorities have experienced. This is true not only from the perspective that most counseling theories were invented by white males and reflect their values and biases, but also that most positions of power and influence have been controlled by men as well. Although this trend is changing (it is now rare for a man to be elected president of the American Counseling Association, one professional group whose members are primarily female), inequalities still exist in many sectors.

## VOICE FROM THE FIELD

I was leading this group mostly composed of women, when one member was discussing her frustrations related to her husband's nonresponsive behavior. I interrupted her several times, essentially saying to her that rather than complaining and blaming, what was she going to do about it? Okay, I admit it: As a man I was identifying with the husband a lot.

The group member ignored me and kept on with her story. I looked around the group and saw a number of female heads nodding in agreement, or perhaps they were just indicating that they were with her. I sure wasn't, because I interrupted her again, this time to ask her where things were going because I was noticing myself (and the other men) becoming bored with the monologue.

She looked me straight in the eyes and said to me: "What is it with you guys—is it so hard for you just to listen to me? I don't want you to fix me. I don't want you to push me or interrupt me. I don't ever feel that men hear what I am saying."

Wow! That sure got my attention. Forever after, I have been considering the multitude of ways that men and women do speak different languages.

---

With a few notable exceptions (Melanie Klein, Anna Freud), men created most of the foundational theories of this field, some showing biases regarding the roles women should play. Certainly Freud's portrayal of the "weaker sex" as dependent, hysterical, and inferior established a precedent. Most of the theories that followed continued to reinforce conventional stereotypes of women as sex objects who need counseling for their boredom.

Women are more likely than men to be diagnosed with major depression, and when they are depressed, they stay depressed longer. The books of Sylvia Plath, Virginia Woolf, Doris Lessing, Alice Walker, and other writers document the depressive episodes all too familiar to women who feel powerless, ignored, abused, and neglected in their lives. Kaplan (1983) claims that one reason why more women than men are labeled and treated as mentally ill is that the diagnostic system is founded on inherently masculine-biased assumptions. The American Psychiatric Association's DSM-IV overemphasizes disorders that are caricatures of traditional female roles—that is, diagnoses that describe women who are overconforming in their efforts to satisfy gender stereotypes. Thus, favorite labels include such terms as *hysterical, passive-dependent,* and *anorexic,* which all describe the symptoms of a woman trying too hard to be subordinate, emotional, dependent, and skinny. Although critics argue that no empirical evidence supports the validity of Kaplan's claims, counselors nevertheless ought to be aware of the danger of creating additional problems for female clients by labeling overconforming behavior as pathological.

Men, as well, suffer the consequences of their own traditional gender roles. When asked what they prefer in a partner, most women might say they'd like a man who is kind, sensitive, caring, expressive, supportive, *and successful.* Very few women would prefer a man as a life partner who may be highly verbal, sensitive, emotionally expressive, yet who is unemployed or working in a job without promise. Now consider what it takes for a man to be successful in the workplace. Most often this requires someone who is ruthless, opportunistic, tough, and emotionally restricted. So the man is expected to act one way at home with his family and quite another way at work, a predicament that is almost impossible to resolve. Of course, the exact same scenario is common for women as well who play a nurturing role at home but are expected to "be like men" in the workplace or they are seen as weak and ineffective.

Then there is the whole concept of body image. Women strive to fulfill some ideal concept of how they should look and in the process often develop distorted images of their body and poor self-concepts. Eating disorders are a particularly dramatic example of the attempts of women to live up to the ideal standards of body image created by Western culture. Almost all models are tall and thin. While striving for this narrow conception of beauty as slimness, some women lose control of their original goal to become thinner and perceive losing weight as a contest. One prevalent problem is anorexia nervosa, or drastic weight loss to the point of starvation. This disorder almost always has its onset in adolescent girls who are overdependent, perfectionistic, and self-critical. Bulimia, or compulsive food gorging, is another way women ruin their bodies through abusive eating habits, often the consequence of rejection and a poor self-concept. Until efforts initiated by Salvador Minuchin (Minuchin, Rosman, & Baker, 1978) and others to treat eating disorders in a family counseling context, the prognosis for these female-oriented problems was not favorable. Now counselors are experiencing successful outcomes by intervening on a structural level within the family unit.

Schlossberg and Kent (1979) present a model for working with women and their special problems that includes an emphasis on developmental transitions. The counselor's role, after becoming aware of transitional crises such as the birth of a child, is to educate the client about universal problems and then to make needed adjustments. A developmental model is often difficult to put into practice, particularly because the traditional theories of Erikson, Freud, Kohlberg, and others are so gender biased. Schlossberg (1984) has attempted to downplay the traditional roles of women as caretakers in an effort to equalize the developmental life cycle for both sexes.

Serious questions are often raised about the validity of counseling interventions with women on the grounds that the personality theories from which they derive are authored by men and focused primarily on male concerns. Concepts such as "penis envy" and "Oedipus complex" and stereotypical portrayals of women as emotional and nurturing make it more difficult for them to attain the autonomy and independence so prized by most psychological theories. Feminist approaches to counseling and therapy provide alternative conceptions to historically limiting theories (Covington & Surrey, 2000; Enns, 1993).

Women are often more frequent victims of poverty and domestic violence. We have witnessed this not only in North American culture but in most countries around the world. Women who live in impoverished conditions are unable to gain access to such support systems as child care, health care, and counseling, so they are more likely to develop serious problems before they receive help. Although women are frequent victims of domestic violence, they are reluctant to reveal their experiences or seek help, in part because victims tend to be viewed as losers (Koss, 1990). Women who survive an abusive relationship often experience grief, depression, and a sense of guilt and shame. The family is not a safeguard against violence for women because violent incidents directed toward women often involve family members.

Current lifestyle issues such as juggling roles, coping with poverty, and responding to violence, combined with developing an identity and positive self-concept in the shadow of theories that discount many aspects of the female experience, demonstrate the importance of acquiring knowledge and insight to counsel women. In particular, female counselors must be careful not to assume that being female correlates with understanding the problems and concerns of all women.

## COUNSELING ETHNIC MINORITIES

The United States is a nation of diverse cultural groups, a few of which control most of the power and resources. A number of traditionally disadvantaged minority groups—notably Latinos, African Americans, Native Americans, and Asian Americans—have been underrepresented not only in positions of prominence but also in opportunities to get help from counselors. There is probably no issue in the field considered more important right now than attention to ways counselors can better serve minority groups in their educational, vocational, and personal pursuits.

Although lip service is often given to this "politically correct" professional issue, it seems that often the changes initiated are cosmetic rather than substantial. I include a chapter in a book such as this one. You take a class and go to a few workshops to increase your multicultural sensitivity. We celebrate Martin Luther King Day or Cinco de Mayo. Employers sponsor workshops in cultural sensitivity. We recognize Black History Month. Certainly this is better than nothing, but it's not nearly enough.

Researchers ascribe much of the failure and ineffectiveness of mental health programs to the lack of recognition given to the needs of minority groups. In their review of the literature pertaining to treatment of minority populations, several conclusions may be reached (Hall and Maloney, 1983; Lee, 2002; Robinson & Howard-Hamilton, 2000):

1. Minority clients are diagnosed as having more severe disturbances and pathological conditions than white persons—a finding that is not surprising considering that most tests of mental illness are culturally biased and most diagnosticians are not members of minority groups.
2. Minority clients will tend to use mental health services only in cases of emergency or severe psychopathology, again skewing the perceptions of clinicians, who may be used to working with normal or neurotic whites

## VOICE FROM THE FIELD

I travel a lot. I try to spend as much time as I can visiting places I've never been before. I used to travel abroad to do this when I was younger, but lately, I've learned that there is so much to see within driving distance. I say that I am visiting places but I'm really far more interested in meeting people, especially those from different cultures. I don't care much for museums or tourist spots; I am drawn to places where people hang out. In fact, lately when I travel I arrange for home-stays rather than antiseptic, homogenous motels. I give up a little privacy, sure, but I learn so much about people living with them for a few days or a week.

My counseling training has served me well during my travels. I have become so skilled at asking the kinds of questions that get people to open up. I listen carefully. I communicate to the people that I meet that I am so interested in their lives, and especially their stories. I think more than anything else I do—workshops I've attended, classes I've taken, supervision—these travels have taught me to be more open and understanding of my clients' experiences.

---

but very disturbed minorities. It is a cultural norm, for instance, among South American populations to handle most psychological problems through the resources of the family and church, relying on counselors or therapists in extreme cases.

3. Minority clients more often drop out of treatment prematurely, usually within the first few sessions. Whether this tendency is a function of poor motivation or a difference in how they are treated is not clear.

4. In inpatient settings, evidence does indicate that African American clients are treated differently from whites, more often receiving stronger medication, seclusion, restraints, and other punitive "therapies" and less often receiving recreational or occupational therapy.

5. Minority group attitudes toward psychological disturbances are markedly different from those of whites, more often stressing the roles of organic factors. Latinos, for example, may have more faith in the power of prayer than in counseling for healing what they believe are inherited illnesses. The expectations of some minority clients may not, therefore, be conducive to success, because so often the faith and hope that are so important are not operating at high levels.

6. Many people feel more comfortable and prefer working with others whom they perceive as similar (particularly with regard to race or ethnic background). Yet there are relatively few trained minority counselors who are available to serve this need.

7. With minority clients, and particularly with those of the lower class, counselors must adapt their strategies and interventions to cultural differences. Eye contact and attention patterns can be interpreted variously as resistance, passivity, or aggression, depending on the client's culture.

8. Counseling can be viewed as a form of social control, because its goals are most often to help deviants better adjust to the cultural norms of the ma-

jority. For the minority client this sort of adjustment presents special problems, because more conflict can result from the clash between subcultural values and those of the majority.

Recognizing your cultural biases is only the first of several steps to ensure effective treatment of minority clients. Counselors must also be highly motivated to educate themselves about other cultural groups. Finally, counselors must develop cross-cultural intervention skills to work with each client as an individual. By endlessly focusing on the differences among various ethnic groups, counselors can fall into the trap of neglecting the uniqueness of each member of the group. A person's ethnic identity is only one of several contextual variables to help counselors understand and work with him or her as a client. Similarly, understanding the cultural heritage of clients is a necessary but insufficient condition for attaining true empathic contact.

A serious need exists not only for increased awareness of racial and ethnic minority groups but also for educational programs to prepare counselors to work with these groups (Abreu, Chung, & Atkinson, 2000; Baruth & Manning, 2003; Casas, Ponterotto, & Gutierrez, 1986). Promoting multicultural development basically involves three stages: awareness, knowledge, and skills (Pedersen, 1988; Pedersen & Carey, 2003). Thus, as students of counseling, you must continue to develop awareness of your own attitudes, acquire knowledge about the different cultures, and develop skills for interacting with persons from various backgrounds. These steps are equally important for all students and practicing counselors, regardless of race or ethnic origin. Belonging to the same race or culture as your client does not mean that you know or understand all the experiences of other members of that group.

In addition to the need for awareness and understanding, counselors must also develop specific skills for working effectively with clients with different backgrounds (Baruth & Manning, 2003). Although the literature on this topic is becoming extensive, there is unfortunately little consensus of the actual behavioral criteria that represent expertise in multicultural counseling. At least a set of multicultural competencies considered desirable if not mandatory for any competent practitioner is beginning to evolve (Ponterotto, Alexander, & Grieger, 1995).

Becoming a competent multicultural practitioner is especially difficult because there are so many diverse populations, each with their own characteristics. Even the grouping of "Latino" or "Asian" is misleading because there are so many differences in subgroups. A Japanese, Vietnamese, Filipino, and Chinese—or Mexcian, Brazilian, Salvadoran, and Cuban—might be greatly offended by some assumptions that they are similar in their cultures. As a student you may consider designing a step-by-step approach that involves first learning about the customs of each and every cultural group that might be represented in your practice. Better yet, arrange immersion experiences in which you "join" the culture on an experiential level. The goal, for each and every one of your clients, is to become an expert on their worlds. Each new client represents an opportunity for you to learn as much as you can about a new culture, including its customs, values, and worldview.

## VOICE FROM THE FIELD

I remember one time I was doing a group that included some Native American participants. I thought I was being so sensitive to their needs and I went to extraordinary lengths to accommodate them as best I could and make them feel welcome.

Then one day I noticed that one of the Native students was absent. She didn't come back the next time either. But I figured it would be intrusive or insensitive of me to push things. Still, I was a bit bewildered by her behavior, just dropping out like that with no courtesy of a phone call. Honestly, I was angry.

I later learned that there had been a death in her family and according to her traditions, she was required to drop out of all normal activities so she could devote herself to a year of mourning. When I asked the other Native participants why she didn't have the courtesy to tell me what had happened, they told me that it wasn't her place to tell me, but my place to ask.

---

Again I want to stress that this is not an additional burden and responsibility of your work—it is a privilege and one of the most satisfying parts of the job. Counselors are not the highest paid professionals around, nor do they receive the same kind of perks as others, but they do enjoy the tremendous benefit of learning so much about different people and their experiences. Some would say that this is the best part of the job.

## COUNSELING THE AGED

When most of you will be at your peak of professional productivity, a disproportionate part of the North American population will be considered elderly citizens. There is little doubt that the single specialty within the helping professions that is most likely to flourish, if not explode, will be counseling older adults. The number of people over 65 has increased sevenfold: from one in thirty Americans in 1900 to an expected one in five Americans by 2020. Life expectancies will continue to lengthen, stretching normal life spans well into the 80s and perhaps 90s. Age 65 will be considered a part of the productive rather than the retirement years. Older citizens will dominate the consumer markets and they will control a significant part of industry, families, and lifestyle. And with these changing roles, opportunities, and expectations will come new problems of adaptation for the aged—and important responsibilities for therapeutic counselors to aid adjustment and resolution of conflicts.

Although there are more similarities than differences in counseling old and young people, the assessment process is more complex with the mature client and specialized competencies are necessary. Not only are there more life experiences to take into account, but the diagnosis may be affected by underlying medical or physiological problems.

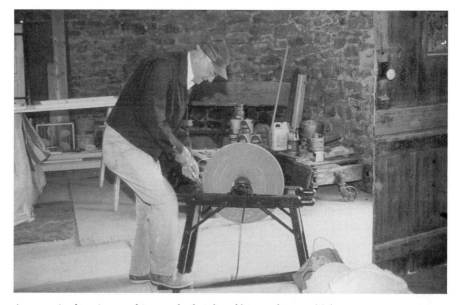

A nonretired senior working at the height of his professional life. For some active and productive people, youth is more a state of mind than chronological age. © Myrleen Ferguson Cate /PhotoEdit.

These special diagnostic problems are more than compensated for by the tremendous satisfaction that geriatric counselors experience in their work. In a sense, you get to hang out with the wise elders of society and learn from their life experiences. Certainly, there are also many challenges such as possibly stirring up all kinds of countertransference feelings.

Some models of aging view older people as helpless, disabled, and burdensome to society. There are special facilities where the aged may be cleaned, clothed, and fed until they die. Institutional environments of this type are often viewed as depressing places where people wander about, forgetting who or where they are. The more agile can play cards, turn the channels on the television, or even shuffle along for walks outside the home.

Alternative conceptions of aging view older persons as senior adults with a wealth of valuable experiences and skills accumulated over a lifetime. Elders used to be considered the wise men and women of the community to whom the young would come for advice and assistance; now they are the elderly—the shuffleboard and Geritol generation. Old age is a time of physical changes—hair thinning and turning white, skin losing its moisture and smoothness, the body actually shrinking in size, muscles becoming flabby and losing their strength. Joints become progressively stiff, bones are fragile, the heart is less efficient, and the arteries that circulate blood work like a slow train. Digestion is slowed, reaction times are diminished, and lungs work at less than peak efficiency and bring less oxygen to provide energy. All the senses lose their precision, and the older person, receiving less information from vision, hearing, taste, touch, and smell, is thus more isolated, irritable, and moody.

## VOICE FROM THE FIELD

Part of my job involves visiting some senior citizen homes, and I'm telling you I had to throw everything I learned out the window. I see the residents in groups, trying to get them to talk about their struggles. Gee, most of them are just so lonely, or at least it looked that way. Later I learned that loneliness is more a problem for younger people, actually.

Anyway, I'd get the group going and it was like a circus. They'd all interrupt one another. This one guy would start rambling all over, which seemed to be okay since nobody was listening anyway. At first, I felt so useless 'cause I couldn't use all my skills I'd been trained in. Once I let go of those expectations, though, I found that I really could help them by just listening to their stories and helping them to do that for one another. Most of these folks didn't want to change; really, they didn't need to. But they did feel a very strong desire to be heard.

---

Yet in spite of these symptoms of physical deterioration, their effects are often slight and the stereotype of the elderly person as slow moving and fragile, with dulled and distorted perceptions, is hardly accurate. From a number of biochemical and physiological changes in the elderly, researchers conclude that slowed intellectual, perceptual, and mental behavior, particularly in those who are free of debilitating diseases, need not necessarily restrict functioning levels in major life areas. That does not mean, however, that you shouldn't make adjustments in the ways you work with this population. In fact, it would probably be advisable to alter assessment techniques, length of sessions, and even the sorts of methods you employ. Still, the aged retain the capacity for self-awareness and insight. They respond to reinforcement. They may be a bit more cautious in their mental and physical movements, but they still think, feel, and act and wish to do so more effectively.

Traditionally, at least at the time Erik Erikson was formulating his theory of psychosocial development, later maturity was a time for resolution of the crisis of despair and for introspective integration of one's life. The elderly were supposed to be giving meaning to their life's work and preparing themselves to accept the inevitability of death. At age 81, himself engaged in this final life stage, Erikson revised many of his thoughts about old age to place much more emphasis on the creative, productive elements supposedly restricted to earlier stages (Hall, 1983). Through their roles in grandparenting, volunteer work, and involvement in intimate relationships, older people can retain the playfulness, joy, and wonder that were so much a part of childhood.

B. F. Skinner, another influential thinker of the twentieth century, also wrote about his own struggle to maintain his desired levels of effectiveness and to avoid growing old as a thinker even though his body stubbornly persisted in its progressive decline. "Old age is like fatigue, except that its effects cannot be corrected by relaxing or taking a vacation" (Skinner, 1983, p. 241). The older adult must learn to accept his or her incapacities and to find alternative ways to accomplish the same goals and to meet the same needs. Death, certain and inevitable, is a difficult issue for the older person as it looms ahead, closer and closer. Some people become crippled by their fears; others welcome their final deliverance. Yet when old persons are given the opportunity to talk through their fears, most are able to resolve the developmental task, accept what they cannot change, and go on about the business of living fully in what time remains. When discomfort arises in confronting the topic of death—with relatives, friends, nurses, doctors, or counselors—it is important to distinguish who exactly is uncomfortable, the older adult or the counselor.

Dying is the last developmental task for everyone. Whether it comes unexpectedly, with or without pain, during sleep or sex, death is patiently waiting. Woody Allen (1976) freely admits, "It's not that I'm afraid to die. I just don't want to be there when it happens" (p. 106). If there is a "process" of dying, even beyond Elizabeth Kubler-Ross' stages of denial, rage, bargaining, depression, and acceptance (assuming death is patient enough to wait for the complete cycle), then certainly counselors could help make the experience easier.

Throughout history the aged have always served the important function of passing on wisdom from one generation to the next. Whether in the role of teacher, guru, shaman, or grandparent, the elders have taught their accumulated knowledge, experience, and skills to youth so that they too might survive life's tests. The aged are responsible, through storytelling and sharing of life experiences, for maintaining family and ethnic traditions. It is through listening to accounts of their own mistakes, failures, and weaknesses that, they hope, their protégés will learn to avoid similar traps.

Publications about adult development and aging are plentiful. So as counseling students you will be able to read and learn much about the issues involved in counseling the elderly. Even if this is not an area of special interest, you will find it necessary to acquire some background knowledge and skills because the number of older people who will be needing and seeking services will continue to grow. Aging is a natural part of the developmental cycle that should not be ignored when you work with this special population.

# COUNSELING LESBIANS AND GAY MEN

Negative social attitudes and a pattern of stigmatization institutionalized in laws and the mental health system have kept gay people an invisible or hidden minority (Dworkin & Gutierrez, 1989; Fassinger, 1991). Homosexuality was viewed by psychiatry as a mental illness until 1973, and it wasn't until the publication of DSM-III-R (1987) that all references to homosexuality were declassified. Thus, the counseling and development needs of gay men and lesbians have not historically been addressed, and the majority of counselor training programs have neglected lesbian and gay issues (Buhrke & Douce, 1991).

There are many issues unique to this population of which you will need to be aware (Barret & Logan, 2002; Murphy, Rawlings, & Howe, 2002).

## VOICE FROM THE FIELD

Homosexuality always went against my basic beliefs and my religious training. I just thought it was wrong. On a personal level, I had even stronger reactions. Then I discovered that one of my clients, whom I already had a very close relationship with, admitted to being lesbian. I tried not to show the shock on my face—or the revulsion. But the strange thing is that I already cared so much for this woman that learning her sexual preferences didn't seem to matter much to me. She was such a good and honorable person.

I learned so much about her history and way of life. Eventually, I'm proud to admit, I even overcame my own biases against people who live alternative lifestyles. I still feel uneasy about the whole thing, but maybe that's because of my own issues related to my own sexuality. What's amazing to me is that, previously, I could never have imagined myself working effectively with this population. Now I quite enjoy the challenge of delving in areas in which I have had little experience.

**Identity Development**    Gay and lesbian clients may often struggle with varying degrees of acceptance and satisfaction with their sexual orientation. A series of developmental stages in this process has been identified that moves from a point of confusion to comparison with others, to acceptance, tolerance, then pride and synthesis (Fassinger, 1991).

**Coming Out**    There are some different issues presented in counseling for those who have publicly disclosed their sexual identity versus those who keep that part of their lives private. Some clients may request support in their efforts to deal with others' reactions to their lifestyle.

**Occupational/Career Issues**    Discrimination in the work arena is a reality for many gay people, and counselors must be sensitive to the special life/career planning issues that arise. Counselors must be aware of occupations or professions that are more tolerant of sexual orientation, be sensitive to the dual-career issues of lesbian and gay couples, and be knowledgeable about the special resources available to gays.

**Racial, Ethnic, and Regional Issues**    Gay men and lesbians have historically experienced discrimination and violence as a result of living in a homophobic and heterosexual society. When social class and racial issues are added, gay individuals may experience double- or triple-minority status with increasing attendant discrimination. Geography and regional differences also affect the gay subculture and may affect the available resources and networking opportunities for gay people. Counselors must be knowledgeable about these issues and be prepared to offer support and encouragement to gay clients experiencing multiple layers of discrimination.

**Isolation**   An openly gay lifestyle in a heterosexist society can result in a feeling of isolation and a fear of discrimination and rejection. Counselors must recognize the dangers of an isolated lifestyle and encourage gay people to develop a full and wide pattern of interaction with both gay and nongay individuals.

**Couple Issues**   Gay individuals need to affirm the validity of their lifestyles and their commitment to their primary partner. In addition to the special issues that confront gay/lesbian couples, there are the typical types of conflicts and stresses inherent in all intimate relationships. Counselors must be cognizant of the special challenges and strengths of the gay/lesbian couple as well as the more traditional problems of all couples.

**HIV**   The role of the counselor in working with AIDS issues has two major focal areas: (1) providing services to HIV-positive individuals and (2) providing education to non-HIV-positive individuals regarding practices designed to prevent AIDS.

This role of health educator is a new and complex one for counselors, yet it is essential because HIV is a largely preventable disease. Counselors must be prepared to discuss sexual practices frankly and to provide information to assist in prevention efforts. AIDS education programs must increase awareness of the risks associated with the disease, promote an understanding of the principles of "safe sex," and encourage the necessary behavioral controls to confront denial and increase the probability of implementing AIDS prevention behaviors.

**Antigay Violence**   Hate crimes against gays and lesbians have been prevalent throughout history. They range from verbal insults and slurs to acts of violence, including murder. This reality exacts a toll on the gay person's self-esteem and can lead to depression and feelings of hopelessness, shame, and guilt. Counselors must provide support to the victims of antigay abuse and work with them to counteract the negative effects on their self-esteem. Counselors can also help their clients to direct their feelings into positive, activist channels to counter antigay violence.

Perhaps the most challenging aspect of working with gay and lesbian as well as transgendered and bisexual clients, is confronting your own biases and prejudices related to these populations (gay and lesbian counselors may have to addresses their own biases and prejudices toward so-called "breeders"). This means addressing your own internalized homophobia, as well as any beliefs or personal convictions that may trigger for you a degree of discomfort talking about this subject (Murphy, Rawlings, & Howe, 2002; Plummer, 1999). You may even hold rather strong ideas about moral issues related to one's sexual orientation. Just as with every other group that is mentioned in this chapter, you can do great harm to people if your personal biases leak into sessions and clients sense your criticism and disdain (Campos & Goldfried, 2001).

■ |    VOICE FROM THE FIELD

When you're working with HIV clients, you have to lose your squeamishness. If a guy recently had sex, for example, you have to ask him very direct questions. Did he use a rubber? Did he protect himself?

With another family I'm seeing how the kids are dealing with their mom's AIDS. She's close to death. As I reflect on my session with them, I see how nervous and unsure I was with them. The simple fact is that I'm afraid to talk about death with them. Death is the enemy. I want to feel differently, but deep down inside there is mostly fear that surrounds a nugget of wonder. It's a small nugget, maybe, but that whisper drives me to search further.

## COUNSELING CLIENTS WHO ARE PHYSICALLY CHALLENGED

Clients who are physically challenged, or disabled, generally become involved in counseling through rehabilitation services provided to assess the needs of the client and establish a program of physical and emotional restoration. Career exploration and establishment of training goals are a major focus of rehabilitation efforts, helping individuals to prepare for alternative forms of meaningful work (Corrigan, Jones, & McWhirter, 2001). Counselors need to recognize, however, that these individuals may have emotional problems not necessarily related to their abilities or disabilities.

People with disabilities are often able to participate fully in life as a result of social, political, and technological developments. Today we are challenged to think of disabled or handicapped people as "differently abled" to remove their stigma. In one sense, we are all "temporarily abled" persons in that the conditions in one's life are variable and likely to change over time. Such a perspective can be discouraging in that it emphasizes lack of control over our individual fate, or it can be reassuring in that it assumes that we can adapt to whatever happens.

When Erik Weihenmayer became the first blind mountaineer to scale Mount Everest, he was attacked by the elite climbing community as being a danger to others. He was considered too handicapped by his lack of sight to assess weather conditions or take care of himself. Responding to one of his critics, Ed Viesturs, one of the premier Everest experts, Erik responded:

> He hadn't seen the 16 years I'd been climbing, learning rope management, crevasse rescue, and avalanche safety; he surely hadn't seen the days spent on big walls when my teammates hung from anchors placed by the blind guy. Or the years I spent becoming independent, learning to build snow walls, cook meals on gas stoves, and set up tents in whiteouts. Viesturs hadn't seen any part of my life except that I was blind (Weihenmayer, 2001, p. 55).

That is one of the major problems that physically challenged people face: they are not seen for who they are, or what they can do: they *are* their handicaps—the blind guy, the dwarf, the lady with no hands, the boy in the wheelchair, the albino. This is really no different from the way that so many of us are labeled or reduced to a single label based on our physical or racial features.

Counselors need to be knowledgeable about and sensitive to the issues faced by clients who are disabled in many various ways. This includes familiarity with the unique cultures of each group that may include language, customs, norms, and rituals just as for any other group we have studied. For example, the deaf community has a complex set of language and cultural dimensions as rich and complex as any ethnic group (Filer & Filer, 2000).

In addition, family members of disabled individuals may experience guilt, anger, resentment, and insecurity because they do not know how to handle problems. These symptoms may be manifested by siblings as well as by spouses and parents. Because the disabled family member requires extra assistance and attention, other family members may not be comfortable asking to have their needs met. The counselor can help the family develop ways to manage time, money, and emotional resources so that everyone can receive appropriate attention and support.

Disabled children, in particular, can provide especially difficult challenges in the family for the parents and the other children. Seligman (1983) points out that, because disabled children need excessive caretaking, other family members must bear the responsibility and burden, often neglecting themselves and one another in the process. But it is certainly not always the case that the presence of a disabled child adversely affects the family. Often the experience encourages brothers and sisters to develop a sensitivity and caring that they will maintain their whole lives. Counselors must realize, however, that the "identified client"—the disabled child—may not be the only one with problems.

This reminder is but a specific application of the principle that holds true for most presenting problems that occur in a family: When one person develops symptoms, they inevitably disrupt the daily lives of everyone else. Particularly when the disabled individual is making a poor psychological adjustment, the added strain and stress place the other children at risk to develop problems. In addition to feeling guilt and resentment, they may also act out as a way to win attention according to family norms that emphasize being taken care of. For all these reasons, it is often advisable to work with the disabled in the context of their families.

# SUMMARY

In one sense, every client you see represents a special population with unique problems and challenges. Nevertheless, some client groups in particular have suffered more than their fair share as a result of discrimination and prejudices. Furthermore, several of the diverse populations discussed in this chapter have tended to underutilize counseling services. That is one reason why the role of being a counselor includes not only prevention and treatment, but also advocacy. Your job is not only to help your individual clients but also to help the world become a more equitable place for people of all backgrounds and experiences.

The complexity of the problems and special considerations for each group is evidenced by the amount of literature detailing the characteristics and methods of treatment. The challenges facing you as a counselor include learning about each of the diverse populations, developing specialized skills to counsel individuals and families, and understanding your own biases and how they affect your thoughts and behavior with clients.

# SELF-GUIDED EXPLORATIONS

1. Describe the cultural, ethnic, religious, gender, and racial influences that have helped to shape your identity. If you were going to work with a counselor, what would you want him or her to know and understand about your cultural background?
2. Your perception of reality is influenced a great deal by how you have been indoctrinated throughout your life by family members, teachers, books, media, and most of all, your cultural identity. List as many of these "social constructions" as you can think of that have shaped who you are and what you most value.
3. Pretend that you wake up tomorrow morning a different race and color than before you went to sleep. After the initial shock wears off and you begin the normal business of resuming your life, what will be most difficult for you to adjust to?
4. In what ways do you feel limited by your gender? What would be different in your life if you were a member of the opposite sex?
5. Describe a time in your life when you felt oppressed by someone. Now imagine going to someone for help who resembles others who have abused you.

# For Homework:

ASSIGNMENT 1

One way to broaden your cultural perspective is through watching certain movies with strong multicultural themes. Examples might include any of the following films: *West Side Story, Birdcage, Joy Luck Club, Philadelphia, White Man's Burden, Once Were Warriors, Hoop Dreams, Priscilla: Queen of the Dessert, Fools Rush In, Six Degrees of Separation, Secrets and Lies, Dangerous Minds, Mi Familia, Black Robe, Songcatcher, American History X, My Left Foot, Hurricane, My Big Fat Greek Wedding.*

Get together with several classmates, friends, or family members and watch a few of these movies (or others you can think of) together. Talk to one another afterwards about what the films stirred up for you. Speak to one another—not as film critics, but as reactors to the cultural themes highlighted.

ASSIGNMENT 2

Explore a culture that you know little about, one that represents a group you may see represented in a future counseling job. Study this culture from several different viewpoints through reading, interviews, observations, and *immersion* experiences. It is crucial that you enter this culture through *direct contact* with as many facets as you have the time and inclination for.

Write in your journal describing what you learned about the culture, and what you learned about yourself during the process. Connect these insights to other themes from class and your text.

ASSIGNMENT 3

Read some novels with strong multicultural themes. For instance in Barbara Kingsolver's book, *Poisonwood Bible*, or in Michael Dorris' book, *A Yellow Raft in Blue Water*, there are prevalent themes dealing with developing a cultural identity.

ASSIGNMENT 4

Take a transformative trip in which you immerse yourself in a different culture. You need not go far from home, just somewhere that presents opportunities for you to experiment with different parts of who you are. Ideally, the most potent environments for personal change are those that:

1. Insulate you from usual influences so you are free to experiment with alternative ways of being.
2. Foster some sort of emotional activation in which you are strongly aroused by what you are experiencing.
3. Force you face some of your fears as well as new challenges.
4. Get you out of your normal routines and comfort zone so that you feel lost and have to find your way.
5. Provide "teachable" moments that are memorable and impactful.
6. Force you to solve problems or overcome obstacles in new ways.
7. Structure opportunities to reflect on the meaning of the experience.
8. Allow you to transfer what you learned to other aspects of your life.

# SUGGESTED READINGS

Axelson, J. A. (1999). *Counseling and development in a multicultural society* (3rd ed.). Pacific Grove, CA: Brooks/Cole.

Barret, B., & Logan, C. (2002). *Counseling gay men and lesbians: A practice primer.* Pacific Grove, CA: Brooks/Cole.

Baruth, L., & Manning, M. L. (2003). *Multicultural counseling and psychotherapy: A lifespan development* (3rd ed). Pacific Grove, CA: Brooks/Cole.

Dorris, M. (1998). *A yellow raft in blue water.* New York: Warner.

Gilbert, L. A., & Scher, M. (1999). *Gender and sex in counseling and psychotherapy.* Boston: Allyn & Bacon.

Ivey, A. E., D'Andrea, M., Ivey, M. B., & Simek-Morgan, L. (2002). *Counseling and psychotherapy: A multicultural perspective.* Boston: Allyn & Bacon.

Kingsolver, B. (1999). *The poisonwood bible*. New York: Harper.

Kiselica, M. S. (1998). *Confronting prejudice and racism during multicultural training*. Alexandria, VA: American Counseling Association.

Lee, C. C. (2002). *Multicultural issues in counseling: New approaches to diversity* (3rd ed.). Alexandria, VA: American Counseling Association.

Pedersen, P., & Carey, J. (2003). *Multicultural counseling in schools: A practical handbook*. Boston: Allyn & Bacon.

Pope-Davis, D. B., & Coleman, H. L. K. (2001). *The interaction of race, class, and gender: Implications for multicultural counseling*. Thousand Oaks, CA: Sage.

Robinson, T. L., & Howard-Hamilton, M. F. (2000). *The convergence of race, ethnicity, and gender*. Upper Saddle River, NJ: Merrill.

Sandhu, D. S., & Aspy, C. B. (1997). *Counseling for prejudice prevention and reduction*. Alexandria, VA: American Counseling Association.

Vontress, C. E., Johnson, J. A., & Epp, L. (1999). *Cross-cultural counseling: A casebook*. Alexandria, VA: American Counseling Association.

# PROFESSIONAL
# PRACTICE

# 14 CHAPTER ETHICAL AND LEGAL ISSUES

## KEY CONCEPTS

Confidentiality

Public welfare

Ethical codes

Divided loyalties

Dual relationships

Sexual misconduct

Clinical misjudgments

Informed consent

Privileged communication

Tarasoff decision

Duty to warn

Mandated reporting

Managed care dilemmas

Counselor impairment

Ethical decision making

Civil, criminal, and mental health law

Client rights

# ETHICAL AND
# LEGAL ISSUES

# CHAPTER 14

You have been working with a young client for three months. He was at first wary, reticent, and cautious. It has taken patience and careful use of your trust and relationship-building skills to break through the resistance.

Finally he is beginning to talk and share something of his life with you in the counseling sessions. Yet each time you begin to make progress, he draws back into his shell with a defensive remark: "You shrink types are all the same. You get your kicks out of prying into other people's lives." You repeatedly reassure him, reminding him of the sanctity and privacy of your office and the confidentiality of your relationship. He has tested your integrity a number of times and has attempted to probe your attitudes and values. You have responded by keeping the focus on him. You have thus spent a disproportionate amount of counseling time reaffirming your trustworthiness.

Finally your persistence and patience pay off. After much hesitation and several false starts, he slowly discloses his secret, meanwhile closely monitoring your reactions to him. He is satisfied as to your neutrality and acceptance of him (which you are consciously controlling) and so continues to describe his problem. This 16-year-old boy has quite a successful career selling various drugs—downers, speed, cocaine, marijuana, and sometimes heroin—to other kids in the junior and senior high school. He has no intention of quitting. In fact, he loves the work. He explains that finally he has power, respect, and friends. He likes the excitement and the risks. He enjoys having his "clients" dependent on him. And he can't complain about the money. No, he certainly has no intention of quitting this lucrative "career."

But he does feel a little guilty, and he wants you to help him soothe his conscience. He reminds you that, if you can't help him, he can always find someone who will. He notices your hesitancy and so, laughingly, throws your own words back in your face: "Remember, everything you say in here is privileged communication, and nothing disclosed will ever leave this room." You have but a moment to respond, to decide on one of several possible courses of action:

1. Because the most sacred principle of counseling is to protect the confidentiality of the client, as well as to act in his best interests, you would have no choice but to honor your commitments. It is, after all, not your purpose to tell people how to live their lives or to judge them.

2. The protection of public welfare (in this case, the young victims of drug abuse) takes precedence over a vow of confidentiality to a single client, especially one who is so irresponsible and unconscionable in his acts. It would be for the greater good of the community, and perhaps, ultimately, for the client's own welfare, to notify the appropriate authorities of his illegal acts so that corrective action may be taken.

3. The young man should be persuaded to stop his predatory behavior and told that, otherwise, you will be forced to notify his parents and the school authorities of his crimes.

4. The boy is obviously disturbed and not responsible for his actions. The counseling relationship ought to continue as it has been developing. It is to be hoped that he will alter his behavior as he gains insight into his self-destructive acts and learns more socially acceptable ways of earning money and social approval.

There are, naturally, myriad other alternatives open to the counselor, according to therapeutic goals, state laws, institutional policies, and even personal feelings toward the particular client. The most difficult aspect of making ethical decisions such as this is that there are rarely single, perfect solutions.

## PROFESSIONAL CODES

Professional codes of ethics are published by a number of organizations that work with therapeutic counselors, such as the American Counseling Association, the Association for Specialists in Group Work, the American Association for Marriage and Family Therapy, the American Psychological Association, the National Academy of Certified Clinical Mental Health Counselors, and the American Association for Sex Educators, Counselors, and Therapists. These guidelines, however, are often difficult to apply to individual cases, are sometimes contradictory, and are challenging for the professional organization to enforce. Furthermore, the field is so fragmented in its various licensures, certifications, and governing bodies that practitioners are often left to sort out the confusion for themselves. To make matters still more confusing, you must not only reconcile various ethical principles but also deal with the often conflicting cultures of the mental health system versus the law (Rowley

## VOICE FROM THE FIELD

Sometimes I'm not sure who my client is. It's supposed to be the children who are part of my caseload, but then the teachers in my school think I should be more accountable to them; they get mad if they think I'm taking the side of a child against them. My principal thinks that I work for her. If I don't please her with what I'm doing, she can make life very difficult for me. Then the parents of my kids feel that they are the ones I should be responding to. So, what do I do when I'm pulled in all these different directions? Everyone has their own agendas.

---

& MacDonald, 2001). For these reasons, ethical rules cannot just be memorized; rather, ethical behavior must be learned and decision-making skills developed to be internally consistent and yet compatible with acceptable societal and professional standards (Corey, Corey, & Callanan, 2003).

Ethics can be particularly frustrating to discuss in relation to the counseling profession. The nature of the field—its young history, conflicting theoretical base, and emphasis on the ambiguous and abstract content of the human mind—makes it difficult to define sanctioned professional behavior, much less enforce such professional standards. Practicing counselors sometimes have conflicting opinions about what constitutes acceptable standards of behavior. Each practitioner uses different labels and terms to describe the processes and has different goals and techniques. Depending on the state or country in which they reside, the institutions in which they work, their training, type of degree, and client needs, they can differ widely in what may be described as "ethical conduct." You would get no such impression from studying the ethical codes of the profession, wherein each point is neatly organized, numbered, and coded and set down in dignified, precise language. Many experienced practitioners have spent their whole careers attempting to set forth these standards of acceptable conduct.

There is a distinction between the ethical decision making of the beginner and that of the experienced practitioner. Whereas the seasoned expert has logged years of therapeutic hours, the beginning counselor is starting out in a haze of confusion. It is difficult enough to track client statements, analyze underlying meanings, plan intervention strategies, and respond effectively without having additionally to contemplate open-ended moral issues and ethical conflicts. It is for this reason that I urge you to read and study your professional ethical codes and follow them to the letter. It is only with vast experience and intensive study that a scholar or practitioner can expect to improvise individual moral decisions based on solid empirical and philosophical grounds. And even those with such wisdom may believe, or publicly announce, something different from what they actually do within the privacy of their offices. The problem is further compounded by the often conflicting demands from a number of sources.

# DIVIDED LOYALTIES

Who exactly does a counselor work for? Counselors learn in school that it is the clients. As professional helpers counselors are to be their advocates, to hold their trust and confidence and protect their rights. However, sometimes loyalties are divided between two or more constituents. If the client is a child, counselors are answerable to the parents for their actions, often a source of conflict when the parties disagree about the best course of action. If counselors were to comply with parental wishes and keep them informed of their work, inevitably they would lose the trust of the child. If they are uncooperative with the parents, the parents may sabotage the child's efforts or remove the child from counseling. To complicate matters further, counselors must answer to their school, agency, or institution for their actions. Counselors are also subject to the personal preferences of supervisors and the norms of the colleagues with whom they work. Then state and federal laws regulate behavior, sometimes against the welfare of clients and the best interests of institutions. As has been previously mentioned, professional codes of various organizations also regulate behavior. And through them all come the urgent whispers of your own inner voice.

Within each invidual are many competing loyalties. The fact that ultimately you answer to yourself for your actions—not to a judge, the government, or your boss—would seem to simplify the matter. Yet it is further confounded by your responsibility to various parts of your own history (for instance, a client you once failed, on whose account you promised yourselves to act differently thereafter) or to the shapers of your values and formulators of your conscience (parents, grandparents, mentors, teachers, and friends).

It is not unusual for a particular agency to dictate to the counselor a rule such as "Any drug use by clients of this agency must be reported to the authorities." Fine. Your first client walks in and casually reports that she smokes marijuana on weekends. You are obligated by contract to report this offense. But if you do, you will surely be betraying the client. Obviously you can't consult your supervisor, who is sworn to uphold the agency's regulations. You desperately want to keep your job and may not believe the offense is serious. The professional dilemma is clear: Do you follow your conscience, or do you abide by the policies you agreed to uphold when you took the job? Some rules are foolish and may be judged as immoral. There comes a time when each person must choose a course of action and live with the consequences.

# AREAS OF ETHICAL DIFFICULTY

Ethics could quite legitimately be discussed under the topic of "fear." The subject is not usually given much thought until the prospect arises that something could go wrong. Ethics is the analysis of good versus bad choices, moral versus immoral motives, helpful versus harmful action. The ethical implications of a problem are considered the last step of therapeutic decision making. Ethical consequences of behavior are usually examined only after a narrowly avoided mishap or the threat of a problem. Ethical discussions are often post-mortem autopsies, analyses of what should have been done or what will be done next time.

It is more useful to consider ethical issues, their implications, and possible resolutions before they occur, during a time when personal and professional needs and beliefs can be rationally thought out and decisions made about behavior. Predicting and identifying the conflicts that are likely to develop in the practice of counseling allow examination of implications, exploration of personal values, and an opportunity to evaluate several preferred responses. This preparation can demystify the process and diminish much of the fear and apprehension that will arise during a crisis.

Right now, what is the ethical conflict *you* fear most? What situation might occur within a session that would create for you a moral nightmare of confusion and frustration? To help stimulate self-exploration, here is a realistic review of some common problems that frequently present themselves in the first year of practice.

## Dual Relationships and Sexual Improprieties

Do you fear being seduced by a client?

F. Scott Fitzgerald's *Tender Is the Night,* a classic in American literature, popularized the theme of the inevitable magnetism between a vulnerable, idolizing young client and her omnipotent therapist, each attracted to the other during the intimacy of a therapeutic encounter. Only within the last few years have many clients had the courage to publicize their experiences of seduction with former and current helping professionals. Before you act indignant and rush to swear that it could never happen to you, first consider the dynamics that operate in a counseling situation: (1) a client who feels helpless, vulnerable, and confused; (2) with few satisfying relationships in his or her life; (3) who feels undying gratitude to the counselor who has provided crucial help at a desperate time; (4) to whom she or he has disclosed the most intimate details of her or his life; (5) whom he or she worships as a professional who at once appears so omnipotent, warm, affectionate, and understanding; and (6) whose attraction is magnified by the inequality in power and control of the relationship. Add to this potent mix the variables of countertransference, involvement, respect, and affection that the counselor will come to feel for some clients, and you have a potentially explosive situation.

This explanation is not meant to excuse or pardon unprofessional conduct that is a dangerous, abusive, and exploitive breach of trust, but rather to encourage a healthy amount of legitimate apprehension about such situations. It is not altogether impossible for a counselor to find that a grateful hug has turned unexpectedly amorous. Often, in such intense situations, emotions don't respond to a half-prepared conscience. A counselor must be constantly aware of the detrimental results that are likely to follow sexually intimate entanglements with clients. The negative consequences will often cancel the previous therapeutic effects and send the client into a tailspin of mistrust for professionals who use their power to their own advantage. It may be helpful to rehearse and role-play sexual encounters, including responses that can be made to initiations from clients. For example: "I have a confession to make. The only reason I keep coming to counseling is that I am so attracted to you. You have helped me so much. I owe it all to you. You are so different from other people I have known. How do you feel about me?"

What is your response?

- "Ah. Our time is about up. Maybe we can continue next time."
- "How would it be helpful to know my feelings?"
- "You're feeling attracted to me because I've been helpful and supportive to you, and you're hoping that I am attracted to you."
- "It is not appropriate for you to think about me personally. We have a professional relationship, and it is necessary that we keep our relationship nonpersonal in order to work together effectively."
- "Since your personal feelings seem to be getting in the way of our professional relationship, perhaps we should discuss the possibility of your working with another counselor."
- "Your place or mine?"

No matter how you look at the situation, with levity or seriousness, this incident may test the resolve of the most experienced counselor. As with all other ethical behaviors, it is insufficient merely to memorize a moral commandment: "Thou shalt not be sexually involved with thy client." You must thoroughly and genuinely believe it as a guiding principle—an internal, personal belief that certain behaviors are crucial to maintaining professional standards. The fear of being caught is not enough to prevent a problem. The counselor must understand the responsibilities, moral obligations, and consequences that come with the territory.

Time after time, research has demonstrated that sexual/romantic entanglements between client and counselor are almost always harmful, no matter what the circumstances or how they are justified (Coleman & Schaefer, 1986; Pope, Keith-Spiegel, & Tabachnick, 1986; Pope & Vasquez, 1991; Rutter, 1989; Taylor & Wagner, 1976). This is true even if the personal relationship begins after the professional one has been formally terminated because there are always lingering dependency and attachment issues. Most licensure laws prohibit romantic relationships between counselors/therapists for a period of two years after treatment has ceased. And there must still be clear indications that such a relationship will not be harmful.

Although sexual entanglements are the most dangerous and destructive kind of dual relationship between a counselor and client, there are other ways that people can be harmed. A number of professional organizations (American Counseling Association, American Psychological Association, American Association of Marriage and Family Therapists) have been debating the potential liabilities of other client/counselor relationships, such as the following cases:

- When a business relationship also exists between the counselor and client
- When the counselor serves in multiple roles in the client's life as a supervisor, colleague, or instructor
- When there is nonerotic physical contact (hugs, stroking) that may be misinterpreted
- When bartering for a fee takes place
- When clients are seen outside the office
- When the counselor becomes friends with a client

These don't necessarily involve ethical violations since making house calls, going on field trips, and hugging are accepted practices in some theoretical orientations. Dual relationships are not necessarily harmful in the first place and may even be helpful in some circumstances (Pearson & Piazza, 1997). Nevertheless, such behaviors are certainly areas of risk in which boundaries may be violated. It is for this reason that Herlihy and Corey (1997) suggest that a number of safeguards be put in place: Setting solid, constructive boundaries in the first place, keeping discussions open if unanticipated issues arise, monitoring your own motivations for initiating actions, and entering any dual or multiple roles should always be for the benefit of clients.

One especially thorny area of discussion is whether students should be asked to participate in experiential activities that require a high degree of personal self-disclosure when they are also to be evaluated and graded on their behavior. Whereas some counselor-educators believe that this is a dual relationship, others think that if certain safeguards are taken, student rights may be protected. These might include such guidelines as the following: Students provided with informed consent about what the risks and consequences are of choosing to participate or not; having the right to pass so that undue pressure is not experienced to say or do more than is comfortable; and not being graded on the behavior in class but rather on more objective products (such as papers).

If you are ever uncertain about whether you are on the verge of violating treatment boundaries or engaging in a dual relationship that may be hazardous to your clients, check with your supervisor, consult with more experienced colleagues, and check with professional ethical codes.

## Clinical Misjudgments and Failures

Are you fearful of making a terrible mistake that might hurt a client and unsure whether you would take responsibility for the consequences?

Making mistakes is inevitable in therapeutic counseling. Some of the time we are working without a clear, detailed map of the desired direction for the counseling process. Clients often don't know themselves what is troubling them, and they frequently mask their true feelings as a defense. Sometimes the deception is even deliberate, part of an elaborate game-playing scheme intended to test the counselor's ability to see through the cover-up.

The counselor's judgment is further subject to error by the relatively low reliability and validity inherent in counseling techniques. Practitioners disagree as often as they agree on the diagnosis of a client; even when they do agree on the diagnosis, they may still choose different treatment plans. Consecutive consultations with different therapeutic helpers might well yield quite different diagnostic assessments. Suppose a client presents symptoms of irritability, listlessness, low energy, failed performance at work, lack of sex drive, and loss of appetite; these symptoms may be diagnosed in a number of ways, ranging from anorexia nervosa to depression to an acute stress reaction. Errors are possible not only in the conclusions drawn about a case but also in the ways chosen for working with the client.

The issue in this discussion is not whether mistakes and misjudgments will occur (many of which will hurt clients), but what can be done about them. What is gained by apologizing to the victim? For example: "I'm awfully sorry. But, ah, remember when I said that it would be best to confront? Well, ah, I've thought about it and think that might not be the best alternative." What would be the likelihood of keeping a job if you rigorously reported every mistake to the supervisor? "Boss, I messed up again. This time, when I should have been supportive, I started confronting. I'm afraid the client won't be coming back." The important part of such ethical conflicts is, first, learning from mistakes to prevent repeating the same errors and, second, minimizing or reversing any negative effects on the client, possibly by seeking counsel from a peer or supervisor or perhaps by admitting to the client the problem and solutions.

It is easy to hide transgressions. No one else will ever know what goes on within the privacy of the office. Clients usually don't challenge a process so mysterious that almost anything can be viewed as potentially therapeutic from at least one theoretical point of view. It becomes all the more essential, then, to develop and internally monitor professional behavior from an ethical perspective. The individual counselor's awareness of and commitment to ethical principles will, in the final analysis, determine the ethical content of interviews.

In processing and working through misjudgments and failures in counseling, several things should be considered (Dillon, 2003; Kottler & Blau, 1989; Kottler & Hazler, 1997; Kottler & Carlson, 2003):

1. Failures are inevitable and unavoidable.
2. Counselors often avoid and deny their mistakes and misjudgments by calling clients resistant, pretending that they have everything under control, and blaming factors outside of their control.
3. Failures are often caused by variables related to the client (unrealistic expectations, toxic personality, poor motivation), counselor (rigidity, arrogance, poor skill execution), therapeutic process (transference, pace, inadequate alliance), and extraneous variables (lack of support, enmeshed family).
4. Mistakes and misjudgments can be worked through by considering the client's secondary gains from remaining stuck, the counselor's personal issues, what has been overlooked, which interventions have been most and least helpful, and what outside resources can be tapped.

5. Failures can provide wonderful opportunities for learning and growth, if processed constructively.

## Deception and Informed Consent

Would you ever deliberately lie to or deceive a client, even if it were for his or her own good?

Counselors stand for truth, honesty, sincerity, and genuineness. But influence is also an important counseling skill. Is it justifiable to manipulate a client into experimenting with a new behavior? Is it ethical to disguise a trap waiting for the unsuspecting client? Is it even appropriate to water down the truth with clients? Although students may respond with a resounding chorus of "NO," most experienced counselors will reluctantly admit that therapeutic deception may be necessary when it is intended for the benefit of the client.

When a client straightforwardly asks a direct question (for instance, a subnormal client asks, "Do you think I'm intelligent?"), we are confronted with the inevitable choice of whether or not to tell the truth. The client might not yet be ready for the truth or, alternatively, might respond poorly to protective lies. The counselor must make a choice representative of his or her ethical standards and live with the consequences of the choice. While you are making your own decisions as to your preferred response, consider the following case.

The client is a young woman, inhibited, rigid, fearful, and shy. She is petrified of anything remotely spontaneous, because the outcome is not 100 percent predictable. She is also terrified of anything that might require her verbal performance, for failure (which she very loosely defines) would certainly crush her already fragile ego.

The counselor quickly (and probably accurately) decides that the vicious cycle of self-defeating beliefs ("I can't do it because I'm_____") can be broken only by encouraging her, just once, to try acting differently from the way she has in the past. If she would pretend, even within the safety of the session, to be somewhat playful and spontaneous, she could not continue to use the excuse "I can't do it," because she would have revealed an exception to her self-defeating behavior.

Role playing would obviously be the technique of choice to encourage the client's creativity and spontaneity, but she is vehement in her refusal to try it. The counselor agrees to back off, and discussion continues in other directions until an opportunity arises. The client, in talking about her mother's endless complaining and cackling, starts to change her voice in imitation of her mother, thus initiating spontaneous role playing. The counselor need only change roles and start imitating the client, knowing that it will provoke her continued performance as her mother. After having previously promised not to pressure her into role playing, the counselor now has an easy chance to trick her into trying it, obviously for her own therapeutic growth. Is the counselor ethically justified in proceeding, when he has said he would not, because the outcomes are so potentially desirable?

In this case the counselor chose to stop the action, disclose aloud the temptation to be manipulative, and then deal with the reactions. The client felt so grateful for the maintenance of trust that she was then able to experiment slowly, not at the same dramatic level as would have been possible in the incident of spontaneous role playing, but well enough to make progress. For every example in which honesty produces the best results, there are also cases in which other, less direct actions might also be defensible.

The principle of informed consent is based on the notion that clients have a right to be protected against any form of coercion, manipulation, and harmful treatment. They have a right to be provided with clear, accurate, and comprehensible information on such things as fee policies, limitations and dangers of treatment approaches, access to records, counselor qualifications training, and the right to refuse treatment (Welfel, 1998).

## Confidentiality and Privileged Communication

Are you worried that you may inadvertently or deliberately violate your client's confidence?

Struggles with maintaining confidentiality are among the most common ethical dilemmas that counselors face. Not a week will go by when you won't be tested in some way—parents wanting to know what their child said to you, another professional calling you for information about a previous case, a current client you are seeing who has AIDS and is sexually active, another client who threatens suicide and may carry out that threat, or even a colleague or a spouse who casually asks you about a client you are seeing. Yet as challenging as these dilemmas seem to you, you can make things easier for yourself by thoughtfully preparing responses to the situations that trouble you the most.

In a situation such as the one presented at the beginning of this chapter, a counselor may quite deliberately decide to break a previous promise because the client is committing a crime. Ethical dilemmas do arise because of a conflict between what is best for the client and what is best for other people. In a landmark court case, now referred to as the Tarasoff decision, a counselor failed to warn a murder victim of potential danger from his client and was held responsible and ordered to pay damages to the victim's parents. Although the judgment was eventually overturned, the case has brought much attention to the limitations of confidentiality. Counselors in most states are now required to do several things if they have direct knowledge of possible harm to an identifiable victim. They must make reasonable efforts to warn the victim and they must notify appropriate authorities.

In addition to a counselor's ethical obligations to uphold a promise of confidentiality, they may have an ethical and legal responsibility to breach the vow (1) when the client is a danger to himself or herself or others, (2) when the client is engaged in some kinds of criminal actions, (3) when the counselor is so ordered by the court, (4) when it is in the best interests of a child who is a victim of abuse, and (5) when case consultation or supervision is needed. Unfortunately, the courts do not offer to counselors the same protection they do to others whose communications are privileged, such as lawyers, physicians, clergy, and spouses. That is one reason why at the beginning of every counseling relationship you are required to inform your clients about the limits of confidentiality. It is also one reason why we are often forced to make painful decisions about times when our previous vow to maintain secrecy with clients should be overruled by an even more pressing moral imperative to protect human life.

Inadvertent slips that reveal confidential information are quite another matter. There is no justifiable excuse. That is not to say that we are not constantly tempted to share information with friends, spouses, or colleagues. But we must endure the isolation of not being able to talk about our work in any revealing detail because clients deserve to have their information protected by professional, ethical behavior.

You should also understand that while confidentiality is an ethical issue to keep the content of communications private, privileged communication is a concept that refers to the legal arena. There are certain exceptions to privilege that you should also know about, meaning certain instances when the client waives or surrenders his or her right to privacy. This can occur in situations such as worker compensation cases, child custody evaluations, sanity hearings, and other legal proceedings. It may also be the case if you are sued for malpractice or if the client is a minor and you believe that his or her rights must be safeguarded.

## Recent Trends

Because ethical and value issues in counseling are reflective of contemporary culture, the standards for professional practice continue to evolve. Some of the most common violations of ethical behavior as well as those dilemmas that are likely to be most salient in the future. The following situations are ones that you should be especially vigilant to monitor closely.

**Duty to Warn**   You will be asked to assess the potential dangerousness of your clients, to determine whether they have the potential to harm themselves or others. This potential can include the threat of physical violence, or it could conceivably apply to the dilemma of working with a client who is HIV infected. If you believe there is imminent danger, you will be required to take action, which could involve warning potential victims, initiating commitment proceedings, or even calling the police. All of those choices, of course, violate your vow of confidentiality, so your assessments must be accurate.

General guidelines recommend the following (Cottone & Tarvydas, 2003; Isaacs, 1997): (1) Take a detailed history, assessing potential dangerousness of a client; (2) document very carefully any progress made in counseling; (3) consult with supervisors for additional input; (4) if necessary and indicated, obtain client's cooperation to warn the potential victim(s); (5) contact authorities if in your professional judgment the client poses a threat to self or others. In addition, it is useful to prepare ahead of time for such challenging cases that, hopefully, you will never have to deal with. This includes having appropriate referrals ready, having informed consent forms that specify the conditions under which confidentiality may be breached, keeping abreast of the laws and policies that govern your practice, and consulting with more experienced colleagues (Standard & Hazler, 1995).

**Reporting Child Abuse**    The law is clear: If you suspect that emotional or physical harm is being inflicted on a child, you must report it to the authorities within 24 hours. The ethical dilemma, however, is not *whether* to report suspected abuse but *when* to report it. In some instances it may be in the child's best interest not to report an incident until after safeguards can be instituted to protect the child from retaliation. More than half the cases of reported child abuse are false claims made by parents involved in custody disputes (Schafer, 1990b). Yet in spite of the possible negative consequences that may result from reporting suspected child abuse inaccurately, most states require you to take action if there is any reasonable evidence (often within 24 hours). It is not your job to assess whether the accusations are true or not, but merely to allow authorities the opportunity to investigate the case. By failing to report suspected abuse, not only do you put yourself at risk for violation of law, but you also may negligently allow children to be harmed.

**Technology Usage**    As more and more client information is stored on computers in schools and agencies, it is becoming increasingly difficult to restrict unauthorized access and guarantee the confidentiality of records. Although computers are making life much easier for counselors as a way to store records, access files, process paperwork, and look up needed information, they are also lacking in safeguards to protect client rights to privacy. A number of ethical and professional hazards have been raised, including compromised confidentiality and validity of information received. Internet communications are hardly secure and most any self-respecting hacker could gain access to the record system to retrieve desired information.

As more and more counselors are engaging in counseling services via the Internet and telephone, and videophone, additional ethical and legal concerns are raised (Masi & Freedman, 2001). In most cases, liability insurance may not cover such professional activity. Additionally, usually you must be licensed in the state in which the client is a resident. Finally, however much more convenient and accessible such services might be, you must be aware of the limits of such professional activity with limited visual cues and information that can only be accessed face-to-face.

**Relationships with Former Clients**    Although ethical codes are quite clear about the inappropriateness of becoming romantically involved with a client, or even conducting a friendship with a client at the same time he or she is in treatment (dual relationship), there is a recent trend to also restrict relationships with former clients. This issue is complicated by confusion as to when counseling actually ends: Is it after the last scheduled session? Or is it when

■ | VOICE FROM THE FIELD

Wait'll you face this one: A kid reports to you that she has been sexually molested before. Before you reach for the phone, though, to report it to CPS [Child Protective Services], you learn some more. It turns out the molestation was relatively mild—light fondling one time when the father was drunk. And then you find out that it happened four years ago and there has never been a reoccurrence. For the sake of argument, let's assume that you believe this is the case.

So now, if you do go ahead and report it, as you are mandated to do, and which you have to do or risk losing your job and license, there's going to be all hell breaking loose in this family, which is now functioning pretty well. You wonder why the kid is reporting it now. You wonder if it really happened. You wonder if it is still going on; maybe she is telling you it stopped but it really didn't.

It's supposed to be an easy call, but sometimes it isn't for me. The solution of calling in the CPS sometimes makes things so much worse, especially if it is a thing in the past. Hell, sometimes I don't know what to do.

---

the client stops thinking of you as a professional (which could take a lifetime)? It is also important to keep in mind that it is not acceptable to end a therapeutic relationship expressly for the purposes of beginning a personal one. This is especially the case because it is so difficult to determine when a therapeutic relationship is really over—not just with the termination of scheduled sessions, but also in the client's fantasies.

Many states specify a time limit for any romantic involvement (anywhere from one to three years), but other sorts of personal relationships, including friendships, are less clear. The situation is compounded by life in rural areas and small towns where it is much more difficult to compartmentalize relationships.

**Managed Care**   "When I first went into private practice it was my dream to have a full caseload. Now I have more clients than I can possibly see but I am making far less money than when I was working for a salary. I feel like an assembly line, turning out stamped products as fast as I can."

As this practitioner complains, insurance carriers, preferred provider organizations, employee assistance programs, and health maintenance organizations are changing the profession into a business. With slashed budgets, even community agencies are being forced to participate in these programs.

All of a sudden, what is best for clients is no longer the only concern; now counselors must consider the realities of what third parties mandate in terms of counseling plans and even length of treatment. Nowhere is this ethical dilemma more prominent than when it comes time to fill in a diagnosis on the appropriate forms.

Assume, for example, that a client presents symptoms that resemble what is known as a personality disorder. In the interests of accuracy, if you should enter a diagnosis of "borderline or narcissistic personality disorder," two things are likely to occur: (1) Your client will not likely have treatment approved because these intractable conditions are not supposed to be amenable to counseling, and (2) your client will be stigmatized for life with a label in the file that can be accessed by any number of sources in the future. This client is also feeling depressed about his condition, so perhaps you might legitimately call the problem "adjustment reaction with depressed mood." Sure it is a bit of a stretch—but aren't you doing this to protect the client's rights?

Ethical dilemmas such as this one are becoming increasingly a part of the ways counselors function. Managed care organizations are forcing them to amend the ways they are used to working. In some cases this is a good thing, because counselors are now required more and more to demonstrate their effectiveness and to operate more efficiently. Yet sacred therapeutic relationships are now intruded on by administrators and review boards, who are telling counselors what they may do and how long they may do it. If they don't follow their instructions, the organization may decide to cut off all support whatsoever.

**Confronting Counselor Impairment**   In spite of best intentions and training, almost all clinicians experience some type of impairment or dysfunction in their lives. These lapses of conduct occur because of drug addictions, life transitions, traumas, poor training, pathological personalities, burnout, or holes in one's conscience (Kottler & Hazler, 1996).

Even as a beginner you have an obligation not only to uphold ethical conduct but also to help other professionals who might be experiencing degrees of impairment. While initially, compassion and empathy should be employed to help an impaired counselor get needed help, at times you may be forced to take more proactive steps that include reporting the ethical breach to licensing boards and professional organizations or even protecting clients who might be in jeopardy.

**Resolving Ethical Conflicts**   Most ethical codes specify that if you become aware of a colleague who is engaging in unethical or unprofessional conduct (or someone perceives you in that way) you must take appropriate steps to intervene and protect the safety of others who may be harmed by this behavior. That guideline seems relatively clear but is, in fact, quite difficult to execute effectively.

Let's say you find out from a client that a former counselor did some things in session that were strange at best, and highly unprofessional at the very least. Do you report this behavior to the local Licensing Board and the practitioner's professional Ethics Board?

The first step is usually to informally resolve the suspected violation by contacting the colleague and communicating your concerns. But in order to do so, you would first need permission of your client to breach confidentiality (and often clients do not want to do that). Once you have attempted this informal resolution, then you may report the violation directly to the proper authorities. They will then investigate the case and make a determination if some sort of action need be taken.

# MAKING ETHICAL DECISIONS

You will be confronted on a regular basis with the necessity of making ethical decisions. When an ethical issue emerges, you will have to make a virtually instantaneous decision; little opportunity will exist for careful analysis and thoughtful reflection. Thus, the first recommendation in making ethical decisions is to anticipate. It is essential to develop a reasonably clear ethical style based on analysis and reflection to guide decision making and a capacity for making sound moral decisions that are compatible with the consensual standards created by the profession and consistent with your own professional identity, sense of personal virtue, and cultural factors (Cohen & Cohen, 1999; Cottone & Tarvydas, 2003; Remley & Herlihy, 2001).

One of the reasons that practitioners are often broadsided by difficult ethical dilemmas is because they fall into one of several traps (Steinman, Richardson, & McEnroe, 1998):

1. *The common sense trap.* This naive orientation is based on the idea that if you merely study the ethical codes you will be well prepared to handle anything that comes up. In truth, while the codes provide guidance, most difficulties arise because of personal interpretations of rules and laws that are not necessarily based on consensual standards.
2. *The values trap.* Some counselors confuse ethical standards with their own values and religious and moral convictions. Under the myth that they are being ethical, they attempt to impose their own strong beliefs on their clients, without respect or sensitivity to their unique cultural values.
3. *The circumstantiality trap.* "You have to understand the situation before you judge whether I was right or wrong." Ah, the old excuse that the reason you ran the red light is that you were . . . There is always some good excuse. Making sound ethical decisions is certainly based on contextual circumstances, but never to the point where a client's rights or safety are compromised.

Keeping these traps in mind, the ethical decision-making process involves a number of sequential steps that would be most helpful for you to study (Corey, Corey, & Callanan, 2003; Forester-Miller & Davis, 1995; Steinman, Richardson, & McEnroe, 1998; Van Hoose & Kottler, 1985; Welfel, 1998).

1. *Recognize that there is an ethical conflict.* In order to make a decision about something you must first be aware that a decision needs to made. Studying ethical issues helps sensitize you to those situations that qualify as a legitimate dilemma in need of some resolution.
2. *Description of problem.* After recognizing that an ethical decision needs to be made, it is useful to specify the parameters of the issue, to figure out what is at stake, what harm can result to whom, what consequences are

## ◼ | VOICE FROM THE FIELD

There's just so little time to think about things when a situation comes up. You're taken by surprise a lot, just not expecting to face some ethical issue. Or at least that's true with me. I've read the codes through and through. I've gone to mandatory refresher courses required to keep my license. I've read books and articles on the subject. Sure, I talk to people about it all the time. Really, I think that's what counselors talk about the most—beside complaining, I mean. But still, I get caught by surprise. You're just kind of in a comfortable position, listening, nodding your head, thinking hard about stuff, then before you know it, there it is: Your client just confessed something, or just told you something, and bells start going off in your head. Like you know you're supposed to do something, but for the life of me, I can't figure out what that should be. I think to myself, "Damn—why me again?"

I usually try to stall for time because I don't do well under pressure like that. I want to buy some time. Then as soon as the client leaves I talk to as many people as I can to find out what I should do or how I should handle the situation. Sometimes that even makes things worse, because everyone has a different answer. But eventually I'm able to sort things out and respond decisively the next time the client comes in.

---

anticipated. Gathering and organizing this information will give you some sense of time parameters involved before a decision must be made and action taken.

3. *Identify appropriate ethical standards involved.* Consult with the ethical codes for guidance. If there is clear and definitive instruction, act accordingly. If the ethical guidelines are ambiguous or unclear, consult with peers and supervisors. If the particular ethical standards fit the situation but the mandated actions seem "wrong," get further supervision and reflect on whether any ethical traps apply.

4. *Review professional literature.* Another source of information, if not wisdom, that you will wish to check out is the scholarship that has been undertaken related to your ethical conflict. It is highly likely that many others before you have struggled with similar issues and have chosen to research various alternatives and their consequences.

5. *Reflect on personal morals and values.* Is your ethical decision in the best interests of your clients, or is it to meet your own needs? Often breaches of ethical conduct and poor decisions are made when counselors fail to recognize the extent to which they are attempting to meet their own needs in the guise of helping others.

6. *Deliberate and decide.* Frame a preliminary course of action. Document the process you followed. Consult with peers and supervisors for feedback. Consider the consequences of your actions and alternative plans if things do not proceed as anticipated.

7. *Take action.* This is where you follow through on your informed, intentional decision that has been well researched and planned intentionally.

8. *Reflection.* Ethical dilemmas are opportunities for systematic growth and moral development. Review the situation as it developed. Consider other ways you could have responded. Identify what you learned from the situation and what you resolve to do differently in the future. If indicated, "publish" the results by informing others (verbally or in writing) what they might learn from your experience.

In addition to the introspective analysis that leads a person to select a defensible moral choice, the decision-making process should also take into account the guidelines established by professional organizations and the legal system. Most of these sources mandate the following actions:

1. *Don't attempt any therapeutic intervention without sufficient knowledge, skills, training, and supervision.* You should never attempt helping actions that are outside the bounds of your qualifications and competence. Workshops, certification programs, postgraduate training, internships, and intensive supervision are the means by which you can legitimately augment your therapeutic skills and continue to grow as a professional. Make referrals to specialists and other helping professionals when appropriate.

2. *You should be free of all biases and prejudices that might interfere with the capacity for objectivity, neutrality, and positive regard in the therapeutic relationship.* This includes sexual and racial biases, as well as those directed toward any ethnic or religious group, special population, or belief system.

3. *Sexual involvement with clients is strictly prohibited.* Under no circumstances should you as a counselor ever engage in erotic contact, act seductively, or respond to overtures made by those who have offered their trust in your professional integrity.

4. *The rights of all participants in research projects should be carefully protected.* All experimental procedures that could conceivably produce side effects must be thoroughly described and informed consent obtained from all subjects.

5. *You are responsible for protecting the privacy and confidentiality of all sessions.* Except in those circumstances wherein human life is endangered, you must preserve the sanctity of the therapeutic encounter. Information regarding a case may be released only with proper client authorization or under legal compulsion.

6. *The focus of counseling is on helping the client to reach self-determined goals.* Except in those instances in which goals appear to be destructive, self-defeating, or in violation of principles of reality, you are committed to working toward the client's greater autonomy and independence. You should therefore avoid manipulating clients, as well as creating dependencies or meeting your own needs in the session.

7. *You are committed to continuing professional training and growth after completing your formal education.* The knowledge and research in the field change so rapidly that practitioners must continually update their expertise. For this reason, many professional organizations and certification/licensing boards require annual continuing-education credits of members.

8. *You have an obligation to confront colleagues engaged in unethical, illegal, or incompetent practices.* As a professional, you have a responsibility to your profession, your community, and the safety of those who seek counseling services. Your duty is to challenge directly the behavior of those who are transcending the bounds of generally accepted principles. If the problem is not sufficiently resolved, you are then required to report such behavior to appropriate authorities.

9. *You are committed to maintaining high standards of integrity, honesty, and moral fiber.* Therapeutic counselors accept their responsibility as professional helpers, recognize their powerful influence, and work toward functioning as effective models for their clients.

10. *As a counselor, you act for the general welfare of clients and society.* You attempt to prevent discrimination, to help the needy and disadvantaged, to promote social justice, and to help all persons become more fully functioning.

As a counselor you must be sensitive to the cultural, ethnic, religious, gender, and philosophical differences among people of diverse backgrounds, all of whom operate by rules, values, and customs that may not be familiar to you. Recognize that, whenever you are dealing with moral issues (and counseling is most certainly a value-laden discipline), there are many different paths to "truth" and many different standards of what is "right."

# LEGAL ISSUES IN COUNSELING

As if it is not complicated enough that you must be familiar with and accountable to the ethical standards of the profession, as well as the standards of professional competence in your work setting, you must also be familiar with how your work intersects with the legal system. You will be expected to apply legal principles and make difficult decisions that may conflict with your own values, the ethical principles of your profession, or the policies of your institution in situations like the following:

- If a client's civil rights are violated, such as in cases involving sex, age, or racial discrimination
- If clients are involved in custody battles or divorce action
- If clients are seeking eligibility for disability or unemployment compensation
- If you believe a client is a danger to himself or herself or to others
- If you receive a court referral
- If you suspect that child abuse has taken place
- If a client you are seeing is engaged in planning or carrying out criminal acts
- If you serve as an expert witness in a case
- If you are subjected to malpractice litigation because of claims that you caused harm or injury to a client or acted negligently

As frightening as these examples might appear, there are several other situations in which counselors may find themselves embroiled in legal disputes: (1) There is a charge of sexual misconduct, (2) there is a breach of confiden-

## VOICE FROM THE FIELD

I'm so tired of being threatened by litigation that I now limit my practice to only those clients I can trust. I know this sounds strange—that we are the ones that are supposed to earn their trust—but I think it goes both ways. Twice already this year I have been threatened by legal action because two very disturbed ex-clients of mine do not want to pay their outstanding bills. They think if they sue me for some imaginary breach they will be able to weasel their way out of their debts.

I will own the part of the problem that I'm not so good at collecting fees for service, but I have to tell you: With both of these cases I worked my butt off for them. I devoted my heart and soul to doing whatever I could to help them. Frankly, I feel betrayed. It's like I need to keep my own attorney on retainer just to deal with all these nuisance suits.

---

tiality, (3) a client has committed suicide, (4) there is a violation of civil rights, (5) there are accusations of libel or slander, (6) there has been a failure to diagnose properly, (7) there is a breach of contract, (8) client abandonment is alleged, (9) the counselor has exerted undue influence, and (10) there has been an accident on the premises.

Practicing counselors are expected to familiarize themselves with three kinds of law that affect their work: *civil law* related to malpractice suits and disputes between parties, *criminal law* in which you may be expected to serve as an expert witness, and *mental health law* that governs the ways that various client groups must be treated (Swenson, 1997). In each of these cases, you will need to have a working mastery of the legal system and how it affects the particular work that you do. Sometime in your career, you are likely to be served a subpoena to show up in court, have your records called, function as a witness on behalf of or against an injured party, or perhaps even be sued yourself for some perceived injustice.

The intention here is not to alarm you to the point where you select a safer occupation, but rather to convince you of the importance that legal and ethical training will have in your work. By familiarizing yourself thoroughly with the legal statutes of your state and the ethical codes of your profession and by learning to apply them in real-life situations, you will protect your clients from harm and also protect yourself from needless vulnerability. In addition, you will guarantee your clients' rights in a number of circumstances:

1. *The right to informed consent.* The client is entitled to receive accurate and clear information regarding the therapeutic process, expected roles, risks and benefits of treatment, costs and contractual arrangements, right to access his or her files, implications of diagnostic labeling, alternative treatment options available, and qualifications and training of the counselor.
2. *The right to privacy.* This involves helping the client to understand the meaning of confidentiality and privileged communication, as well as the

circumstances under which they may be breached. It also means keeping records secure and protecting the content of counseling sessions.

3. *The right to protection against harm.* This means following the major dictum of all helping professions: Do no harm! But it involves more than not hurting a client through negligence; it also means protecting the client against himself or herself. There are certain circumstances—notably when clients are suicidal or otherwise self-destructive—that require intervention to avoid a disaster.

4. *The right to refuse treatment.* At one time, mentally ill inpatients were forced to undergo shock and chemical treatments against their will. A number of new laws were enacted to protect people from being subjected to "chemical straitjackets," especially with regard to being medicated and "medically managed" to the point where they lost their free will. Except in emergency situations, or when someone is in imminent danger of inflicting harm, laws now offer limited protection against forcible mental health treatments.

5. *The right to competent treatment.* The client is entitled to a counselor who is well trained in the profession and in any specialties that are practiced (for example, substance-abuse counseling, family therapy, hypnosis, and so on). In legal language this means that you will abide by the usual and customary standards of care that are agreed on by members of the profession. You can familiarize yourself with these "standards of care" by carefully reading the ethical codes and consulting a knowledgeable supervisor when you have questions.

It is the perceived violation of this last client's right that most often embroils counselors in the legal system, usually in the form of a malpractice suit. When a client's rights are compromised or, more specifically, when the counselor's actions may be deemed as negligent, malpractice may be claimed. Such a charge must meet several criteria: (1) A professional relationship existed between the client and counselor, (2) a demonstrable standard of care was breached, (3) the client suffered harm, and (4) the counselor's behavior was the probable cause of the client's injury (Bennett, Bryant, Vanden Bos, & Greenwood, 1990).

Let's apply these factors to a particular case. A client comes to you complaining of anxiety and poor self-esteem. He has trouble sleeping at night and feels agitated. You attempt to treat him with weekly counseling, but his condition worsens to the point where he requires hospitalization. During routine tests at admission, it is discovered that his symptoms are not psychologically based but were, in fact, caused by an underlying neurological disease. Does this situation constitute negligence on your part and justify a malpractice suit against you?

1. No. You were not the cause of his injury—the neurological disease was.

2. No. Because you are not a physician, you are not qualified or expected to diagnose neurological problems.

3. Yes. You violated the standard of customary care. Through your negligence in not referring the client for a medical consultation, he suffered un-

due pain and hardship.

This last choice is the correct answer. It illustrates the kinds of professional challenges you will face and the fact that you must safeguard your client's welfare by getting adequate consultation and supervision when you even suspect the possibility of problems outside your specialty.

As frightening as these situations may be for you to consider (and as tragic as they may be for some clients), the risks can be significantly decreased by following several guidelines:

1. Study the ethical codes, state laws, and standards of care for your profession very carefully. Review some of the "casebooks" that are available (Herlihy & Corey, 1996; Huber, 1994) to help you to reason through professional decision making.
2. Make sure that you carry liability insurance to protect yourself from malpractice claims (as a student you are eligible for coverage at very reasonable rates).
3. As a beginner in the field, do not attempt any treatments without adequate supervision by qualified experts.
4. Document carefully your case records. Be especially prudent in checking out suicidal/homicidal ideation, history, and intent.
5. Consult frequently with medical personnel and make appropriate referrals when there is a possibility of some underlying organic problem.
6. Take steps to improve your level of competence by pursuing continuing education and advanced training.
7. Alert yourself to signs of fatigue and burnout that may lead you to miss important information or make needless mistakes.
8. Avoid those high-risk situations that are most likely to result in litigation: Failure to treat a needy client, sexual involvement with a client, breach of confidentiality, failure to warn someone of potential harm, negligence leading to suicide, inadequate record keeping, collecting unpaid fees, and failure to diagnose or treat properly.
9. If you believe you might be engaging in some ethical or legal violation, get some help for yourself. Often remedial therapy alone is not enough and other forms of rehabilitation may be required to counteract the chronic boundary violation, especially in the case of sexual contact.
10. Make yourself more knowledgeable about the differences and commonalities between ethical codes, the legal system, and the realities of everyday practice.

Keep in mind that this is an introductory course so it is only appropriate to cover general principles of ethical and legal conduct. As you gain more experience, and work in more specialized areas, you will be expected to apply sound ethical decision making to particular kinds of situations and cases. There are, for instance, more detailed guidelines for practitioners working with minors in the mental health system (Isaacs & Stone, 2001), older adults (Schwiebert, Myers, & Dice, 2000), gay and lesbian clients (Davison, 2001), family counseling modalities (Gladding, Remley, & Huber, 2001), Internet-based treatments

(Houston, 2002; Hsiung, 2001), addictions (Cottone & Tarvydas, 2003), and managed care settings (Cooper & Gottlieb, 2000; Daniels, 2001). In each case, and in every setting, you will required to assess the potential ethical and legal risks that could occur as a result of your actions—or inaction (Falvey, 2002). If you are ever called on to appear in court, seek legal counsel as well as sources that prepare you for depositions and appearances as a witness (see Barsky & Gould, 2002).

Remember, as a beginner to this field you are not expected to know everything and be able to do everything perfectly. Making mistakes is part of your growth and crucial to your learning. You are, however, responsible for making certain that you find the best possible training and supervision so that you can become the most proficient and responsible professional possible.

## SUMMARY

The first step in making ethically sound decisions is to anticipate some possible dilemmas and to think through alternatives and preferred responses in an objective and analytical manner. These personal resolutions must be congruent with professional standards, state and federal laws, and institutional policies in order to be useful.

A systematic approach will yield ethical decisions that are personally meaningful, have a specific rationale for behavior, and are objectively defensible. It will also enable the counselor to respond to challenges, legal or personal, with a sense of integrity and a clear rationale for any behavior. The counselor should maintain an open, questioning attitude toward ethical decision making, recognizing the need to challenge and question decisions, values, and attitudes.

Ethical decision making is not a state counselors achieve but an ongoing process of learning, growth, and maturation. Ethical decision making means that counselors take responsibility for functioning at the highest possible level of moral behavior, both to serve clients better and to avoid legal entanglements. Periodic reflection and a full examination of ethically challenging situations are essential factors in this process. It is often helpful to consult with colleagues and supervisors. Yet in this profession, confusion has its healthy side; it helps counselors avoid rigidity and forces them to personalize the meaning of their behavior.

## SELF-GUIDED EXPLORATIONS

1. List some of your strongest beliefs and values regarding how you and other people should live their lives. Include those related to religion, premarital and extramarital sex, abortion, children's discipline, drug use, war, divorce, and any others that come to mind. Then describe the values of a person who feels the opposite that you do. Now, imagine that your opposite walks in the door to see you as a client. How will you work with him or her?

2. List three of the most important moral rules that guide your life. Meet with several others to share your individual principles. Come to a consensus as to which three moral rules you can all agree with. Describe your personal reactions to this dialogue and negotiation.

3. Think of a time in your life when you faced a major ethical dilemma. Trace the internal process you went through to reach a decision. What helped you along the way to reach a satisfactory resolution?

4. Which is the ethical conflict that you fear the most? Describe a real-life example in which you are confronted by this very issue. Talk through how you would come to some decision as to what you should do.

## For Homework:

Carefully read through the *Ethical Codes* of the profession. Jot down a few notes of areas that you think are particularly confusing or about which you have questions. Check with a few experienced counselors to sort out your areas of concern.

## SUGGESTED READINGS

Barsky, A. E., & Gould, J. W. (2002). *Clinicians in court: A guide to subpoenas, depositions, testifying, and everything else you need to know*. New York: Guilford.

Cohen, E. D., & Cohen, G. S. (1999). *The virtuous therapist: Ethical practice of counseling and psychotherapy*. Pacific Grove, CA: Brooks/Cole.

Corey, G., Corey, M. S., & Callanan, P. (2003). *Issues and ethics in the helping professions* (6th ed.). Pacific Grove, CA: Brooks/Cole.

Cottone, R., & Tarvydas, V. M. (2003). *Ethical and professional issues in counseling* (2nd ed.). Columbus, OH: Merrill.

Dillon, C. (2003). *Learning from mistakes in clinical practice*. Pacific Grove, CA: Brooks/Cole.

Falvey, J. E. (2002). *Managing clinical supervision: Ethical practice and legal risk management*. Pacific Grove, CA: Brooks/Cole.

Gladding, S. T., Remley, T. P., & Huber, C. H. (2001). *Ethical, legal, and professional issues in the practice of marriage and family therapy*. Upper Saddle River, NJ: Prentice-Hall.

Jones, C., Shillito-Clark, C., & Syme, G. (2001). *A question of ethics in counseling and therapy*. Buckingham, GB: Open University Press.

Kottler, J. A., & Carlson, J. (2003). *Bad therapy: Master therapists share their worst failures*. New York: Brunner/Routledge.

Remley, T. P., & Herlihy, B. (2001). *Ethical, legal, and professional issues in counseling*. Upper Saddle River, NJ: Prentice-Hall.

Welfel, E. R. (2002). *Ethics in counseling and psychotherapy: Standards, research, and emerging issues* (2nd ed.). Pacific Grove, CA: Brooks/Cole.

# 15 TOWARD CLOSURE: ADVICE FOR THE PASSIONATELY COMMITTED COUNSELING STUDENT

# TOWARD CLOSURE: ADVICE FOR THE PASSIONATELY COMMITTED COUNSELING STUDENT

CHAPTER 15

This chapter is for those dedicated individuals who, after completing their introductory course in counseling, have decided to devote their lives to helping other people. Your commitment to the counseling profession is not to be taken lightly, nor can you realistically expect to treat your career as a mere job in which you just put in your time. Counselors are passionately committed to helping their clients to become more productive, fully functioning beings. The counseling student, too, must be intensely motivated to pursue a path of lifelong learning. It is only through your own hunger to understand, your thirst to know, your craving to find truth, and your skill in communicating your ideas that you become able to influence people in constructive ways.

In the spirit of enthusiasm for the mission of counselors, I offer the following advice to students.

## Be Self-Directed

The best way to become passionate about learning is to follow your own natural curiosity to make sense of the world. So much of counseling deals with abstractions and complex queries that defy understanding. Your teachers, supervisors, and authors you read will only begin to tantalize you with answers to the questions that plague you the most. How does counseling work? Why does counseling work? Your assigned readings, lectures, and class discussions are but stimuli for you to begin resolving many of these difficult issues. It is through personal reflection, self-directed study, and leisurely wandering through the library and Internet that you can really begin to educate yourself.

## Read

I would encourage you, in your self-directed study, to research systematically the works that have had the most impact in the counseling profession. Make a list of classic books in the field—and read them. Solicit nominations from teachers and peers. Notice in the literature those titles that are most frequently cited. Most of all, find a few reliable persons whose opinions you respect (such as a mentor) and read everything they recommend. Don't restrict yourself to just the books in counseling, but become familiar with the literature in related fields such as psychology, social work, psychiatry, education, nursing, sociology, and philosophy.

There are some who believe (and I am among them) that reading fiction can offer as much insight into the inner workings of the human condition as any professional book. Indeed, Michael Dorris' novel *The Yellow Raft in Blue Water* offers as much deep exploration into the experience of being marginalized in an oppressed minority as any book on the subject. Likewise, the novels of Jonathan Kellerman teach us about the intricacies of child assessment, just as those by Pat Conroy bring dysfunctional families to life. By all means, ask for recommendations about instructive novels, as well as professional books.

## Find a Mentor

In all chosen professions—the arts, sciences, law, medicine, business—and especially in a people-oriented career such as counseling, it is important to have a model to emulate. A mentor, usually a teacher, senior colleague, or other benevolent friend/coach, helps the neophyte to learn the ropes during the period of apprenticeship. A mentor does more, much more, than give homespun advice or recommend books; she or he becomes an advocate. It is through this relationship that the beginning counselor receives support, encouragement, constructive feedback, and a guiding hand.

Select a mentor whom you admire, who has skills and knowledge you respect and wish to acquire for yourself, and who has a genuine, nonpossessive interest in you. Find someone you can trust and confide in, yet one who does not feel that such a commitment is a burden. A mentor can be a source not only of nurturance and wisdom during the formative years of professional development but also of invaluable assistance in securing a job.

## Volunteer to Do Research

Getting actively involved in a research project is helpful in a number of obvious ways. It allows you to apply learning to the solution of real-life problems and personalizes the usefulness of the scientific method. Upon publication, a writing credit can be a marketable commodity for gaining entrance to a doctoral program or a competitive job. Doing research also permits interaction with professors and colleagues on a level that would not be possible in the classroom. Finally, research gives you practical experience in exploring the issues, problems, and methodology of the profession. It is an opportunity to advance the growth of counseling and your own knowledge.

## Ask Questions

When you don't know the answer to a question, *ask!*

Many of the questions students ask in class are posed less to learn new ideas than to win brownie points, demonstrate what they already know, or express opinions in diplomatic ways; for example, "Aren't you saying that students are afraid to take risks by displaying their ignorance?"

Unfortunately, yes—that's what I'm saying. In my experience, it is rare that a student really feels comfortable enough to ask the questions that she or he would most like to have answered. As I flash back to my school days, I recall that there were scores of things I didn't understand, but I felt too timid to admit my uncertainty—as if by questioning the professors, I might reveal to others that I was not so bright and didn't really belong in class. It was only much later, when I was playing "I'll show you mine (ignorance) if you show me yours" that I discovered the universal passivity.

I therefore encourage you to take risks in class and ask about those things you don't understand. How, after all, can you expect your future clients to open up if you feel such reluctance? Right at this moment, make a list of the questions you never got around to asking. Good news! There are still many opportunities left in future classes.

## Challenge Your Teachers

Challenging those ideas presented in class with which you disagree is even riskier than questioning—but potentially more fun too. This style of learning is critical to the development of your own ideas, especially with those teachers who don't react defensively.

There are many concepts central to the core of therapeutic counseling that some beginning students accept with great difficulty. For example, the notion of avoiding absolutes, shoulds, and other moralistic "rights" and "wrongs" cannot be internalized except through active dialogue with others who have reflected on the implications and tested the principles. It is through interesting debates and challenging new ideas that these principles can be understood and personalized.

## Challenge Yourself

The most difficult task of a student is to maintain an openness to new ideas while simultaneously retaining a critical perspective. When ideas, concepts, and theories are presented that at first seem threatening, rather than immediately leaping to defend yourself against other classmates or professors, first challenge

## VOICE FROM THE FIELD

I pick my supervisor's brain constantly. I talk to other professionals all the time—on the phone, at lunch, on e-mail, at conferences. I subscribe to every publication I can afford. I continuously consult Web sites and list servers I can check for information. I read. I survey and watch other people all the time. I question people: "So tell me, you seem to be a happy person. How do you manage that?"

Based on all this study, I try new things in my work. Right now I'm working on a new drawing technique and a different approach to use with this one adolescent who is giving me a hard time. I'm always searching for new metaphors and stories to use.

---

yourself to explore the merits of the point of view. Ask yourself why you are responding so emotionally to the subject. What would it mean for you if you had to change your ideas to conform to this added information?

A related danger is that of too enthusiastically embracing a particular point of view, sowing the seeds of terminal rigidity and closing out the possibility of other ideas. Initially it is helpful to be suspicious and tentative. After exploring a theory that seems attractive and useful, do not fall into the destructive trap of confusing it with ultimate truth.

## Experience Counseling as a Client

In the process of challenging yourself, there is no vehicle more appropriate than experiencing counseling as a client. Many programs encourage participation in a form of counseling prior to graduation. For anyone who hopes to do counseling, it is important to know intimately the fears, joys, and apprehensions that clients experience.

Participating in counseling as a client allows you to work through inhibitions, distracting conflicts, and unresolved problems that may interfere with the ability to remain objective, focused, and therapeutic. It also helps you to believe fervently in the power of the process when you have experienced firsthand its beneficial effects.

I urge you to seek out both individual and group counseling experiences for another reason. Clearly, while a counseling student is engaged in a therapeutic relationship, there is always a part of him or her that is closely observing the process, noting the interventions that work best, and knowing—really knowing—how the process works. If we truly believe that counseling is for everyone, then it is most certainly for us—all of us.

## Personalize Everything

Counseling is a joy to study because all the abstract ideas, theoretical constructs, research hypotheses, clinical interpretations, class lectures, and textbook discourses can be personalized and applied to your own life. All of a sudden the behavior of those around you no longer appear the same. As counselors, we seem more critical yet more forgiving.

The novels we read, movies we see, and conversations we participate in become wonderful opportunities to think, act, and feel differently. Learning has more meaning to us if we can make it more relevant. And that, primarily, is the student's job—to take the nucleus of an idea from one's teacher, mentor, counselor, or colleague and apply it in such a way that it becomes personally useful.

## Expand Your World

The people who most likely need help the most are not like you. They come from different backgrounds, subscribe to different values, and may even have a different color of skin. They come from a variety of different religions and spiritual belief systems. Many of them have led impoverished or disadvantaged lives or suffered abuse and neglect that is unimaginable. All of them bring a unique cultural context to their worlds and their problems, shaped by their ethnicity, gender, identity, and life experiences.

A course or two in multicultural counseling or diverse populations can't put a dent in all the things you need to know in order to be helpful to clients who need you the most. All the reading in the world can't substitute either for what you can learn in the real world. While clients will help to educate you about their cultures and values, you can't depend on them to do your work for you; there is so much to learn and so little time.

One of the best ways to expand your world is through travel, not just to foreign lands but also to any novel environment that exposes you to diverse peoples, new customs and language, different values and beliefs. Push yourself, whenever possible, to explore as much of the planet as you can. More importantly, don't travel like a tourist who is only interested in souvenirs, taking photographs, and seeing sanctioned sites. Interact with people and find out about their worlds. Take risks to venture into unknown territory. Monitor the judgments you have internally about the ways people act differently. Notice how critical you are of different customs you don't fully understand. Then take this learning home with you. Apply it to your work in such a way that you become more sensitive and responsive to those who are most unlike you.

## Become Active in Professional Organizations

The American Counseling Association, the American Association for Marriage and Family Therapy, and the American Psychological Association are a few of the groups that advance the profession of therapeutic counseling. Through their lobbying activities, public relations and consumer education programs, and professional development courses, these organizations help support practitioners. They also develop written ethical codes, work toward certification and training standards, provide referral services, sponsor national and regional conventions, fund research projects, publish professional journals, run job search programs, and provide social activities for their members.

## VOICE FROM THE FIELD

It's a funny thing, travel. The best things you find are those you're not really looking for. I used to think in going to conferences that the important stuff was in the programs. I was so compulsive about following a schedule, collecting handouts, hitting as many different presentations as I could. I had this misguided belief that if only I could soak up all this knowledge that I could serve my clients best when I got home.

Then I discovered one day when I skipped going to the conference that a whole new world opened up to me by trying to learn about the place that I was at from the people. I rode a subway in a big city for the first time. I talked to everyone I could. And I learned so much that I could never have found out any other way.

There are many opportunities for students to get actively involved in the organizations by attending conventions, contributing articles to journals, serving on committees, presenting papers and workshops, and working on special projects of interest. Participating in state, regional, and national conventions is especially interesting because of the opportunities to make lifelong friendships with colleagues around the world. Conventions are also ideal places to receive specialized training and find jobs, because many employers are present to interview for positions.

Organizational activities help you to identify with the counseling profession as a whole, as well as a number of specialty areas. The American Counseling Association or the American Psychological Association offer members a number of divisions they can join, each with its own journal and networking opportunities. Within ACA, for example, students can join, for reduced rates, specialty groups that focus on dozens of different areas, including adult development and aging, college counseling, multicultural counseling, mental health counseling, rehabilitation counseling, school counseling, and many others. You can join as many of these divisions as you have the time and inclination for, each one offering a unique perspective of the field.

## Develop a Flexible Specialty

As I have already said, a degree in counseling does not guarantee employment in a specific career. Graduates may have to market themselves in such a way that they will fit a particular position or even tailor a job to fit their own unique skills, training, and interests.

Practically everyone knows what the psychologist, psychiatrist, or social worker can and cannot do. Counseling practitioners, however, now function in many diverse settings. Five students in the same program, with the same course work, may eventually find employment in five different settings: school counseling, industrial relations, consumer education, rehabilitation counseling, and mental health counseling. The counseling degree, then, reflects education for the generalist who, through specialized training and interests, develops a unique professional identity.

I therefore suggest to the beginning student the following course of action to find eventual employment in a desired area:

1. Talk to counselors in the field about what they do and how they feel about their jobs.
2. Find excuses to talk to prospective employers to determine what they are looking for in candidates.
3. Discover a few particular types of client populations (disabled, gifted), age groups (preschoolers, older adults), settings (hospitals, schools), and counseling skills (consultation, group interventions) in which you can gain specialized experience.
4. Use elective courses, workshop experiences, and your internship sites to become expert in a few flexible specialties.
5. Volunteer your time at local community agencies to accumulate additional professional experiences.

## Resist Burnout

In recent years there has developed a considerable body of literature describing the burnout phenomenon, especially as it relates to counselors, psychologists, social workers, teachers, and other human services personnel (see Kottler, 1993; Skovholt, 2001). Symptoms of this insidious condition include fatigue, irritation, reduced work performance, apathy, boredom, and negative attitudes. In its earliest forms you will notice more subtle signs of feeling dispirited and disillusioned.

The condition is caused, in part, by such factors as an excessive workload, monotony, a lack of control, and isolation in your work. Belson (1992) facetiously recommends several tried-and-true methods to achieve burnout, if that is your goal:

1. Work long hours, especially weekends and evenings. Tell yourself this doesn't really interfere with the quality of your relationships with family and friends.
2. Think about your hardest cases even when you are not working. Worry about what you aren't doing that you should be doing.
3. Blame your clients, their families, your colleagues, your boss, or the system for the reasons why things are not going as smoothly as you would prefer.
4. Believe that you can help everyone you see, and cure them within a very short time.

The only antidotes for burnout are renewed enthusiasm or a job change. Those counselors who are most committed to their jobs and to the profession may be less likely to experience the effects of burnout and disillusionment. They also tend to be practitioners who, despite having high standards of

## VOICE FROM THE FIELD

When I go home, I go home. I have come to value the ambiguity of the work that I do. But I have to have an anchored place to retreat from it. For me, that anchor is my home, my husband, and my son. After a tough day, I answer no calls at home. I cancel any evening appointments.

Although I have learned to tolerate—even appreciate—the ambiguous, stressful nature of my work, I can't let it permeate all my life. I must be able to say, "This far, no farther!" I've just got to have my haven, my safe boundary line.

---

excellence for their work, are accepting of their limitations. They are able to let go of those aspects of their jobs that they can't control and focus instead on what is within their power to change.

The time to prevent burnout is now, not when you are already experiencing negative symptoms. Begin structuring your professional life so that you are surrounded by a good support system. Most importantly: Practice what you preach and take care of yourself!

## Confront Your Fears of Failure

I recall sitting in my first counseling class, looking around the room, and feeling utterly despondent because everyone else seemed so much brighter and more talented than I was. Doubts assailed me: "Am I smart enough to get through this program?" "Do I have what it takes to be a counselor?" "What will my professors think when they find out how weird I really am?"

These doubts, and many others like them, are not only a normal part of most students' inner thoughts, but also continue to plague practitioners in the field. Counselors often worry about failure. What if they inadvertently harm a client? What if they are confronted with a situation in which they don't know what to do? What if they are caught making a mistake? Yet these doubts become unmanageable only when they are avoided and denied; it is by confronting your fears that you are able to work through them.

I therefore urge you to find a support group of peers in which you can confide your doubts and fears, disclose your fantasies of being an imposter, and talk about your imperfections and misunderstandings. I can confidently reassure you that, although it is difficult to recruit confidants who are compatible in any walk of life, you are definitely not alone in your apprehensions. Even after several decades of practicing and teaching counseling, I still continue to confront my own fears of failure.

The implications for the beginning counselor are clear. You must work diligently to develop a sense of professional commitment to clients, colleagues, the profession, and ultimately yourselves as professional counselors. This sense of commitment will result in renewal and provide the energy base necessary to perform creatively and enthusiastically. The time to begin developing that sense of commitment is now.

## Get the Most from Supervision

Just as it takes some practice and skill to be a "good" client in counseling, that is, to get the most from the experience, so too does it take a certain resolve, trust, perseverance, and commitment to get the most from your supervision experience. Much will depend, of course, on whether you trust and respect your supervisor, whether you think and feel that he or she is competent and has your best interests at heart. But even when you are forced to work with supervisors you would never have chosen, you can still gain much from their experience. Under the best circumstances, you may be fortunate to work with someone who is not only highly skilled, sensitive, and caring, but who is also well trained in the special nuances of conducting supervisory relationships.

In order to get the most from supervision, you will need to work hard on the relationship. This means doing solid preparation. It means reflecting on your cases and professional struggles, defining where you are having the most difficulty, and articulating your concerns and needs. More than anything, supervisors appreciate working with students who talk about what is working and what is not working. I don't just mean with your own cases but also in your supervision relationship. Your supervisor cannot better meet your needs or address your major concerns if you don't take responsibility for communicating what is most and least helpful.

## Seize the Day

Try to be a model of the person you would like your clients to be. If you think that people are happiest, most satisfied, and most productive when they are loving and caring—when they live in the present as much as possible—then strive to do the same in your own life. Be who you want your clients to be by the way you live your life—with honesty and integrity, with compassion, with hunger to experience as much as you can in the brief time you will be residing on this planet.

My coauthor on previous editions of this textbook, Bob Brown, died several years ago. I interviewed him just a few weeks before he died of cancer, and this is the advice he offered to new counselors in the field:

> What do I have to say to counselors in the field who are trying to find their way, to create meaning in their own lives? Don't take yourself seriously, but take yourself measurably. Don't take yourself in a manner that is cavalier, but take yourself in a manner that has sincerity and thoughtfulness about it.

What Bob was struggling to grasp in his last days was what meaning his career had. He had spent decades as a science teacher, a school counselor, a psychologist, and a counselor-educator. He had devoted his life to helping others, yet felt regretful about the time he wasted not allowing himself to give and receive love to those who mattered the most to him.

"Dying is not that big a deal," Bob said. "I know how to die. Now I want to die with a sense of enjoyment and laughter and happiness and contentment. I want to be filled with the excitement of every precious moment I have left."

We are all dying—right this moment. The question remains, what do *you* want to do with the time you have left? That is the question you will help your clients struggle with. You will be a lot better prepared to do so if you have the answers for yourself.

# WHAT MOST STUDENTS DON'T LEARN UNTIL IT IS WAY TOO LATE

There are some secrets to this profession that are not ordinarily discussed in your training. Perhaps the reasoning is that there is no sense depressing, discouraging, or otherwise overwhelming you with realities of practice before you've had a chance to really get your feet wet—and get hooked to the point you can't let go if you wanted to.

My feeling on the matter is that you are better off knowing what you are likely to face so you can take steps to prepare yourself for certain challenges. If you prefer surprise endings, then read no further.

Stop reading now if you are faint of heart.

No? I didn't think so. Courage, after all, is an important attribute for counselors.

In all honesty (and I intend to be very honest with you), I believe the following material will actually make you more intrigued with this work, more committed to doing what you can to flourish in spite of some difficult issues that lay ahead.

A friend and I (Kottler & Hazler, 1997) decided to catalogue some of the things that we never learned in our training, plus a few more that most programs don't cover in great detail. I've added to the list over the years, including other secrets that are rarely spoken aloud.

As a very dramatic example, one concept you have already been exposed to is the idea of "informed consent." This means that you provide people with the accurate information they need, including risks and contraindications, so that they can make good decisions about whether to undergo a particular procedure or therapeutic experience. For instance, if you were going to take a medication prescribed by your doctor she would first tell you about possible side effects that might occur. Then you decide whether you want to go ahead with the treatment.

In therapy and counseling, we follow this standard procedure as well, letting our clients know what they might face so that they can decide if they wish to follow our lead in that area. I was thinking that if we were truly to practice informed consent with respect to your training as a counselor or therapist, there are a lot of things we would tell you that might very well scare you away. For instance, are you aware that there is a decent possibility that as a result of training to be a therapist you may leave your spouse or partner behind? Just consider the consequences to a relationship when one person—you—makes a major commitment to work on yourself in a significant way. You read, study, attend classes, complete assignments, all of which are designed to change not only your professional demeanor but your whole being. If your loved one continues with the usual things and does not make a parallel commitment to personal growth, what effect do you think that might have on the relationship? If you guess a fairly negative one, you'd be correct. Not only is there a risk that your loved one might get left behind, but he or she may become quite threatened by your new friends, new growth, and "strange" transformations. And if you think you can get through your training without changing who you are, then you haven't been paying very close attention.

Must relationships always be left in the dust? Of course not. In fact, your education actually prepares you to make your most important relationships even more satisfying. But I'd be negligent if I didn't warn you about the risks involved.

Likewise, another probable consequence of your educational experience is that all your relationships will change—with your friends, your family members, your neighbors, and co-workers. You may find yourself bored with superficial conversations. You may feel a greater need for deeper intimacy in relationships. In some ways, you will become spoiled. After practicing your new skills, learning to get inside people's heads and hearts, working hard on developing closeness with others, you will also want to apply all this to the relationships that matter most.

Just watch a bunch of therapists hanging out together and you can immediately see that we are a strange breed. It is not that we don't enjoy talking about sports and weather and politics, it is just that because we spend our lives dealing with very deep issues, talking about the most private and intimate topics imaginable, it raises the bar considerably as far as what we like to talk about when we are off duty. Others who have not been exposed to this stuff may very well flee in terror. As you've already discovered, people are a little afraid and in awe of therapists. They think we can read minds, and in a sense we can, and do. Based on our training and experience, we can predict what people will do before they are even aware that they are headed in that direction. We are highly skilled at influencing people; we can get them to do things they don't particularly want to do. What all this adds up to is that we are treated like gods, we act like gods, and sometimes even believe we have superpowers not granted to mortal beings.

Listed below are several other secrets that are not often revealed to beginners:

- *There are very personal reasons why you entered this profession.* As I mentioned in the beginning of this book, newcomers to this field not only want to heal others but also heal themselves. Some of us have been victims of abuse, neglect, traumas, or just plain old self-doubt. We are voyeurs. We yearn for power or control. We enjoy the one-way intimacy that is part of therapeutic relationships. There is a dark side to our own narcissism.

- *Life isn't a multiple-choice exam.* The problem you will face is not a scarcity of options but far too many from which to choose. This class, or others, may offer multiple-choice exams in which you are presented with four choices, one of which is obviously the wrong one, but counseling practice overwhelms you with so many options that it often feels whichever action you take there were a hundred others you could have chosen that might have been better.

- *The answers you need most are not found in books.* You don't really learn counseling by reading about it, or listening to people talking about it. You've got to experience it yourself, from both ends. You have to immerse yourself more fully in life, explore other cultures, take constructive risks, engage more completely in relationships.

- *What we do is often absurd.* A lot about therapy doesn't make sense. We don't fully understand how and why it works. We don't agree on the best way to approach this craft. And even when we do help people, we can't always explain why it happened, or why the effects did or didn't last.

- *Your family still won't listen to you.* One of the reasons I studied to be a counselor, and then attained more advanced degrees, is because I wanted the respect and approval of my family, especially my father. Even with a masters degree, then a Ph.D., then being a professor, then an author, my family still doesn't take me any more seriously than they did before.

- *People don't want what you are selling.* Even the clients who seem cooperative and motivated may have hidden agendas. The honest ones tell you directly they don't trust you. The really difficult clients will pretend they want counseling, and even report that they are improving, but secretly they just want to keep you from getting close.

- *You will never know enough.* You will never get it right. No matter how hard you study, how compulsively you strive for perfection, how many books you read, how many degrees you attain, or workshops you attend, you will still not know as much as you need to do the job. That is one of the burdens of this profession but also one of the most exciting aspects— you could study counseling your whole life, or a dozen lifetimes, and you will still never master the discipline.

- *Failure is more important than success.* It is interesting how when things go well, we put the incident out of our minds; it is when we fail that we are forever haunted by our mistakes. There is no shame in failing with your clients; this is inevitable. The most important thing, however, is to learn from these experiences so you can process them constructively and not make the same mistakes again.

- *Who you are is as important as what you do.* As much as you want to learn all the content and skills and fancy techniques of counseling, to fill up your bag of tricks, your essential kindness and caring and commitment are as important as what you can do. I don't mean to say that being knowledgeable and highly skilled are not important, because they are, but rather that they are not enough. You must also work hard to make yourself into the best kind of person you can be—someone who is compassionate and dedicated to making the world a better place.

- *Many changes don't last.* As hard as it seems to help people to change, that is only the first step. Look at how many times in your own life that you have started to make changes you said were important—losing weight, starting an exercise program, calling your mother regularly, saving your money, studying two hours per day. You really meant it when you promised yourself to do those things. You may have even made solid efforts to get things going. But how long did the changes last? Never forget that your job does not only involve helping people to get started on their personal transformations but to make those changes permanent.

- *You will be haunted by those you helped, and those you didn't.* The relationships you develop with clients will become so intimate, so moving, so challenging at times, that their memories will stay in your head as long as you live. For better or worse, you will be irrevocably changed as a result of these encounters. You will smile and feel all warm inside thinking about some of the people you really helped, and who were so grateful for your efforts. Then there will be others who will leave your services dissatisfied, angry, and determined to make your life miserable. What distinguishes those who do well in our field are those who accept their mistakes, learn from them, and then move on, readily able to forgive themselves for being less than perfect.

- *You won't have enough time to do what you want, or what needs to be done.* You have to pace yourself. You have to set limits. You can't possibly do everything that needs to be done, especially in the time constraints that you must live with. In many jobs, you will be understaffed and overworked. If you hope to stay in this profession long and enjoy the work you do, you must find ways to set limits, to accept your limitations, and do what you can.

- *Supervision isn't always available when you need it most.* A lot of the time you're on your own. Even with the best possible supervision available, you will still find yourself having to figure out many things on your own. Almost every session will present you with questions that you can't answer. Every day you will feel flooded by challenges and internal conflicts. Even if you had the opportunity to talk to a supervisor about all of them, you will still have unanswered questions. Somehow, some way, you are going to have to learn to live with the complexity and ambiguity of what you do.

- *Counselors are not just trained, or educated; they are grown.* You must remain committed to your own growth and development. This does not mean simply taking more classes or going to continuing education workshops. It means seeking help for yourself when you need it. Most of all, it means practicing in your own life what you ask of your clients.

# VARIATIONS ON A THEME

Naturally, I wish to leave you with the appropriate balance of healthy confusion and eager enthusiasm to grow, to learn more, to find your own truth, and to continue in a profession that helps others to clarify their directions. One consequence of doing counseling that is often observed by experienced practitioners is an increase in their own self-awareness, self-assurance, and psychological sensitivity. This phenomenon is, perhaps, the best reason of all for feeling passionate about and committed to the role.

In the sixteenth century, a Samurai warrior and master of kendo ("he who wields the sword") wrote a manual of instruction for those who wished to learn his strategy. Musashi's *Book of Five Rings* (1982) has since become a bible for Japanese business people. I believe that his wisdom also speaks to prospective counselors—to those who wish to learn "the Way of Water," to become calm, unbiased, with a settled spirit, and to those who follow "the Way of Fire," who research and train diligently. Musashi prescribes the following advice for those who want to follow his way:

- Do not think dishonestly.
- The Way is in training.
- Become acquainted with every art.
- Know the Ways of all professions.
- Distinguish between gain and loss in worldly matters.
- Develop intuitive judgment and understanding for everything.
- Perceive those things which cannot be seen.
- Pay attention to trifles.
- Do nothing which is of no use.

The greatest obstacle to any significant discovery is the illusion of knowledge. Boorstein (1983) explains that it was not ignorance that precipitated our descent into the Dark Ages of history, but rather those imaginative bold strokes that temporarily pacified fears and served hopes for simple solutions. True knowledge always advances slowly, with contradictions, conflicts, and controversy. And it is precisely these furiously passionate debates among discrepant views that produce an approximation of truth. With each course you take, with each book you read, with each workshop you attend, with each supervision session you complete, and with each client you see, greater wisdom and competence will evolve if (1) you learn from mistakes, (2) you passionately search for greater mastery in personal and professional skills, and (3) you retain sufficient humility to continue asking questions that have no simple answers.

## A Closing Voice from the Field

In a supervision conference, one counselor lamented her frustrations and confusions about a particular case in which she felt lost, inept, and discouraged. "How, after all," she pleaded, "can I work with this client when I have no idea what is going on?"

The supervisor softly responded in a voice that rose above the chatter of advice directed to the counselor.

"Don't worry when you don't know what you're doing," he said. "Worry when you think you do."

# SELF-GUIDED EXPLORATIONS

1. What are some of your most perplexing questions about counseling that you would like to be able to answer before you graduate?
2. By challenging material presented in your textbook and by your instructor, you are able to develop your own ideas and internalize novel concepts. Write down at least three ideas presented in the textbook and three ideas presented by your instructor in class that you disagree with. Explain your reasoning.
3. Make a list of the goals that you have for yourself that you wish to accomplish in the next year. Sign and date this commitment.
4. As you look back on all the things that you have reflected on and written about in these Self-Guided Explorations, what stands out for you as being most significant?
5. Describe how you intend to educate yourself to be the best possible counselor that you can be.

## Personal Reflections

These exercises represent the beginning, not the end, of your self-explorations and reflections on what it means for you to be a counselor. In a journal, continue writing follow-up entries about the lingering effects from this class. Make yourself accountable to all the previous things you declared and committed yourself to during the course of the semester. Make sure you write to yourself at least once per week for the next dozen or so weeks. After that you may wish to continue this intensive search in your own unstructured journal.

# SUGGESTED READINGS

Bradley, L. J., & Ladany, N. (2001). *Counselor supervision*. New York: Brunner/Routledge.

Corey, M. S., & Corey, G. (2003). *Becoming a helper* (4th ed.). Pacific Grove, CA: Brooks/Cole.

Kottler, J. A. (1999). *The therapist's workbook*. San Francisco: Jossey-Bass.

Kottler, J. A. (2001). *Making changes last*. New York: Brunner/Routledge.

Morrissette, P. J. (2001). *Self-supervision: A primer for counselors and helping professionals*. New York: Brunner/Routledge.

Ram Dass & Gorman, P. (1985). *How can I help? Stories and reflections on service*. New York: Knopf.

Rosenthal, H. (1998). *Before you see your first client: 55 things counselors and human service providers need to know*. Holmes Beach, CA: Learning Publications.

Skovholt, T. M. (2001). *The resilient practitioner: Burnout prevention and self-care strategies for counselors, therapists, teachers, and health professionals.* Boston: Allyn & Bacon.

Yalom, I. (2001). *Gift of therapy: An open letter to a new generation of therapists and their patients.* New York: HarperCollins.

*NOTE TO THE READER:* If you would like to contribute a "voice from the field" describing in a few paragraphs a reality-based opinion or experience, or would like to make a suggestion for the next edition, send your comments to me at: jk@jeffreykottler.com.

# AMERICAN COUNSELING ASSOCIATION

## Code of Ethics
## and Standards of Practice

(Approved by the Governing Council, April 1995)

## PREAMBLE

The American Counseling Association is an educational, scientific, and professional organization whose members are dedicated to the enhancement of human development throughout the life span. Association members recognize diversity in our society and embrace a cross-cultural approach in support of the worth, dignity, potential, and uniqueness of each individual.

The specification of a code of ethics enables the association to clarify to current and future members, and to those served by members, the nature of the ethical responsibilities held in common by its members. As the code of ethics of the association, this document establishes principles that define the ethical behavior of association members. All members of the American Counseling Association are required to adhere to the *Code of Ethics* and the *Standards of Practice*. The *Code of Ethics* will serve as the basis for processing ethical complaints initiated against members of the association.

# CODE OF ETHICS

## Section A: The Counseling Relationship

### A.1.  CLIENT WELFARE

a. *Primary Responsibility*. The primary responsibility of counselors is to respect the dignity and to promote the welfare of clients.

b. *Positive Growth and Development*. Counselors encourage client growth and development in ways that foster the clients' interest and welfare; counselors avoid fostering dependent counseling relationships.

c. *Counseling Plans*. Counselors and their clients work jointly in devising integrated, individual counseling plans that offer reasonable promise of success and are consistent with abilities and circumstances of clients. Counselors and clients regularly review counseling plans to ensure their continued viability and effectiveness, respecting clients' freedom of choice. (See A.3.b.)

d. *Family Involvement*. Counselors recognize that families are usually important in clients' lives and strive to enlist family understanding and involvement as a positive resource when appropriate.

e. *Career and Employment Needs*. Counselors work with their clients in considering employment in jobs and circumstances that are consistent with the clients' overall abilities, vocational limitations, physical restrictions, general temperament, interest and aptitude patterns, social skills, education, general qualifications, and other relevant characteristics and needs. Counselors neither place nor participate in placing clients in positions that will result in damaging the interest and the welfare of clients, employers, or the public.

### A.2.  RESPECTING DIVERSITY

a. *Nondiscrimination*. Counselors do not condone or engage in discrimination based on age, color, culture, disability, ethnic group, gender, race, religion, sexual orientation, marital status, or socioeconomic status. (See C.5.a., C.5.b., and D.1.i.)

b. *Respecting Differences*. Counselors will actively attempt to understand the diverse cultural backgrounds of the clients with whom they work. This includes, but is not limited to, learning how the counselor's own cultural/ethnic/racial identity impacts her/his values and beliefs about the counseling process. (See E.8. and F.2.i.)

### A.3.  CLIENT RIGHTS

a. *Disclosure to Clients*. When counseling is initiated, and throughout the counseling process as necessary, counselors inform clients of the purposes, goals, techniques, procedures, limitations, potential risks and benefits of services to be performed, and other pertinent information. Counselors take steps to ensure that clients understand the implications of diagnosis, the intended use of tests and reports, fees, and billing arrangements. Clients have the right to expect confidentiality and to be provided with an explanation of its limitations, including supervision and/or treatment team professionals; to obtain clear information about their case records; to participate in the ongoing counseling plans; and to refuse any recommended services and be advised of the consequences of such refusal. (See E.5.a. and G.2.)

b. *Freedom of Choice.* Counselors offer clients the freedom to choose whether to enter into a counseling relationship and to determine which professional(s) will provide counseling. Restrictions that limit choices of clients are fully explained. (See A.1.c.)

c. *Inability to Give Consent.* When counseling minors or persons unable to give voluntary informed consent, counselors act in these clients' best interests. (See B.3.)

A.4.   CLIENTS SERVED BY OTHERS

If a client is receiving services from another mental health professional, counselors, with client consent, inform the professional persons already involved and develop clear agreements to avoid confusion and conflict for the client. (See C.6.c.)

A.5.   PERSONAL NEEDS AND VALUES

a. *Personal Needs.* In the counseling relationship, counselors are aware of the intimacy and responsibilities inherent in the counseling relationship, maintain respect for clients, and avoid actions that seek to meet their personal needs at the expense of clients.

b. *Personal Values.* Counselors are aware of their own values, attitudes, beliefs, and behaviors and how these apply in a diverse society and avoid imposing their values on clients. (See C.5.a.)

A.6.   DUAL RELATIONSHIPS

a. *Avoid When Possible.* Counselors are aware of their influential positions with respect to clients, and they avoid exploiting the trust and dependency of clients. Counselors make every effort to avoid dual relationships with clients that could impair professional judgment or increase the risk of harm to clients. (Examples of such relationships include, but are not limited to, familial, social, financial, business, or close personal relationships with clients.) When a dual relationship cannot be avoided, counselors take appropriate professional precautions, such as informed consent, consultation, supervision, and documentation, to ensure that judgment is not impaired and no exploitation occurs. (See F.1.b.)

b. *Superior/Subordinate Relationships.* Counselors do not accept as clients superiors or subordinates with whom they have administrative, supervisory, or evaluative relationships.

A.7.   SEXUAL INTIMACIES WITH CLIENTS

a. *Current Clients.* Counselors do not have any type of sexual intimacies with clients and do not counsel persons with whom they have had a sexual relationship.

b. *Former Clients.* Counselors do not engage in sexual intimacies with former clients within a minimum of two years after terminating the counseling relationship. Counselors who engage in such relationship after two years following termination have the responsibility to thoroughly examine and document that such relations did not have an exploitative nature, based on factors such as duration of counseling, amount of time since counseling, termination circumstances, client's personal history and mental status, adverse impact on the client, and actions by the counselor suggesting a plan to initiate a sexual relationship with the client after termination.

A.8.  MULTIPLE CLIENTS

When counselors agree to provide counseling services to two or more persons who have a relationship (such as husband and wife, or parents and children), counselors clarify at the outset which person or persons are clients and the nature of the relationships they will have with each involved person. If it becomes apparent that counselors may be called upon to perform potentially conflicting roles, they clarify, adjust, or withdraw from roles appropriately. (See B.2. and B.4.d.)

A.9.  GROUP WORK

a. *Screening*. Counselors screen prospective group counseling/therapy participants. To the extent possible, counselors select members whose needs and goals are compatible with goals of the group, who will not impede the group process, and whose well-being will not be jeopardized by the group experience.

b. *Protecting Clients*. In a group setting, counselors take reasonable precautions to protect clients from physical or psychological trauma.

A.10. FEES AND BARTERING

(See D.3.a. and D.3.b.)

a. *Advance Understanding*. Counselors clearly explain to clients, prior to entering the counseling relationship, all financial arrangements related to professional services including the use of collection agencies or legal measures for nonpayment. (A.11.c.)

b. *Establishing Fees*. In establishing fees for professional counseling services, counselors consider the financial status of clients and locality. In the event that the established fee structure is inappropriate for a client, assistance is provided in attempting to find comparable services of acceptable cost. (See A.10.d., D.3.a., and D.3.b.)

c. *Bartering Discouraged*. Counselors ordinarily refrain from accepting goods or services from clients in return for counseling services because such arrangements create inherent potential for conflicts, exploitation, and distortion of the professional relationship. Counselors may participate in bartering only if the relationship is not exploitive, if the client requests it, if a clear written contract is established, and if such arrangements are an accepted practice among professionals in the community. (See A.6.a.).

d. *Pro Bono Service.* Counselors contribute to society by devoting a portion of their professional activity to services for which there is little or no financial return (pro bono).

## A.11. TERMINATION AND REFERRAL

a. *Abandonment Prohibited.* Counselors do not abandon or neglect clients in counseling. Counselors assist in making appropriate arrangements for the continuation of treatment, when necessary, during interruptions, such as vacations, and following termination.

b. *Inability to Assist Clients.* If counselors determine an inability to be of professional assistance to clients, they avoid entering or immediately terminate a counseling relationship. Counselors are knowledgeable about referral resources and suggest appropriate alternatives. If clients decline the suggested referral, counselors should discontinue the relationship.

c. *Appropriate Termination.* Counselors terminate a counseling relationship, securing client agreement when possible, when it is reasonably clear that the client is no longer benefiting, when services are no longer required, when counseling no longer serves the client's needs or interests, when clients do not pay fees charged, or when agency or institution limits do not allow provision of further counseling services. (See A.10.b. and C.2.g.)

## A.12. COMPUTER TECHNOLOGY

a. *Use of Computers.* When computer applications are used in counseling services, counselors ensure that (1) the client is intellectually, emotionally, and physically capable of using the computer application; (2) the computer application is appropriate for the needs of the client; (3) the client understands the purpose and operation of the computer applications; and (4) a follow-up of client use of a computer application is provided to correct possible misconceptions, discover inappropriate use, and assess subsequent needs.

b. *Explanation of Limitations.* Counselors ensure that clients are provided information as a part of the counseling relationship that adequately explains the limitations of computer technology.

c. *Access to Computer Applications.* Counselors provide for equal access to computer applications in counseling services. (See A.2.a.)

# Section B: Confidentiality

## B.1. RIGHT TO PRIVACY

a. *Respect for Privacy.* Counselors respect their clients' right to privacy and avoid illegal and unwarranted disclosures of confidential information. (See A.3.a. and B.6.a.)

b. *Client Waiver.* The right to privacy may be waived by the client or their legally recognized representative.

c. *Exceptions.* The general requirement that counselors keep information confidential does not apply when disclosure is required to prevent clear and imminent danger to the client or others or when legal requirements demand that confidential information be revealed. Counselors consult with other professionals when in doubt as to the validity of an exception.

d. *Contagious, Fatal Diseases.* A counselor who receives information confirming that a client has a disease commonly known to be both communicable and fatal is justified in disclosing information to an identifiable third party, who by his or her relationship with the client is at a high risk of contracting the disease. Prior to making a disclosure the counselor should ascertain that the client has not already informed the third party about his or her disease and that the client is not intending to inform the third party in the immediate future. (See B.1.c. and B.1.f.)

e. *Court Ordered Disclosure.* When court ordered to release confidential information without a client's permission, counselors request to the court that the disclosure not be required due to potential harm to the client or counseling relationship. (See B.1.c.)

f. *Minimal Disclosure.* When circumstances require the disclosure of confidential information, only essential information is revealed. To the extent possible, clients are informed before confidential information is disclosed.

g. *Explanation of Limitations.* When counseling is initiated and throughout the counseling process as necessary, counselors inform clients of the limitations of confidentiality and identify foreseeable situations in which confidentiality must be breached. (See G.2.a.)

h. *Subordinates.* Counselors make every effort to ensure that privacy and confidentiality of clients are maintained by subordinates including employees, supervisees, clerical assistants, and volunteers. (See B.1.a.)

i. *Treatment Teams.* If client treatment will involve a continued review by a treatment team, the client will be informed of the team's existence and composition.

B.2.   GROUPS AND FAMILIES

a. *Group Work.* In group work, counselors clearly define confidentiality and the parameters for the specific group being entered, explain its importance, and discuss the difficulties related to confidentiality involved in group work. The fact that confidentiality cannot be guaranteed is clearly communicated to group members.

b. *Family Counseling.* In family counseling, information about one family member cannot be disclosed to another member without permission. Counselors protect the privacy rights of each family member. (See A.8., B.3. and B.4.d.)

B.3.   MINOR OR INCOMPETENT CLIENTS

When counseling clients who are minors or individuals who are unable to give voluntary, informed consent, parents or guardians may be included in the counseling process as appropriate. Counselors act in the best interests of clients and take measures to safeguard confidentiality. (See A.3.c.)

B.4.    RECORDS

a. *Requirement of Records.* Counselors maintain records necessary for rendering professional services to their clients and as required by laws, regulations, or agency or institution procedures.

b. *Confidentiality of Records.* Counselors are responsible for securing the safety and confidentiality of any counseling records they create, maintain, transfer, or destroy whether the records are written, taped, computerized, or stored in any other medium. (See B.1.a.)

c. *Permission to Record or Observe.* Counselors obtain permission from clients prior to electronically recording or observing sessions. (See A.3.a.)

d. *Client Access.* Counselors recognize that counseling records are kept for the benefit of clients and, therefore, provide access to records and copies of records when requested by competent clients unless the records contain information that may be misleading and detrimental to the client. In situations involving multiple clients, access to records is limited to those parts of records that do not include confidential information related to another client. (See A.8., B.1.a., and B.2.b.)

e. *Disclosure or Transfer.* Counselors obtain written permission from clients to disclose or transfer records to legitimate third parties unless exceptions to confidentiality exist as listed in Section B.1. Steps are taken to ensure that receivers of counseling records are sensitive to their confidential nature.

B.5.    RESEARCH AND TRAINING

a. *Data Disguise Required.* Use of data derived from counseling relationships for purposes of training, research, or publication is confined to content that is disguised to ensure the anonymity of the individuals involved. (See B.1.g. and G.3.d.)

b. *Agreement for Identification.* Identification of a client in a presentation or publication is permissible only when the client has reviewed the material and has agreed to its presentation or publication. (See G.3.d.)

B.6. CONSULTATION

a. *Respect for Privacy.* Information obtained in a consulting relationship is discussed for professional purposes only with persons clearly concerned with the case. Written and oral reports present data germane to the purposes of the consultation, and every effort is made to protect client identity and avoid undue invasion of privacy.

b. *Cooperating Agencies.* Before sharing information, counselors make efforts to ensure that there are defined policies in other agencies serving the counselor's clients that effectively protect the confidentiality of information.

## Section C: Professional Responsibility

C.1.  STANDARDS KNOWLEDGE

Counselors have a responsibility to read, understand, and follow the *Code of Ethics* and the *Standards of Practice*.

C.2.  PROFESSIONAL COMPETENCE

a. *Boundaries of Competence.* Counselors practice only within the boundaries of their competence, based on their education, training, supervised experience, state and national professional credentials, and appropriate professional experience. Counselors will demonstrate a commitment to gain knowledge, personal awareness, sensitivity, and skills pertinent to working with a diverse client population.

b. *New Specialty Areas of Practice.* Counselors practice in specialty areas new to them only after appropriate education, training, and supervised experience. While developing skills in new specialty areas, counselors take steps to ensure the competence of their work and to protect others from possible harm.

c. *Qualified for Employment.* Counselors accept employment only for positions for which they are qualified by education, training, supervised experience, state and national professional credentials, and appropriate professional experience. Counselors hire for professional counseling positions only individuals who are qualified and competent.

d. *Monitor Effectiveness.* Counselors continually monitor their effectiveness as professionals and take steps to improve when necessary. Counselors in private practice take reasonable steps to seek out peer supervision to evaluate their efficacy as counselors.

e. *Ethical Issues Consultation.* Counselors take reasonable steps to consult with other counselors or related professionals when they have questions regarding their ethical obligations or professional practice. (See H.1)

f. *Continuing Education.* Counselors recognize the need for continuing education to maintain a reasonable level of awareness of current scientific and professional information in their fields of activity. They take steps to maintain competence in the skills they use, are open to new procedures, and keep current with the diverse and/or special populations with whom they work.

g. *Impairment.* Counselors refrain from offering or accepting professional services when their physical, mental or emotional problems are likely to harm a client or others. They are alert to the signs of impairment, seek assistance for problems, and, if necessary, limit, suspend, or terminate their professional responsibilities. (See A.11.c.)

C.3.  ADVERTISING AND SOLICITING CLIENTS

a. *Accurate Advertising.* There are no restrictions on advertising by counselors except those that can be specifically justified to protect the public from deceptive practices. Counselors advertise or represent their services to the public by identifying their credentials in an accurate manner that is not false, misleading, deceptive, or fraudulent. Counselors may only advertise the highest degree earned which is in counseling or a closely related field from a college or university that was accredited when the degree was awarded by one of the regional accrediting bodies recognized by the Council on Postsecondary Accreditation.

b. *Testimonials.* Counselors who use testimonials do not solicit them from clients or other persons who, because of their particular circumstances, may be vulnerable to undue influence.

c. *Statements by Others.* Counselors make reasonable efforts to ensure that statements made by others about them or the profession of counseling are accurate.

d. *Recruiting Through Employment.* Counselors do not use their places of employment or institutional affiliation to recruit or gain clients, supervisees, or consultees for their private practices. (See C.5.e.)

e. *Products and Training Advertisements.* Counselors who develop products related to their profession or conduct workshops or training events ensure that the advertisements concerning these products or events are accurate and disclose adequate information for consumers to make informed choices.

f. *Promoting to Those Served.* Counselors do not use counseling, teaching, training, or supervisory relationships to promote their products or training events in a manner that is deceptive or would exert undue influence on individuals who may be vulnerable. Counselors may adopt textbooks they have authored for instruction purposes.

g. *Professional Association Involvement.* Counselors actively participate in local, state, and national associations that foster the development and improvement of counseling.

## C.4.  CREDENTIALS

a. *Credentials Claimed.* Counselors claim or imply only professional credentials possessed and are responsible for correcting any known misrepresentations of their credentials by others. Professional credentials include graduate degrees in counseling or closely related mental health fields, accreditation of graduate programs, national voluntary certifications, government-issued certifications or licenses, ACA professional membership, or any other credential that might indicate to the public specialized knowledge or expertise in counseling.

b. *ACA Professional Membership.* ACA professional members may announce to the public their membership status. Regular members may not announce their ACA membership in a manner that might imply they are credentialed counselors.

c. *Credential Guidelines.* Counselors follow the guidelines for use of credentials that have been established by the entities that issue the credentials.

   d. *Misrepresentation of Credentials.* Counselors do not attribute more
      to their credentials than the credentials represent and do not imply
      that other counselors are not qualified because they do not possess
      certain credentials.
   e. *Doctoral Degrees from Other Fields.* Counselors who hold a mas-
      ter's degree in counseling or a closely related mental health field but
      hold a doctoral degree from other than counseling or a closely
      related field do not use the title, "Dr." in their practices and do not
      announce to the public in relation to their practice or status as a
      counselor that they hold a doctorate.

C.5.   PUBLIC RESPONSIBILITY
   a. *Nondiscrimination.* Counselors do not discriminate against clients,
      students, or supervisees in a manner that has a negative impact based
      on their age, color, culture, disability, ethnic group, gender, race, reli-
      gion, sexual orientation, or socioeconomic status, or for any other
      reason (See A.2.a.)
   b. *Sexual Harassment.* Counselors do not engage in sexual harassment.
      Sexual harassment is defined as sexual solicitation, physical ad-
      vances, or verbal or nonverbal conduct that is sexual in nature, that
      occurs in connection with professional activities or roles, and that
      either (1) is unwelcome, is offensive, or creates a hostile workplace
      environment, and counselors know or are told this; or (2) is suffi-
      ciently severe or intense to be perceived as harassment to a reason-
      able person in the context. Sexual harassment can consist of a single
      intense or severe act or multiple persistent or pervasive acts.
   c. *Reports to Third Parties.* Counselors are accurate, honest, and unbi-
      ased in reporting their professional activities and judgments to appro-
      priate third parties including courts, health insurance companies, those
      who are the recipients of evaluation reports, and others. (See B.1.g.)
   d. *Media Presentations.* When counselors provide advice or comment
      by means of public lectures, demonstrations, radio or television pro-
      grams, prerecorded tapes, printed articles, mailed material, or other
      media, they take reasonable precautions to ensure that (1) the state-
      ments are based on appropriate professional counseling literature
      and practice; (2) the statements are otherwise consistent with the
      *Code of Ethics* and the *Standards of Practice;* and (3) the recipients
      of the information are not encouraged to infer that a professional
      counseling relationship has been established. (See C.6.b.)
   e. *Unjustified Gains.* Counselors do not use their professional positions
      to seek or receive unjustified personal gains, sexual favors, unfair ad-
      vantage, or unearned goods or services. (See C.3.d.)

C.6.   RESPONSIBILITY TO OTHER PROFESSIONALS
   a. *Different Approaches.* Counselors are respectful of approaches to
      professional counseling that differ from their own. Counselors know
      and take into account the traditions and practices of other profes-
      sional groups with which they work.

b. *Personal Public Statements.* When making personal statements in a public context, counselors clarify that they are speaking from their personal perspectives and that they are not speaking on behalf of all counselors or the profession. (See C.5.d.)

c. *Clients Served by Others.* When counselors learn that their clients are in a professional relationship with another mental health professional, they request release from clients to inform the other professionals and strive to establish positive and collaborative professional relationships. (See A.4.)

# Section D: Relationships with Other Professionals

D.1.   RELATIONSHIPS WITH EMPLOYERS AND EMPLOYEES

a. *Role Definition.* Counselors define and describe for their employers and employees the parameters and levels of their professional roles.

b. *Agreements.* Counselors establish working agreements with supervisors, colleagues, and subordinates regarding counseling or clinical relationships, confidentiality, adherence to professional standards, distinction between public and private material, maintenance and dissemination of recorded information, workload, and accountability. Working agreements in each instance are specified and made known to those concerned.

c. *Negative Conditions.* Counselors alert their employers to conditions that may be potentially disruptive or damaging to the counselor's professional responsibilities or that may limit their effectiveness.

d. *Evaluation.* Counselors submit regularly to professional review and evaluation by their supervisor or the appropriate representative of the employer.

e. *In-Service.* Counselors are responsible for in-service development of self and staff.

f. *Goals.* Counselors inform their staff of goals and programs.

g. *Practices.* Counselors provide personal and agency practices that respect and enhance the rights and welfare of each employee and recipient of agency services. Counselors strive to maintain the highest levels of professional services.

h. *Personnel Selection and Assignment.* Counselors select competent staff and assign responsibilities compatible with their skills and experiences.

i. *Discrimination.* Counselors, as either employers or employees, do not engage in or condone practices that are inhumane, illegal, or unjustifiable (such as considerations based on age, color, culture, disability, ethnic group, gender, race, religion, sexual orientation, or socioeconomic status) in hiring, promotion, or training. (See A.2.a. and C.5.b.)

j. *Professional Conduct.* Counselors have a responsibility both to clients and to the agency or institution within which services are performed to maintain high standards of professional conduct.

k. *Exploitive Relationships.* Counselors do not engage in exploitive relationships with individuals over whom they have supervisory, evaluative, or instructional control or authority.

l. *Employer Policies.* The acceptance of employment in an agency or institution implies that counselors are in agreement with its general policies and principles. Counselors strive to reach agreement with employers as to acceptable standards of conduct that allow for changes in institutional policy conducive to the growth and development of clients.

D.2. CONSULTATION (See B.6.)

a. *Consultation as an Option.* Counselors may choose to consult with any other professionally competent persons about their clients. In choosing consultants, counselors avoid placing the consultant in a conflict of interest situation that would preclude the consultant being a proper party to the counselor's efforts to help the client. Should counselors be engaged in a work setting that compromises this consultation standard, they consult with other professionals whenever possible to consider justifiable alternatives.

b. *Consultant Competency.* Counselors are reasonably certain that they have or the organization represented has the necessary competencies and resources for giving the kind of consulting services needed and that appropriate referral resources are available.

c. *Understanding with Clients.* When providing consultation, counselors attempt to develop with their clients a clear understanding of problem definition, goals for change, and predicted consequences of interventions selected.

d. *Consultant Goals.* The consulting relationship is one in which client adaptability and growth toward self-direction are consistently encouraged and cultivated. (See A.1.b.)

D.3. FEES FOR REFERRAL

a. *Accepting Fees from Agency Clients.* Counselors refuse a private fee or other remuneration for rendering services to persons who are entitled to such services through the counselor's employing agency or institution. The policies of a particular agency may make explicit provisions for agency clients to receive counseling services from members of its staff in private practice. In such instances, the clients must be informed of other options open to them should they seek private counseling services. (See A.10.a., A.11.b., and C.3.d.)

b. *Referral Fees.* Counselors do not accept a referral fee from other professionals.

D.4. SUBCONTRACTOR ARRANGEMENTS

When counselors work as subcontractors for counseling services for a third party, they have a duty to inform clients of the limitations of confidentiality that the organization may place on counselors in providing counseling services to clients. The limits of such confidentiality ordinarily are discussed as part of the intake session. (See B.1.e. and B.1.f.)

## Section E: Evaluation, Assessment, and Interpretation

E.1.   GENERAL
   a. *Appraisal Techniques.* The primary purpose of educational and psychological assessment is to provide measures that are objective and interpretable in either comparative or absolute terms. Counselors recognize the need to interpret the statements in this section as applying to the whole range of appraisal techniques including test and nontest data.
   b. *Client Welfare.* Counselors promote that welfare and best interests of the client in the development, publication, and utilization of educational and psychological assessment techniques. They do not misuse assessment results and interpretations and take reasonable steps to prevent others from misusing the information these techniques provide. They respect the client's right to know the results, the interpretations made, and the basis for their conclusions and recommendations.

E.2.   COMPETENCE TO USE AND INTERPRET TESTS
   a. *Limits of Competence.* Counselors recognize the limits of their competence and perform only those testing and assessment services for which they have been trained. They are familiar with reliability, validity, related standardization, error of measurement, and proper application of any technique utilized. Counselors using computer-based test interpretations are trained in the construct being measured and the specific instrument being used prior to using this type of computer application. Counselors take reasonable measures to ensure the proper use of psychological assessment techniques by persons under their supervision.
   b. *Appropriate Use.* Counselors are responsible for the appropriate application, scoring, interpretation, and use of assessment instruments whether they score and interpret such tests themselves or use computerized or other services.
   c. *Decisions Based on Results.* Counselors responsible for decisions involving individuals or policies that are based on assessment results have a thorough understanding of educational and psychological measurement, including validation criteria, test research, and guidelines for test development and use.
   d. *Accurate Information.* Counselors provide accurate information and avoid false claims or misconceptions when making statements about assessment instruments or techniques. Special efforts are made to avoid unwarranted connotations of such terms as IQ and grade equivalent scores. (See C.5.c.)

E.3.  INFORMED CONSENT

  a. *Explanation to Clients.* Prior to assessment, counselors explain the nature and purposes of assessment and the specific use of results in language the client (or other legally authorized person on behalf of the client) can understand unless an explicit exception to this right has been agreed upon in advance. Regardless of whether scoring and interpretation are completed by counselors, by assistants, or by computer or other outside services, counselors take reasonable steps to ensure that appropriate explanations are given to the client.

  b. *Recipients of Results.* The examinee's welfare, explicit understanding, and prior agreement determine the recipients of test results. Counselors include accurate and appropriate interpretations with any release of individual or group test results. (See B.1.a. and C.5.c.)

E.4.  RELEASE OF INFORMATION TO COMPETENT PROFESSIONALS

  a. *Misuse of Results.* Counselors do not misuse assessment results, including test results, and interpretations, and take reasonable steps to prevent the misuse of such by others. (See C.5.c.)

  b. *Release of Raw Data.* Counselors ordinarily release data (e.g., protocols, counseling or interview notes, or questionnaires) in which the client is identified only with the consent of the client or the client's legal representative. Such data are usually released only to persons recognized by counselors as competent to interpret the data. (See B.1.a.)

E.5.  PROPER DIAGNOSIS OF MENTAL DISORDERS

  a. *Proper Diagnosis.* Counselors take special care to provide proper diagnosis of mental disorders. Assessment techniques (including personal interview) used to determine client care (e.g., locus of treatment, type of treatment, or recommended follow-up) are carefully selected and appropriately used. (See A.3.a. and C.5.c)

  b. *Cultural Sensitivity.* Counselors recognize that culture affects the manner in which clients' problems are defined. Clients' socioeconomic and cultural experience is considered when diagnosing mental disorders.

E.6.  TEST SELECTION

  a. *Appropriateness of Instruments.* Counselors carefully consider the validity, reliability, psychometric limitations, and appropriateness of instruments when selecting tests for use in a given situation or with a particular client.

  b. *Culturally Diverse Populations.* Counselors are cautious when selecting tests for culturally diverse populations to avoid inappropriateness of testing that may be outside of socialized behavioral or cognitive patterns.

E.7.  CONDITIONS OF TEST ADMINISTRATION

  a. *Administration Conditions.* Counselors administer tests under the same conditions that were established in their standardization. When tests are not administered under standard conditions or when unusual behavior or irregularities occur during the testing session, those conditions are noted in interpretation, and the results may be designated as invalid or of questionable validity.

b. *Computer Administration.* Counselors are responsible for ensuring that administration programs function properly to provide clients with accurate results when a computer or other electronic methods are used for test administration. (See A.12.b.)

c. *Unsupervised Test-Taking.* Counselors do not permit unsupervised or inadequately supervised use of tests or assessments unless the tests or assessments are designed, intended, and validated for self-administration and/or scoring.

d. *Disclosure of Favorable Conditions.* Prior to test administration, conditions that produce most favorable test results are made known to the examinee.

E.8. DIVERSITY IN TESTING

Counselors are cautious in using assessment techniques, making evaluations, and interpreting the performance of populations not represented in the norm group on which an instrument was standardized. They recognize the effects of age, color, culture, disability, ethnic group, gender, race, religion, sexual orientation, and socioeconomic status on test administration and interpretation and place test results in proper perspective with other relevant factors. (See A.2.a.)

E.9. TEST SCORING AND INTERPRETATION

a. *Reporting Reservations.* In reporting assessment results, counselors indicate any reservations that exist regarding validity or reliability because of the circumstances of the assessment or the inappropriateness of the norms for the person tested.

b. *Research Instruments.* Counselors exercise caution when interpreting the results of research instruments possessing insufficient technical data to support respondent results. The specific purposes for the use of such instruments are stated explicitly to the examinee.

c. *Testing Services.* Counselors who provide test scoring and test interpretation services to support the assessment process confirm the validity of such interpretations. They accurately describe the purpose, norms, validity, reliability, and applications of the procedures and any special qualifications applicable to their use. The public offering of an automated test interpretations service is considered a professional-to-professional consultation. The formal responsibility of the consultant is to the consultee, but the ultimate and overriding responsibility is to the client.

E.10. TEST SECURITY

Counselors maintain the integrity and security of tests and other assessment techniques consistent with legal and contractual obligations. Counselors do not appropriate, reproduce, or modify published tests or parts thereof without acknowledgment and permission from the publisher.

### E.11.  OBSOLETE TESTS AND OUTDATED TEST RESULTS

Counselors do not use data or test results that are obsolete or outdated for the current purpose. Counselors make every effort to prevent the misuse of obsolete measures and test data by others.

### E.12.  TEST CONSTRUCTION

Counselors use established scientific procedures, relevant standards, and current professional knowledge for test design in the development, publication, and utilization of educational and psychological assessment techniques.

## Section F: Teaching, Training, and Supervision

F.1    COUNSELOR EDUCATORS AND TRAINERS

a. *Educators as Teachers and Practitioners.* Counselors who are responsible for developing, implementing, and supervising educational programs are skilled as teachers and practitioners. They are knowledgeable regarding the ethical, legal, and regulatory aspects of the profession, are skilled in applying that knowledge, and make students and supervisees aware of their responsibilities. Counselors conduct counselor education and training programs in an ethical manner and serve as role models for professional behavior. Counselor educators should make an effort to infuse material related to human diversity into all courses and/or workshops that are designed to promote the development of professional counselors.

b. *Relationship Boundaries with Students and Supervisees.* Counselors clearly define and maintain ethical, professional, and social relationship boundaries with their students and supervisees. They are aware of the differential in power that exists and the student's or supervisee's possible incomprehension of that power differential. Counselors explain to students and supervisees the potential for the relationship to become exploitive.

c. *Sexual Relationships.* Counselors do not engage in sexual relationships with students or supervisees and do not subject them to sexual harassment. (See A.6. and C.5.b.)

d. *Contributions to Research.* Counselors give credit to students or supervisees for their contributions to research and scholarly projects. Credit is given through coauthorship, acknowledgment, footnote statement, or other appropriate means in accordance with such contributions. (See G.4.b. and G.4.c.)

e. *Close Relatives.* Counselors do not accept close relatives as students or supervisees.

f. *Supervision Preparation.* Counselors who offer clinical supervision services are adequately prepared in supervision methods and techniques. Counselors who are doctoral students serving as practicum or internship supervisors to master's level students are adequately prepared and supervised by the training program.

g. *Responsibility for Services to Clients.* Counselors who supervise the counseling services of others take reasonable measures to ensure that counseling services provided to clients are professional.

h. *Endorsement.* Counselors do not endorse students or supervisees for certification, licensure, employment, or completion of an academic or training program if they believe students or supervisees are not qualified for the endorsement. Counselors take reasonable steps to assist students or supervisees who are not qualified for endorsement to become qualified.

F.2.   COUNSELOR EDUCATION AND TRAINING PROGRAMS

a. *Orientation.* Prior to admission, counselors orient prospective students to the counselor education or training program's expectations including but not limited to the following: (1) the type and level of skill acquisition required for successful completion of the training, (2) subject matter to be covered, (3) basis for evaluation, (4) training components that encourage self-growth or self-disclosure as part of the training process, (5) the type of supervision settings and requirements of the sites for required clinical field experiences, (6) student and supervisee evaluation and dismissal policies and procedures, and (7) up-to-date employment prospects for graduates.

b. *Integration of Study and Practice.* Counselors establish counselor education and training programs that integrate academic study and supervised practice.

c. *Evaluation.* Counselors clearly state to students and supervisees, in advance of training, the levels of competency expected, appraisal methods, and timing of evaluations for both didactic and experiential components. Counselors provide students and supervisees with periodic performance appraisal and evaluation feedback throughout the training program.

d. *Teaching Ethics.* Counselors make students and supervisees aware of the ethical responsibilities and standards of the profession and the students' and supervisees' ethical responsibilities to the profession. (See C.1. and F.3.e.)

e. *Peer Relationships.* When students or supervisees are assigned to lead counseling groups or provide clinical supervision for their peers, counselors take steps to ensure that students and supervisees placed in these roles do not have personal or adverse relationships with peers and that they understand they have the same ethical obligations as counselor educators, trainers, and supervisors. Counselors make every effort to ensure that the rights of peers are not compromised when students or supervisees are assigned to lead counseling groups or provide clinical supervision.

f. *Varied Theoretical Positions.* Counselors present varied theoretical positions so that students and supervisees may make comparisons and have opportunities to develop their own positions. Counselors provide information concerning the scientific basis of professional practice. (See C.6.a.)

g. *Field Placements.* Counselors develop clear policies within their training program regarding field placement and other clinical experiences. Counselors provide clearly stated roles and responsibilities for the student or supervisee, the site supervisor, and the program supervisor. They confirm that site supervisors are qualified to provide supervision and are informed of their professional and ethical responsibilities in this role.

h. *Dual Relationships as Supervisors.* Counselors avoid dual relationships, such as performing the role of site supervisor and training program supervisor in the student's or supervisee's training program. Counselors do not accept any form of professional services, fees, commissions, reimbursement, or remuneration from a site for student or supervisee placement.

i. *Diversity in Programs.* Counselors are responsive to their institution's and program's recruitment and retention needs for training program administrators, faculty, and students with diverse backgrounds and special needs. (See A.2.a.)

F.3.    STUDENTS AND SUPERVISEES

a. *Limitations.* Counselors, through ongoing evaluation and appraisal, are aware of the academic and personal limitations of students and supervisees that might impede performance. Counselors assist students and supervisees in securing remedial assistance when needed and dismiss from the training program supervisees who are unable to provide competent service due to academic or personal limitations. Counselors seek professional consultation and document their decision to dismiss or refer students or supervisees for assistance. Counselors assure that students and supervisees have recourse to address decisions made, to require them to seek assistance, or to dismiss them.

b. *Self-Growth Experiences.* Counselors use professional judgment when designing training experiences conducted by the counselors themselves that require student and supervisee self-growth or self-disclosure. Safeguards are provided so that students and supervisees are aware of the ramifications their self-disclosure may have on counselors whose primary role as teacher, trainer, or supervisor requires acting on ethical obligations to the profession. Evaluative components of experiential training experiences explicitly delineate predetermined academic standards that are separate and not dependent on the student's level of self- disclosure. (See A.6.)

c. *Counseling for Students and Supervisees.* If students or supervisees request counseling, supervisors or counselor educators provide them with acceptable referrals. Supervisors or counselor educators do not serve as counselor to students or supervisees over whom they hold administrative, teaching, or evaluative roles unless this is a brief role associated with a training experience. (See A.6.b.)

d. *Clients of Students and Supervisees.* Counselors make every effort to ensure that the clients at field placements are aware of the services rendered and the qualifications of the students and supervisees rendering those services. Clients receive professional disclosure information and are informed of the limits of confidentiality. Client permission is obtained in order for the students and supervisees to use any information concerning the counseling relationship in the training process. (See B.1.e.)

e. *Standards for Students and Supervisees.* Students and supervisees preparing to become counselors adhere to the *Code of Ethics* and the *Standards of Practice.* Students and supervisees have the same obligations to clients as those required of counselors. (See H.1.)

## Section G: Research and Publication

G.1.   RESEARCH RESPONSIBILITIES

a. *Use of Human Subjects.* Counselors plan, design, conduct, and report research in a manner consistent with pertinent ethical principles, federal and state laws, host institutional regulations, and scientific standards governing research with human subjects. Counselors design and conduct research that reflects cultural sensitivity appropriateness.

b. *Deviation from Standard Practices.* Counselors seek consultation and observe stringent safeguards to protect the rights of research participants when a research problem suggests a deviation from standard acceptable practices. (See B.6.)

c. *Precautions to Avoid Injury.* Counselors who conduct research with human subjects are responsible for the subjects' welfare throughout the experiment and take reasonable precautions to avoid causing injurious psychological, physical, or social effects to their subjects.

d. *Principal Researcher Responsibility.* The ultimate responsibility for ethical research practice lies with the principle researcher. All others involved in the research activities share ethical obligations and full responsibility for their own actions.

e. *Minimal Interference.* Counselors take reasonable precautions to avoid causing disruptions in subjects' lives due to participation in research.

f. *Diversity.* Counselors are sensitive to diversity and research issues with special populations. They seek consultation when appropriate. (See A.2.a. and B.6)

G.2.   INFORMED CONSENT

a. *Topics Disclosed.* In obtaining informed consent for research, counselors use language that is understandable to research participants and that (1) accurately explains the purpose and procedures to be followed; (2) identifies any procedures that are experimental or relatively untried; (3) describes the attendant discomforts and risks; (4) describes the benefits or changes in individuals or organizations that might be reasonably expected; (5) discloses appropriate alternative procedures that would be advantageous for subjects; (6) offers to answer any inquiries concerning the procedures; (7) describes any limitations on confidentiality; and (8) instructs that subjects are free to withdraw their consent and to discontinue participation in the project at any time. (See B.1.f.)

b. *Deception.* Counselors do not conduct research involving deception unless alternative procedures are not feasible and the prospective value of the research justifies the deception. When the methodological requirements of a study necessitate concealment or deception, the investigator is required to explain clearly the reasons for this action as soon as possible.

c. *Voluntary Participation.* Participation in research is typically voluntary and without any penalty for refusal to participate. Involuntary participation is appropriate only when it can be demonstrated that participation will have no harmful effects on subjects and is essential to the investigation.

d. *Confidentiality of Information.* Information obtained about research participants during the course of an investigation is confidential. When the possibility exists that others may obtain access to such information, ethical research practice requires that the possibility, together with the plans for protecting confidentiality, be explained to participants as a part of the procedure for obtaining informed consent. (See B.1.e.)

e. *Persons Incapable of Giving Informed Consent.* When a person is incapable of giving informed consent, counselors provide an appropriate explanation, obtain agreement for participation, and obtain appropriate consent from a legally authorized person.

f. *Commitments to Participants.* Counselors take reasonable measures to honor all commitments to research participants.

g. *Explanations After Data Collection.* After data are collected, counselors provide participants with full clarification of the nature of the study to remove any misconceptions. Where scientific or human values justify delaying or withholding information, counselors take reasonable measures to avoid causing harm.

h. *Agreements to Cooperate.* Counselors who agree to cooperate with another individual in research or publication incur an obligation to cooperate as promised in terms of punctuality of performance and with regard to the completeness and accuracy of the information required.

i. *Informed Consent for Sponsors.* In the pursuit of research counselors give sponsors, institutions, and publication channels the same respect and opportunity for giving informed consent that they accord to individual research participants. Counselors are aware of their obligation to future research workers and ensure that host institutions are given feedback information and proper acknowledgment.

G.3.  REPORTING RESULTS

a. *Information Affecting Outcome.* When reporting research results counselors explicitly mention all variables and conditions known to the investigator that may have affected the outcome of a study or the interpretation of data.

b. *Accurate Results.* Counselors plan, conduct, and report research accurately and in a manner that minimizes the possibility that results will be misleading. They provide thorough discussions of the limitations of their data and alternative hypotheses. Counselors do not engage in fraudulent research, distort data, misrepresent data, or deliberately bias their results.

c. *Obligation to Report Unfavorable Results.* Counselors communicate to other counselors the results of any research judged to be of professional value. Results that reflect unfavorably on institutions, programs, services, prevailing opinions, or vested interests are not withheld.

d. *Identity of Subjects.* Counselors who supply data, aid in the research of another person, report research results, or make original data available take due care to disguise the identity of respective subjects in the absence of specific authorization from the subjects to do otherwise. (See B.1.g. and B.5.a.)

e. *Replication Studies.* Counselors are obligated to make available sufficient original research data to qualified professionals who may wish to replicate the study.

G.4.  PUBLICATION

a. *Recognition of Others.* When conducting and reporting research, counselors are familiar with and give recognition to previous work on the topic, observe copyright laws, and give full credit to those to whom credit is due. (See F.1.d. and G.4.c.)

b. *Contributors.* Counselors give credit through joint authorship, acknowledgment, footnote statements, or other appropriate means to those who have contributed significantly to research or concept development in accordance with such contributions. The principal contributor is listed first and minor technical or professional contributions are acknowledged in notes or introductory statements.

c. *Student Research.* For an article that is substantially based on a student's dissertation or thesis, the student is listed as the principal author. (See F.1.d. and G.4.a.)

d. *Duplicate Submission.* Counselors submit manuscripts for consideration to only one journal at a time. Manuscripts that are published in whole or in substantial part in another journal or published work are not submitted for publication without acknowledgment and permission from the previous publication.

e. *Professional Review.* Counselors who review material submitted for publication, research, or other scholarly purposes respect the confidentiality and proprietary rights of those who submitted it.

# Section H: Resolving Ethical Issues

H.1.  KNOWLEDGE OF STANDARDS

Counselors are familiar with the *Code of Ethics* and the *Standards of Practice* and other applicable ethics codes from other professional organizations of which they are member or from certification and licensure bodies. Lack of knowledge or misunderstanding of an ethical responsibility is not a defense against a charge of unethical conduct. (See F.3.e.)

H.2.  SUSPECTED VIOLATIONS

a. *Ethical Behavior Expected.* Counselors expect professional associates to adhere to *Code of Ethics*. When counselors possess reasonable cause that raises doubts as to whether a counselor is acting in an ethical manner, they take appropriate action. (See H.2.d. and H.2.e.)

b. *Consultation.* When uncertain as to whether a particular situation or course of action may be in violation of *Code of Ethics*, counselors consult with other counselors who are knowledgeable about ethics, with colleagues, or with appropriate authorities.

c. *Organization Conflicts.* If the demands of an organization with which counselors are affiliated pose a conflict with *Code of Ethics*, counselors specify the nature of such conflicts and express to their supervisors or other responsible officials their commitment to *Code of Ethics*. When possible, counselors work toward change within the organization to allow full adherence to *Code of Ethics*.

d. *Informal Resolution.* When counselors have reasonable cause to believe that another counselor is violating an ethical standard, they attempt to first resolve the issue informally with the other counselor if feasible providing that such action does not violate confidentiality rights that may be involved.

e. *Reporting Suspected Violations.* When an informal resolution is not appropriate or feasible, counselors, upon reasonable cause, take action, such as reporting the suspected ethical violation to state or national ethics committees, unless this action conflicts with confidentiality rights that cannot be resolved.

f. *Unwarranted Complaints.* Counselors do not initiate, participate in, or encourage the filing of ethics complaints that are unwarranted or intend to harm a counselor rather than to protect clients or the public.

H.3.  COOPERATION WITH ETHICS COMMITTEES

Counselors assist in the process of enforcing *Code of Ethics*. Counselors cooperate with investigations, proceedings, and requirements of the ACA Ethics Committee or ethics committees of other duly constituted associations or boards having jurisdiction over those charged with a violation. Counselors are familiar with the ACA Policies and Procedures and use it as a reference in assisting the enforcement of the *Code of Ethics*.

# REFERENCES

Abreu, J. M., Chung, R. H. G., & Atkinson, D. R. (2000). Multicultural counseling training: Past, present, and future directions. *Counseling Psychologist, 28*(5), 641–656.

Adler, A. (1958). *What life should mean to you.* New York: Putnam.

Alexander, F. G., & Selesnick, S. T. (1966). *The history of psychiatry.* New York: Mentor.

Allen, W. (1976). *Without feathers.* New York: Warner.

Altekruse, M. K., Harris, H. L., & Brandt, M. A. (2001). The role of the professional counselor in the 21st century. *Counseling and Human Development, 34*(4), 1–10.

American Psychiatric Association. (2000). *Diagnostic and statistical manual of mental disorders* (4th ed.). Washington, DC: American Psychiatric Association.

Anastasi, A. (1997). *Psychological testing* (7th ed.). New York: Macmillan.

Anderson, H., & Goolishian, H. (1992). The client is the expert: A not knowing approach to therapy. In S. McNamee & K. J. Gergen (Eds.), *Therapy as social construction* (pp. 7–24). Newbury Park, CA: Sage.

Anderson, W. T. (1990). *Reality isn't what it used to be.* San Francisco: HarperCollins.

Argyris, C. (1974). *Theory in practice: Increasing professional effectiveness.* San Francisco: Jossey-Bass.

Association for Specialists in Group Work. (1992). Professional standards for the training of group leaders. *Journal for Specialists in Group Work, 17*(1), 12–19.

Atkinson, G., Jr., & Murrell, P. H. (1988). Kolb's experiential learning theory: A meta-model for career exploration. *Journal of Counseling and Development, 66,* 374–377.

Bacaigalupe, G. (2002). Reflecting teams: Creative, integrative, and collaborative practices. *Journal of Systemic Therapies, 21*(1), 78.

Bandura, A. (1977). *Social learning theory.* Englewood Cliffs, NJ: Prentice-Hall.

Bankart, C. P. (1997). *Talking cures: A history of Western and Eastern psychotherapies.* Pacific Grove, CA: Brooks/Cole.

Barak, A. (1994). A cognitive-behavioral educational workshop to combat sexual harassment in the workplace. *Journal of Counseling and Development, 72*, 595–602.

Barret, B., & Logan, C. (2002). *Counseling gay men and lesbians: A practice primer.* Pacific Grove, CA: Brooks/Cole.

Barsky, A. E., & Gould, J. W. (2002). *Clinicians in court: A guide to subpoenas, depositions, testifying, and everything else you need to know.* New York: Guilford.

Baruth, L. G., & Manning, M. L. (2003). *Multicultural counseling and psychotherapy.* Upper Saddle River, NJ: Prentice-Hall.

Bass, E. (1988). *The courage to heal.* New York: HarperPerennial.

Basow, S. A. (1992). *Gender: Stereotypes and roles.* Pacific Grove, CA: Brooks/Cole.

Beck, A. T. (1976). *Cognitive therapy and the emotional disorders.* New York: International Universities Press.

Beers, C. (1945). *A mind that found itself.* New York: Doubleday.

Belson, R. (1992, September/October). Ten tried-and-true methods to achieve therapist burnout. *Family Therapy Networker, 22.*

Bemak, F., & Epp, L. R. (1996). The 12th curative factor: Love as an agent of healing in group psychotherapy. *Journal for Specialists in Group Work, 21*, 118–127.

Bemak, F., & Epp, L. R. (2001). Countertransference in the development of graduate student group counselors. *Journal for Specialists in Group Work, 26*(4), 305–318.

Berg-Cross, L. (2001). *Couples therapy* (2nd ed.). New York: Haworth.

Beutler, L. E., & Hardwood, T. M. (2000). *Prescriptive psychotherapy: A practical guide to systematic treatment selection.* New York: Oxford University Press.

Beutler, L. E., Machado, P. P., & Neufeldt, S. A. (1994). Therapist variables. In A. E. Bergin & S. L. Garfield (Eds.), *Handbook of psychotherapy and behavior change* (4th ed., pp. 229–269). New York: Wiley.

Biancoviso, A. N., Fuertes, J. N., & Bishop-Towle, W. (2001). Planned group counseling: A single session intervention for reluctant, chemically dependent individuals. *Journal for Specialists in Group Work, 26*(4), 319–338.

Blake, R. (1990). Mental health counseling and older problem drinkers. *Journal of Mental Health Counseling, 12*, 354–367.

Blocher, D. H. (2000). *Counseling: A developmental approach* (4th ed.). New York: Wiley.

Bloom, B. L. (1997). *Planned short-term psychotherapy: A clinical handbook.* Boston: Allyn & Bacon.

Boer, P. M. (2001). *Career counseling over the Internet.* Mahwah, NJ: Lawrence Erlbaum Associates.

Bongar, B. (2002). *The suicidal patient: Clinical and legal standards of care.* Washington, DC: American Psychological Association.

Book, H. E. (1998). *How to practice brief, psychodynamic psychotherapy.* Washington, DC: American Psychological Association.

Boorstein, D. (1983). *The discoverers.* New York: Random House.

Boy, A. V. (1989). Psychodiagnosis: A person-centered perspective. *Person-Centered Review, 4*(2), 132–151.

Boy, A. V., & Pine, G. J. (1982). The effectiveness of a counseling theory. *Michigan Personnel and Guidance Journal, 4*, 39–42.

Boy, A. V., & Pine, G. I. (1990). *A person-centered foundation for counseling and psychotherapy.* Springfield, IL: Charles C. Thomas.

Bradley, L. J., Parve, G., & Gould, L. J. (1995). Counseling and psychotherapy: An integrative perspective. In D. Capuzzi & D. R. Gross (Eds.), *Counseling and psychotherapy: Theories and interventions.* Columbus, OH: Merrill.

Brammer, L., Abrego, P. J., & Shostrom, E. L. (1998). *Therapeutic counseling and psychotherapy* (7th ed.). Englewood Cliffs, NJ: Prentice-Hall.

Brilhart, J., & Jochern, L. (1964). Effects of different patterns on outcomes of problem-solving discussions. *Journal of Applied Psychology, 48,* 175–179.

Brooks, D. K., & Gerstein, L. H. (1990). Counselor credentialing and interpersonal collaboration. *Journal of Counseling and Development, 68,* 477–484.

Brown, J. H., & Brown, C. S. (2002). *Marital therapy: Concepts and skills for effective practice.* Pacific Grove, CA: Brooks/Cole.

Brown, M. T., Lum, J. L., & Voyle, K. (1997). Roe revisited: A call for the reappraisal of the theory of personality development and career choice. *Journal of Vocational Behavior, 51,* 283–294.

Bugental, J. F. T. (1991). Outcomes of an existential-humanistic psychotherapy. *Humanistic Psychologist, 19,* 2–9.

Bugental, J. F. T., Peirson, J. F., & Schneider, K. J. (2001). Closing statements. In K. J. Schneider, J. F. T. Bugental, & J. F. Peirson (Eds.), *The Handbook of Humanistic Psychology.* Thousand Oaks, CA: Sage.

Buhrke, R. A., & Douce, L. A. (1991). Training issues for counseling psychologists in working with lesbian women and gay men. *Counseling Psychologist, 19,* 216–234.

Burks, H. M., Jr., & Steffire, B. (1979). *Theories of counseling* (3rd ed.). New York: McGraw-Hill.

Burstow., B. (1992). *Radical feminist therapy.* Newbury Park, CA: Sage.

Butcher, J. N., Perry, J. N., & Atlis, M. M. (2000). Validity and utility of computer-based test interpretation. *Psychological Assessment, 12*(1), 6–18.

Campos, P. E., & Goldfried, M. R. (2001). Perspectives on therapy with gay, lesbian, and bisexual clients. *Journal of Clinical Psychology, 57*(5), 609–613.

Caplow, T. (1954). *The sociology of work.* Minneapolis: University of Minnesota Press.

Capuzzi, D. (2003). *Approaches to group work: A handbook for practitioners.* Upper Saddle River, NJ: Prentice-Hall.

Capuzzi, D., & Gross, D. R. (Eds.). (2001). *Counseling and psychotherapy.* Englewood Cliffs, NJ: Merrill.

Capuzzi, D., & Gross, D. R. (2002). *Introduction to group counseling* (3rd ed.). Denver: Love.

Carkhuff, R. R., & Anthony, W. A. (1979). *The skills of helping: An introduction to counseling.* Amherst, MA: Human Resources Development Press.

Carkhuff, R. R., & Berenson, B. G. (1977). *Beyond counseling and therapy* (2nd ed.). New York: Holt, Rinehart & Winston.

Carlson, J., & Kjos, D. (2001). *Theories and strategies of family therapy.* Boston: Allyn & Bacon.

Carlson, J., & Sperry, L. (2000). *Brief therapy with individuals and couples.* Phoenix: Zeig, Tucker.

Carlson, J., Sperry, L, & Lewis, J. (2003). *Family therapy techniques.* New York: Brunner/Routledge.

Carroll, M., Bates, M., & Johnson, C. (1997). *Group leadership* (3rd ed.). Denver: Love.

Casas, J. M., Ponterotto, J. G., & Gutierrez, J. M. (1 986). An ethical indictment of counseling research and training: The cross-cultural perspective. *Journal of Counseling and Development, 64,* 347–349.

Chrisler, J. C., & Ulsh, H. M. (2001). Feminist bibliotherapy: Report on a survey of feminist therapies. *Women and Therapy, 23*(4), 71–84.

Christensen, T. M., & Kline, W. B. (2001). Anxiety as a condition for learning in group supervision. *Journal for Specialists in Group Work, 26*(4), 385–396.

Chung, R., & Bemak, F. (2002). The relationship of culture and empathy in cross-cultural counseling. *Journal of Counseling and Development, 80,* 154–159.

Claiborn, C. D. (1979). Counselor verbal intervention, non-verbal behavior, and social power. *Journal of Counseling Psychology, 26,* 378–383.

Claiborn, C. D. (1987). Science and practice: Reconsidering the Pepinskys. *Journal of Counseling and Development, 65,* 286–288.

Cochran, L. (1997). *Career counseling: A narrative approach*. Thousand Oaks, CA: Sage.

Cochran, S. D., & Mays, V. M. (1989). Women and AIDS-related concerns: Roles for psychologists in helping the worried well. *American Psychologist, 44*, 529–535.

Coleman, E., & Schaefer, S. (1986). Boundaries of sex and intimacy between client and counselor. *Journal of Counseling and Development, 64*(5), 341–344.

Combs, A. W., & Gonzalez, D. W. (1994). *Helping relationships* (4th ed.). Boston: Allyn & Bacon.

Conyne, R., Rapin, L., & Rand, J. (1997). A model for leading task groups. In H. Forester-Miller & J. Kottler (Eds.), *Issues and challenges for group practitioners*. Denver: Love.

Cook, E. P. (Ed.). (1993). *Woman, relationships, and power*. Alexandria, VA: American Counseling Association.

Cooper, C. C., & Gottlieb, M. C. (2000). Ethical issues in managed care: Challenges facing counseling psychology. *Counseling Psychologist, 28*(2), 179–236.

Corey, G. (2000). *Theory and practice of counseling and psychotherapy* (6th ed.). Pacific Grove, CA: Brooks/Cole.

Corey, G., Corey, M. S., & Callanan, P. (2003). *Issues and ethics in the helping professions* (6th ed.). Pacific Grove, CA: Brooks/Cole.

Corey, M. S., & Corey, G. (2000). *Groups: Process and practice* (5th ed.). Pacific Grove, CA: Brooks/Cole.

Cormier, W. H., & Cormier, L. S. (1998). *Interviewing strategies for helpers* (4th ed.). Pacific Grove, CA: Brooks/Cole.

Corrigan, M. J., Jones, C. A., & McWhirter, J. J. (2001). College students with disabilities: An access employment group. *Journal for Specialists in Group Work, 26*(4), 339–349.

Cottone, R. R. (1992). *Theories and paradigms of counseling and psychotherapy*. Boston: Allyn & Bacon.

Cottone, R., & Tarvydas, V. M. (2003). *Ethical and professional issues in counseling* (2nd ed.). Columbus, OH: Merrill.

Covington, S. S., & Surrey, J. (2000). *The relational model of women's psychological development: Implications for substance abuse*. Wellesley, MA: Stone Center For Developmental Services and Studies.

D'Andrea, M. Postmodernism, constructivism, and multiculturalism: Three forces reshaping and expanding our thoughts about counseling. *Journal of Mental Health Counseling, 22*(1), 1–16.

Daniels, J. A. (2001). Managed care, ethics, and counseling. *Journal of Counseling and Development, 79*, 119–122.

Daniels, J. A. (2002). Assessing threats of school violence: Implications for counselors. *Journal of Counseling and Development, 80*, 215–218.

Das, A. K. (1996). Rethinking multicultural counseling: Implications for counselor education. *Journal of Counseling and Development, 74*, 45–74.

Davanloo, H. (1978). *Basic principles and techniques in short-term dynamic psychotherapy*. New York: Spectrum.

Davis, K. M. (2001). Structural-strategic family counseling: A case study in elementary school counseling. *Professional School Counseling, 4*(3), 180–186.

Davison, G. C. (2001). Conceptual and ethical issues in therapy for the psychological problems of gay men, lesbians, and bisexuals. *Journal of Clinical Psychology, 57*(5), 695–704.

De Jong, P., & Berg, I. K. (2002). *Interviewing for solutions* (2nd ed.). Pacific Grove, CA: Brooks/Cole.

de Shazer, S. (1991). *Putting difference to work*. New York: W. W. Norton.

Dies, R. R. (1992). The future of group therapy. *Psychotherapy, 29*, 58–64.

Dillon, C. (2003). *Learning from mistakes in clinical practice*. Pacific Grove, CA: Brooks/Cole.

Dinkmeyer, D., & Sperry, L. (2000). *Counseling and psychotherapy: An integrated, individual psychology approach*. Upper Saddle River, NJ: Merrill.

Dollard, J., & Miller, N. (1950). *Personality and psychotherapy.* New York: McGraw-Hill.

Donigian, J., & Malnati, R. (1999). *Critical incidents in group therapy* (2nd ed.). Pacific Grove, CA: Brooks/Cole.

Dorn, F. J. (1986). Needed: Competent, confident, and committed career counselors. *Journal of Counseling and Development, 65,* 216–217.

Doweiko, H. F. (1996). *Concepts of chemical dependency* (3rd ed.). Pacific Grove, CA: Brooks/Cole.

Doyle, R. E. (1998). *Essential skills and strategies in the helping process* (2nd ed.). Pacific Grove, CA: Brooks/Cole.

Dreikurs, R. (1950). *Fundamentals of Adlerian psychology.* Chicago: Alfred Adler Institute.

Dworkin, S. H., & Gutierrez, F. (1989). Introduction to the special issue. Counselors be aware: Clients come in every size, shape, color, and sexual orientation. *Journal of Counseling and Development, 68,* 6–8.

Dye, A. (1980). Thoughts on training. *Journal for Specialists in Group Work, 5,* 5–7.

Dyer, W. W., & Vriend, J. (1975). *Counseling techniques that work.* Alexandria, VA: American Counseling Association.

Ecker, B., & Hulley, L. (1996). *Depth oriented brief therapy.* San Francisco: Jossey-Bass.

Edwards, R. B. (1982). Mental health as rational autonomy. In R. B. Edwards (Ed.), *Psychiatry and ethics* (pp. 68–78). Buffalo: Prometheus.

Efran, J. S., Lukens, M. D., & Lukens, R. J. (1990). *Language, structure, and change.* New York: W. W. Norton.

Egan, G. (2002). *The skilled helper: A systematic approach to effective helping* (7th ed.). Pacific Grove, CA: Brooks/Cole.

Ellis, A. (1962). *Reason and emotion in psychotherapy.* New York: Lyle Stuart.

Ellis, A. (1988, September). Albert Ellis on the essence of RET. *Psychology Today,* 5–8.

Ellis, A. (1991). The revised ABC's of rational-emotive therapy. *Journal of Rational-Emotive and Cognitive-Behavior Therapy, 9,* 139–177.

Ellis, A. (1995). *Better, deeper, and more enduring brief therapy: The rational emotive behavior therapy approach.* New York: Brunner/Mazel.

Ellis, A. (1996). The humanism of rational emotive behavior therapy and other cognitive therapies. *Journal of Humanistic Education and Development, 35,* 69–88.

Ellis, A. (2001). *Overcoming destructive beliefs, feelings, and behaviors: New directions for rational emotive behavior therapy.* New York: Prometheus.

Ellis, A., & Grieger, R. (Eds.). (1986). *Handbook of rational-emotive therapy.* New York: Springer.

Ellis, A., & Harper, R. (1975). *A new guide to rational living.* Hollywood: Wilshire.

Ellis, A., & Whiteley, J. M. (Eds.). (1979). *Theoretical and empirical foundations of rational emotive therapy.* Pacific Grove, CA: Brooks/Cole.

Ellis, A., & Wilde, J. (2002). *Case studies in rational emotive behavior therapy with children and adolescents.* Upper Saddle River, NJ: Prentice-Hall.

Enns, C. Z. (1993). Twenty years of feminist counseling and therapy. *Counseling Psychologist, 21*(1), 3–87.

Enns, C. Z. (1997). *Feminist theories and feminist psychotherapies.* New York: Harrington Park.

Epston, D., White, M., & Murray, K. (1992). A proposal for a re-authoring therapy: Rose's revisioning of her life and commentary. In S. McNamee & K. J. Gergen (Eds.), *Therapy as social construction* (pp. 96–115). Newbury Park, CA: Sage.

Erikson, E. (1950). *Childhood and society.* New York: W. W. Norton.

Erlanger, M. A. (1990). Using the genogram with the older client. *Journal of Mental Health Counseling, 12*(3), 321–331.

Evans, W. P., & Carter, M. J. (1997). Urban school-based family counseling. *Journal of Counseling and Development, 75,* 366–374.

Faller, K. C. (1993). *Guidelines for determining the likelihood child sexual abuse occurred.* Washington, DC: U.S. Government Printing Office.

Falvey, J. E. (2002). *Managing clinical supervision: Ethical practice and legal risk management.* Pacific Grove, CA: Brooks/Cole.

Fassinger, R. E. (1991). The hidden minority: Issues and challenges in working with lesbian women and gay men. *Counseling Psychologist, 19,* 157–176.

Fearing, J. (1996, March). New addiction finds people hooked on the Net. *Counseling Today,* 26.

Filer, R. D., & Filer, P. A. (2000). Practical considerations for counselors working with hearing children of deaf parents. *Journal of Counseling and Development, 78,* 38–43.

Fisch, R., Weakland, J. H., & Segal, L. (1982). *The tactics of change.* San Francisco: Jossey-Bass.

Fish, J. (1973). *Placebo therapy.* San Francisco: Jossey-Bass.

Flores, L. Y., & Heppner, M. J. (2002). Multicultural career counseling: Ten essentials for training. *Journal of Career Development, 28*(3), 181–202.

Forester-Miller, H., & Davis, T. E. (1995). *A practitioner's guide to ethical decision making.* Alexandria, VA: American Counseling Association.

Forester-Miller, H., & Gressard, C. F. (1997). The tao of group work. In H. Forester-Miller & J. Kottler (Eds.), *Issues and challenges for group practitioners.* Denver: Love.

Frager, S. (2000). *Managing managed care.* New York: Wiley.

Frank, J. D. (1973). *Persuasion and healing.* Baltimore: Johns Hopkins University Press.

Frankl, V. (1962). *Man's search for meaning.* Boston: Beacon.

Frankl, V. (1978). *The unheard cry for meaning.* New York: Simon and Schuster.

Freeny, M. (2001, March/April). Better than being there. *Psychotherapy Networker,* 31–39.

French, T. M. (1933). Interrelations between psychoanalysis and the experimental work of Pavlov. *American Journal of Psychiatry, 89,* 1165–1203.

Freud, S. (1912). The dynamics of transference. In J. Strachey (Ed.), *The standard edition of the complete psychological works of Sigmund Freud* (Vol. 12, p. 97–108). London: Hogarth.

Freud, S. (1924). *A general introduction to psychoanalysis.* New York: Washington Square.

Freud, S. (1954). *The origins of psychoanalysis.* New York: Basic Books.

Fukuyama, M. A., Probert, B. S., Neimeyer, G. J., Nevill, D. D., & Metzler, A. E. (1988). Effects of discovery on career self-efficacy and decision making of undergraduates. *Career Development Quarterly, 37,* 56–62.

Garb, H. N. (2000). Computers will become increasingly important for psychological assessment: Not that there's anything wrong with that! *Psychological Assessment, 12*(1), 31–39.

Gazda, G. M., Ginter, E. J., & Horne, A. M. (2001). *Group counseling and group psychotherapy.* Boston: Allyn & Bacon.

Geis, H. J. (1973). Effectively leading a group in the present moment. *Educational Technology, 13*(1), 76–88.

Gergen, K. J. (1991). *The saturated self.* New York: Basic Books.

Gergen, K. J., & Kaye, J. (1992). Beyond narrative in the negotiation of therapeutic meaning. In S. McNamee & K. J. Gergen (Eds.), *Therapy as a social construction* (pp. 166–185). Newbury Park, CA: Sage.

Gergen, K. J. (1994). *Toward transformation in social knowledge* (3rd ed.). Thousand Oaks, CA: Sage.

Geroski, A. M., Rodgers, K. A., & Breen, D. T. (1997). Using the DSM-IV to enhance collaboration among school counselors, clinical counselors, and primary care physicians. *Journal of Counseling and Development, 75,* 231–239.

Gill, M. (1982). *The analysis of transference.* New York: International Universities Press.

Gilligan, C. (1982). *In a different voice.* Cambridge, MA: Harvard University Press.

Ginzberg, E. (1972). Toward a theory of occupational choice: A restatement. *Vocational Guidance Quarterly, 20,* 169–176.

Gladding, S. T. (1997c). *Community and agency counseling.* Columbus: Merrill.

Gladding, S. T. (2000). *Counseling: A comprehensive profession* (4th ed.). Upper Saddle River, NJ: Merrill.

Gladding, S. T. (2003). *Group work: A counseling specialty* (4th ed.). Englewood Cliffs, NJ: Merrill.

Gladding, S. T., Remley, T. P., & Huber, C. H. (2001). *Ethical, legal, and professional issues in the practice of marriage and family therapy.* Upper Saddle River, NJ: Prentice-Hall.

Glantz, K., & Pearce, J. K. (1989). *Exiles from Eden: Psychotherapy from an evolutionary perspective.* New York: W. W. Norton.

Glasser, W. (1965). *Reality therapy.* New York: Harper and Row.

Glasser, W. (1990). *The quality school.* New York: HarperCollins.

Glasser, W. (1998). *Choice theory: A new psychology of personal freedom.* New York: HarperCollins.

Glasser, W., & Breggin, P. R. (2001).*Counseling with choice theory.* New York: Quill.

Glosoff, H. L. (2001). Early historical perspectives. In D. Capuzzi & D. R. Gross (Eds.), *Introduction to the Counseling Profession.* Boston: Allyn & Bacon.

Godzki, L. (2002). *The new private practice: Therapist-coaches share stories, strategies, and advice.* New York: W. W. Norton.

Goldfried, M. R. (Ed.). (1982). *Converging themes in psychotherapy.* New York: Springer.

Goodyear, R. K., Cortese, J. R., Guzzardo, C. R., Allison, R. D., Claiborn, C. D., & Packard, T. (2000). Factors, trends, and topics in the evolution of counseling psychology training. *Counseling Psychologist, 28*(5), 603–621.

Gordon, T. G. (1970). *Parent effectiveness training.* New York: Peter Wyden.

Gordon, T. G. (1974). *Teacher effectiveness training.* New York: Peter Wyden.

Gottman, J. M. (1999). *The marriage clinic: A scientifically-based marital therapy.* New York: W. W. Norton.

Gottman, J. M., & Leiblum, S. R. (1974). *How to do psychotherapy and how to evaluate it.* New York: Holt, Rinehart & Winston.

Green, S. L., & Hansen, J. C. (1989). Ethical dilemmas faced by family therapists. *Journal of Marital and Family Therapy, 15*(2), 149–158.

Greenberg, L. S. (2002). *Emotion-focused therapy: Coaching clients to work through feelings.* Washington, DC: American Psychological Association.

Greenberg, L. S., & Safran, J. D. (1987). *Emotion in psychotherapy.* New York: Guilford.

Greenspan, S. L., & Wieder, S. (1984). Dimensions and levels of the therapeutic process. *Psychotherapy: Theory, Research, and Practice, 21*(1), 5–23.

Gross, D. R., & Robinson, S. E. (1987). Ethics, violence, and counseling: Hear no evil, see no evil, speak no evil? *Journal of Counseling and Development, 65,* 340–344.

Hackney, H., & Cormier, S. (1996). *The professional counselor.* Boston: Allyn & Bacon.

Haley, J. (1973). *Uncommon therapy.* New York: W. W. Norton.

Haley, J. (1976). *Problem solving therapy.* New York: Harper and Row.

Haley, J. (1980). How to be a marriage therapist without knowing practically anything. *Journal of Marital and Family Counseling, 6*(4), 385–392.

Haley, J. (1984). *Ordeal therapy: Unusual ways to change behavior.* San Francisco: Jossey-Bass.

Haley, J. (1989). *The first therapy session.* San Francisco: Jossey-Bass.

Haley, J., & Zeig, J. (2001). *Changing directives: The strategic psychotherapy of Jay Haley.* Phoenix, AZ: Zeig, Tucker.

Halford, W. K. (2001). *Brief therapy for couples.* New York: Guilford.

Hall, E. (1983, June). A conversation with Erik Erikson. *Psychology Today, 22–30.*

Hall, G. C. N., & Maloney, H. N. (1983). Cultural control in psychotherapy with minority clients. *Psychotherapy: Theory, Research, and Practice, 20*(2), 131–142.

Hare-Mustin, R. (1978). A feminist approach to family therapy. *Family Process, 17,* 181–194.

Hare-Mustin, R. (1994). Discourses in the mirrored room: A postmodern analysis of therapy. *Family Process, 33,* 19–35.

Hays, P. A. (1996). Addressing the complexities of culture and gender in counseling. *Journal of Counseling and Development, 74,* 332–338.

Hazler, R. J., Stanard, R., Conkey, V., & Granello, P. (1997). Mentoring group leaders. In H. Forester-Miller & J. Kottler (Eds.), *Issues and challenges for group practitioners.* Denver: Love.

Heitzman, D., Schmidt, A. K., & Hurley, F. W. (1986). Career encounters: Career decision making through on-site visits. *Journal of Counseling and Development, 66,* 209–210.

Held, B. S. (1984). Toward a strategic eclecticism. *Psychotherapy: Theory, Research, and Practice, 21*(2), 232–241.

Helwig, A. A., & Holicky, R. (1994). Substance abuse in persons with disabilities: Treatment considerations. *Journal of Counseling and Development, 72,* 227–233.

Heppner, P. P., & Anderson, W. P. (1985). On the perceived non-utility of research in counseling. *Journal of Counseling and Development, 63,* 545–547.

Heppner, P. P., Kivlighan, D. M., & Wampold, B. E. (1998). *Research design in counseling.* Pacific Grove, CA: Wadsworth.

Herlihy, B., & Corey, G. (1996). *Ethical standards casebook.* Alexandria, VA: American Counseling Association.

Herlihy, B., & Corey, G. (1997). *Boundary issues in counseling: Multiple roles and responsibilities.* Alexandria, VA: American Counseling Association.

Herron, W. G., & Rouslin, S. (1984). *Issues in psychotherapy.* Washington, DC: Oryn.

Hill, C. E. (1990). Is individual therapy process really different from group therapy process? The jury is still out. *Counseling Psychologist, 18,* 126–130.

Hill, C. L., & Ridley, C. R. (2001). Diagnostic decision making: Do counselors delay final judgments. *Journal of Counseling and Development, 79,* 98–104.

Ho, B. S. (2001). Family-centered, integrated services: Opportunities for school counselors. *Professional School Counseling 4*(5), 357–361.

Hohenshil, T. H. (2000). High tech counseling. *Journal of Counseling and Development, 78,* 365–368.

Holland, J. (1966). *The psychology of vocational choice.* Waltham, MA: Blaisdell.

Holland, J. (1973). *Making vocational choices: A theory of careers.* Englewood Cliffs, NJ: Prentice-Hall.

Hoppock, R. (1976). *Occupational information* (4th ed.). New York: McGraw-Hill.

Horowitz, D. L. (1985). *Ethnic groups in conflict.* Berkeley, CA: University of California Press.

Hoshmand, L. T., & Polkinghorne, D. E. (1992). Redefining the science-practice relationship and professional training. *American Psychologist, 47,* 55–66.

Houston, C. J. (2001, August). The perils of email. *Counseling Today,* 7–8.

Hoyt, M. F. (2000). *Some stories are better than others: Doing what works best in brief therapy and managed care.* New York: Brunner/Routledge.

Hsiung, R. C. (2001). *E-therapy: Case studies, guiding principles, and the clinical potential of the Internet.* New York: W. W. Norton.

Huber, C. H. (1994). *Ethical, legal, and professional issues in the practice of marriage and family therapy.* New York: Merrill.

Hubble, M. A., Duncan, B. L., & Miller, S. D. (1999). *The heart and soul of change.* Washington, DC: American Psychological Association.

Impara, J. C. (Ed.). (2001). *The fourteenth mental measurements yearbook*. Buros Institute.

Isaacs, M. L. (1997). The duty to warn and protect: Tarasoff and the elementary school counselor. *Elementary School Guidance and Counseling, 31,* 326–342.

Isaacs, M. L., & Stone, C. (2001). Confidentiality with minors: Mental health counselors' attitudes toward breaching or preserving confidentiality. *Journal of Mental Health Counseling, 23*(4), 342–356.

Ivey, A. (1991). *Developmental strategies for helpers*. Pacific Grove, CA: Brooks/Cole.

Ivey, A. (1998). *Intentional interviewing and counseling* (4th ed.). Pacific Grove, CA: Brooks/Cole.

Ivey, A., & Authier, J. (1978). *Micro-counseling* (2nd ed.). Springfield. IL: Charles C. Thomas.

Jacobs, E. E., Masson, R. L., & Harvill, R. L. (1998). *Group counseling: Strategies and skills* (3rd ed.). Pacific Grove, CA: Brooks/Cole.

Jackson, A. P., & Scharman, J. S. (2002). Constructing family-friendly careers: Mothers' experiences. *Journal of Counseling and Development, 80,* 180–187.

James, O. O. (1997). *Play therapy: A comprehensive guide*. New York: Jason Aronson.

James, W. (1907). *Pragmatism*. New York: New American Library.

Jennings, L. & Skovholt, T. M. (1999). The cognitive, emotional, and relational characteristics of master therapists. *Journal of Counseling Psychology, 46*(1), 3–11.

Jensen, J. P., Bergin, A. E., & Greaves, D. W. (1990). The meaning of eclecticism: New survey and analysis of components. *Professional Psychology: Research and Practice, 21,* 124–130.

Johnson, D. W., & Johnson, F. P. (2003). *Joining together: Group theory and group skills*. Boston: Allyn & Bacon.

Johnson, S., & Lebow, J. (2000). The coming of age of couple therapy: A decade review. *Journal of Marital and Family Therapy, 26*(1), 23–38.

Jones, B. E., & Gray, B. A. (1986). Problems in diagnosing schizophrenia and affective disorders among blacks. *Hospital and Community Psychiatry, 37,* 61–65.

Joshua, J., & DeMenna, D. (2000). *Read two books and let's talk next week: Using bibliotherapy in clinical practice*. New York: Wiley.

Josselson, R. (1992). *The space between us: Exploring the dimensions of human relationships*. San Francisco: Jossey-Bass.

Kagan, N. (1973). Can technology help us toward reliability in influencing human interaction? In J. Vriend & W. Dyer (Eds.), *Counseling effectively in groups*. Englewood Cliffs, NJ: Educational Technology.

Kahn, M. (1997). *Between therapist and client: The new relationship* (rev. ed.). New York: W. H. Freeman.

Kaiser, H. (1965). *Effective psychotherapy: The contribution of Hellmuth Kaiser* (L. Fierman, Ed.). New York: Free Press.

Kanfer, F. H., & Goldstein, A. P. (1991). *Helping people change* (4th ed.). New York: Pergamon.

Kanfer, F. H., & Phillips, J. S. (1970). *Learning foundations of behavior therapy*. New York: Wiley.

Kaplan, H. S. (1974). *The new sex therapy*. New York: Brunner/Mazel.

Kaplan, M. (1983). A woman's view of DSM-III. *American Psychologist, 38*(7), 786–792.

Katkin, E. S., & Goldband, S. (1980). Biofeedback. In F. H. Kanfer & A. P. Goldstein (Eds.), *Helping people change* (pp. 537–578). New York: Pergamon.

Kelly, E. W., Jr. (1997). Relationship-centered counseling: A humanistic model of integration. *Journal of Counseling and Development, 75,* 337–345.

Kernberg, O. (1984). *Severe personality disorders*. New Haven, CT: Yale University Press.

Kiselica, M. S. (1998). *Confronting prejudice and racism during multicultural training*. Alexandria, VA: American Counseling Association.

Kleinke, C. L. (1994). *Common principals of psychotherapy*. Pacific Grove, CA: Brooks/Cole.

Kleinplatz, P. J. (Ed.). (2001). *New directions in sex therapy: Innovations and alternatives*. New York: Brunner/Routledge.

Kline, W. B. (2003). *Interactive group counseling and therapy.* Upper Saddle River, NJ: Prentice-Hall.

Koffka, K. (1935). *Principles of Gestalt psychology.* New York: Harcourt Brace & World.

Kohlberg, L. (1969). *Stages in the development of moral thought and action.* New York: Holt, Rinehart & Winston.

Kohler, W. (1929). *Gestalt psychology.* New York: Liveright.

Koss, M. P. (1990). The women's mental health research agenda: Violence against women. *American Psychologist, 45,* 374–380.

Kottler, J. A. (1991). *The compleat therapist.* San Francisco: Jossey-Bass.

Kottler, J. A. (1992). *Compassionate therapy: Working with difficult clients.* San Francisco: Jossey-Bass.

Kottler, J. A. (1993). *On being a therapist* (rev. ed.). San Francisco: Jossey-Bass.

Kottler, J. A. (1994a). *Beyond blame: A new way of resolving conflicts in relationships.* San Francisco: Jossey-Bass.

Kottler, J. A. (1994b). *Advanced group leadership.* Pacific Grove, CA: Brooks/Cole.

Kottler, J. A. (1995). *Growing a therapist.* San Francisco: Jossey-Bass.

Kottler, J. A. (1997b). *What's really said in the teachers' lounge.* Thousand Oaks, CA: Corwin.

Kottler, J. A. (2000). *Doing good: Passion and commitment for helping others.* New York: Brunner/Routledge.

Kottler, J. A. (2001). *Making changes last.* New York: Brunner/Routledge.

Kottler, J. A., & Blau, D. (1989). *The imperfect therapist: Learning from failures in therapeutic practice.* San Francisco: Jossey-Bass.

Kottler, J. A., & Carlson, J. (2003). *Bad therapy: Master therapists share their worst failures.* New York: Brunner/Routledge.

Kottler, J. A., & Hazler, R. (1996). Impaired counselors: The dark side brought into light. *Journal of Humanistic Education and Development, 34,* 98–107.

Kottler, J. A., & Hazler, R. (1997). *What you never learned in graduate school.* New York: W. W. Norton.

Kottler, J. A., & Markos, P. (1997). The group leader's uses of self. In H. Forester-Miller & J. Kottler (Eds.), *Issues and challenges for group practitioners.* Denver: Love.

Kottler, J. A., Sexton, T., & Whiston, S. (1994). *The heart of healing: Relationships in therapy.* San Francisco: Jossey-Bass.

Kovacs, A. L. (1982). Survival in the 1980s on the theory and practice of brief psychotherapy. *Psychotherapy: Theory, Research, and Practice, 19*(2), 142–159.

Kroll, J. (1988). *The challenge of the borderline patient.* New York: W. W. Norton.

Krumboltz, J. D. (1965). Behavioral counseling: Rationale and research. *Personnel and Guidance Journal, 44,* 373–387.

Krumboltz, J. D. (Ed.). (1966). *Revolution in counseling: Implications of behavioral science.* Boston: Houghton Mifflin.

Krumboltz, J. D. (1978). A social learning theory of career selection. In J. M. Whiteley & A. Resnikoff (Eds.), *Career counseling.* Pacific Grove, CA: Brooks/Cole.

Kubie, L. S. (1934). Relation of the conditioned reflex to psychoanalytic technique. *Archives of Neurology and Psychiatry, 32,* 1137–1142.

Lafountain, R. M., & Bartos, R. B. (2001). Research and statistics made meaningful in counseling and student affairs with Infotrac. Pacific Grove, CA: Brooks/Cole.

Layman, M. J., & McNamara, J. R. (1997). Remediation for ethics violations: Focus on psychotherapists' sexual contact with clients. *Professional Psychology: Research and Practice, 28,* 281–292.

Lazarus, A. A. (1981). *The practice of multi-modal therapy.* New York: McGraw-Hill.

Lazarus, A. A. (1993). Tailoring the therapeutic relationship, or being an authentic chameleon. *Psychotherapy, 30.*

Lazarus, A. A. (1995). Multimodal therapy. In R. J. Corsini & D. Wedding (Eds.), *Current psychotherapies* (5th ed.). Itasca, IL: F. E. Peacock.

Lazarus, A. A., & Beutler, L. E. (1993). On technical eclecticism. *Journal of Counseling and Development, 71,* 381–385.

Lee, C. C. (2002). *Multicultural issues in counseling: New approaches to diversity* (3rd ed.). Alexandria, VA: American Counseling Association.

Lega, L. I., & Ellis, A. (2001). Rational emotive behavior therapy in the new millennium: A cross-cultural approach. *Journal of Rational Emotive and Cognitive Behavior Therapy, 19*(4), 201–222.

Leiblum, S. R., & Rosen, R. C. (Eds.). (2000). *Principles and practices of sex therapy* (3rd ed.). New York: Guilford.

Levenson, H. (1995). *Time limited dynamic psychotherapy.* New York: Basic Books.

Lewis, J. A., Dana, R. G., & Blevins, G. A. (2002). *Substance abuse counseling: An individualized approach* (3rd ed.). Pacific Grove, CA: Brooks/Cole.

Lieberman, M., Yalom, L., & Miles, M. (1973). *Encounter groups: First facts.* New York: Basic Books.

Littrel, J. M. (1998). *Brief counseling in action.* New York: W. W. Norton.

Loevinger, J. (1976). *Ego development.* San Francisco: Jossey-Bass.

Long, V. (1996). *Communication skills in helping relationships.* Pacific Grove, CA: Brooks/Cole.

Lum, D. (2003). *Culturally competent practice.* Pacific Grove, CA: Brooks/Cole.

Lum, W. (2002). The use of the self of the therapist. *Contemporary Family Therapy, 24*(1), 181–197.

Lundin, R. W. (1989). *Alfred Adler's basic concepts and implications.* Muncie, IN: Accelerated Development.

MacDougall, C. (2002). Rogers's person-centered approach: Consideration for use in multicultural counseling. *Journal of Humanistic Psychology, 42*(2), 48–65.

Madanes, C. (1983). *Strategic family therapy.* San Francisco: Jossey-Bass.

Madanes, C. (1984). *Beyond the one-way mirror.* San Francisco: Jossey-Bass.

Mahoney, M. J. (1974). *Cognition and behavior modification.* Cambridge, MA: Ballinger.

Mahrer, A. R. (1987). These are the components of any theory of psychotherapy. *Journal of Integrative and Eclectic Psychotherapy, 6*(1), 28–31.

Maione, P. V., & Chenail, R. J. (1999). Qualitative inquiry in psychotherapy: Research on common factors. In M. A. Hubble, B. L. Duncan, & S. D. Miller (Eds.), *The heart and soul of change: What works in therapy.* Washington, DC: American Psychological Association.

Malgady, R. G. (1996). The question of cultural bias in assessment and diagnosis of ethnic minority clients: Let's reject the null hypothesis. *Professional Psychology: Research and Practice, 27,* 73–77.

Mander, G. (2000). *Psychodynamic approach to brief therapy.* Thousand Oaks, CA: Sage.

Mann, J. (1973). *Time limited psychotherapy.* Cambridge, MA: Harvard University Press.

Masi, D., & Freedman, M. (2001). The use of telephone and on-line technology in assessment, counseling, and therapy. *Employee Assistance Quarterly, 16*(3), 49–63.

Maultsby, M. C. (1984). *Rational behavior therapy.* Englewood Cliffs, NJ: Prentice-Hall.

May, R. (1958). *Existence.* New York: Simon & Schuster.

May, R. (1967). *The art of counseling.* Nashville: Abingdon.

May, R. (1981). *Freedom and destiny.* New York: W. W. Norton.

May, R. (1983). *The discovery of being.* New York: W. W. Norton.

May, R., & Yalom, I. (1995). Existential psychotherapy. In R. J. Corsini & D. Wedding, *Current psychotherapies* (5th ed.). Itasca, IL: F. E. Peacock.

McGoldrick, M., & Gerson, R. (1985). *Genograms in family assessment.* New York: W. W. Norton.

McRae, B. (1998). *Negotiating and influencing skills.* Thousand Oaks, CA: Sage.

McWhirter, P. T., & McWhirter, J. J. (1996). Transition-to-work group: University students with learning disabilities. *Journal for Specialists in Group Work, 21,* 144–148.

Meadow, A., Parnes, S., & Reese, J. (1959). Influence of brainstorming instructions and problem sequence on creative problem solving. *Journal of Applied Psychology, 43,* 413–436.

Meichenbaum, D. H. (1977). *Cognitive-behavior modification: An integrative approach.* New York: Plenum.

Mikulas, W. L. (2002). *The integrative helper: Convergence of Eastern and Western traditions.* Pacific Grove, CA: Brooks/Cole.

Miller, G. M. (1982). Deriving meaning from standarized tests: Interpreting results to clients. *Measurement and Evaluation in Guidance, 15,* 87–94.

Miller, T. W., Veltkamp, L. J., Lane, T., Bilyeu, J., & Elzie, N. (2002). Care pathway guidelines for assessment and counseling for domestic violence. *The Family Journal, 10*(1), 41–48.

Miller, W. R., & Hester, R. (1986). Inpatient alcoholism treatment: Who benefits? *American Psychologist, 41,* 794–805.

Miller, W. R., Meyers, R. J., & Tonigan, J. S. (1999). Engaging the unmotivated in treatment for alcohol problems. *Journal of Consulting and Clinical Psychology, 67*(5), 688–697.

Minuchin, S. (1974). *Families and family therapy.* Cambridge, MA: Harvard University Press.

Minuchin, S., & Fishman, H. C. (1981). *Family therapy techniques.* Cambridge, MA: Harvard University Press.

Minuchin, S., Rosman, B., & Baker, L. (1978). *Psychosomatic families: Anorexia nervosa in context.* Cambridge, MA: Harvard University Press.

Mitchell, L. K., & Krumboltz, J. D. (1987). The effects of cognitive restructuring and decision making training on career indecision. *Journal of Counseling and Development, 66,* 171–174.

Monk, G., Winslade, J., Crocket, K., & Epston, D. (1997). *Narrative therapy in practice.* San Francisco: Jossey-Bass.

Moore, T. (1994). *Soul mates: Honoring the mysteries of love and relationships.* New York: HarperCollins.

Morrison, J. (1994). *The first interview.* New York: Guilford.

Murphy, B. C., & Dillon, C. (1998). *Interviewing in action: Process and practice.* Pacific Grove, CA: Brooks/Cole.

Murphy, J. A., Rawlings, E. I., & Howe, S. R. (2002). A survey of clinical psychologists on treating lesbian, gay, and bisexual clients. *Professional Psychology: Research and Practice, 33*(2), 183–189.

Murphy, J. J. (1997). *Solution-focused counseling in middle and high schools.* Alexandria, VA: American Counseling Association.

Musashi, M. (1982). *A book of five rings.* Woodstock, NY: Overlook Press.

National Institute on Alcohol Abuse and Alcoholism. (2001). *Alcohol alert: New advances in alcohol treatment.* No. 49–2000. Rockville, MD: NIAAA.

Neimeyer, R. A. (2002). *Lessons of loss: A guide to coping* (2nd ed.). New York: Brunner/ Routledge.

Neimeyer, R. A., & Mahoney, M. J. (Eds.). (1999). *Constructivism in psychotherapy.* Washington, DC: American Psychological Association.

Nelson, J. R., Dykeman, C., Powell, S., & Petty, D. (1996). The effects of a group counseling intervention on students with behavioral adjustment problems. *Elementary School Guidance and Counseling, 31,* 21–33.

Nelson, M. L. (1996). Separation versus connection, the gender controversy: Implications for counseling women. *Journal of Counseling and Development, 74,* 339–344.

Neugarten, B. (1968). *Middle age and aging.* Chicago: University of Chicago Press.

Nevels, L. A., & Coche, J. M. (1993). *Powerful wisdom.* San Francisco: Jossey-Bass.

Newman, B., & Newman. P. (1999). *Development through life* (7th ed.). Pacific Grove, CA: Brooks/Cole.

Nichols, M. P., & Schwartz, R. C. (2001). *Family therapy: Concepts and methods* (5th ed.). Boston: Allyn & Bacon.

Nolan, E. J. (1978). Leadership interventions for promoting personal mastery. *Journal for Specialists in Group Work, 3*(3), 132–138.

Norcross, J. C., Prochaska, J. O., & Gallagher, K. M. (1989). Clinical psychologists in the 1980s. *Clinical Psychologist, 42*(2).

Nugent, F. A. (2000). *An introduction to the profession of counseling.* Upper Saddle River, NJ: Merrill.

Ogles, B. M., Lunnen, K. M., & Bonesteel, K. (2001). Clinical significance: History, application, and current practice. *Clinical Psychology Review, 21*(3), 421–446.

O'Hanlon, W. H. (1994, November/December). The third wave. *Family Therapy Networker,* 18–26.

O'Hanlon, W. H., & Weiner-Davis, M. (1989). *In search of solutions.* New York: W. W. Norton.

Okun, B. F. (2002). *Effective helping: Interviewing and counseling techniques* (6th ed.). Pacific Grove, CA: Brooks/Cole.

O'Leary, J. V. (2001). The postmodern turn in group therapy. *International Journal of Group Psychotherapy, 51*(4), 473–487.

Paniagua, F. A. (2001). *Diagnosis in a multicultural context: A casebook for mental health professionals.* Thousand Oaks, CA: Sage.

Pardeck, J. T., & Pardeck, J. A. (1993). *Bibliotherapy: A clinical approach for helping children.* New York: Gordon & Breach.

Parloff, M. (1956). Some factors affecting the quality of therapeutic relationships. *Journal of Abnormal and Social Psychology, 52,* 5–10.

Parsons, F. (1909). *Choosing a vocation.* Boston: Houghton Mifflin.

Parsons, R. D. (1996). *The skilled consultant.* Boston: Allyn & Bacon.

Pascarelli, E. F. (1981). Drug abuse and the elderly. In J. H. Lowinson & P. Ruiz (Eds.), *Substance abuse: Clinical problems and perspectives.* Baltimore: Williams & Wilkins.

Patterson, L. E., & Welfel, E. R. (1999). *The counseling process* (5th ed.). Pacific Grove, CA: Brooks/Cole.

Pearson, B., & Piazza, N. (1997). Classification of dual relationships in the helping professions. *Counselor Education and Supervision, 37,* 89–99.

Pedersen, P. (1988). *A handbook for developing multicultural awareness.* Alexandria, VA: American Counseling Association.

Pedersen, P. (1991). Multiculturalism as a generic approach to counseling. *Journal of Counseling and Development, 70,* 6–12.

Pedersen, P., & Carey, J. C. (2003). *Multicultural counseling in the schools.* Boston: Allyn & Bacon.

Perls, F. (1969a). *Gestalt therapy verbatim.* Lafayette, CA: Real People Press.

Perls, F. (1969b). *In and out of the garbage pail.* Lafayette, CA: Real People Press.

Perosa, S. L., & Perosa, L. M. (1987). Strategies for counseling midcareer changers: A conceptual framework. *Journal of Counseling and Development, 65,* 558–561.

Phillips, S. D., Christopher-Sisk, E. K., & Gravino, K. L. (2001). Making career decisions in a relational context. *Counseling Psychologist, 29*(2), 193–213.

Phinney, J. S. (1996). When we talk about American ethnic groups, what do we mean? *American Psychologist, 51,* 918–927.

Piaget, J. (1926). *The language and thought of the child.* New York: Harcourt Brace Jovanovich.

Plummer, D. (1999). *One of the boys: Masculinity, homophobia, and modern manhood.* New York: Haworth.

Ponterotto, J. G., Alexander, C. M., & Grieger, I. (1995). A multicultural competency checklist for counseling training programs. *Journal of Multicultural Counseling and Development, 23,* 11–20.

Pope, K. S., Keith-Spiegel, P., & Tabachnick, B. O. (1986). Sexual attraction to clients. *American Psychologist, 41*(2), 147–158.

Pope, K. S., & Vasquez, M. J. (1991). *Ethics in psychotherapy and counseling.* San Francisco: Jossey-Bass.

Posthuma, B. W. (2001). *Small groups in counseling and therapy* (4th ed.). Boston: Allyn & Bacon.

Prediger, D. J. (1993). *Multicultural assessment standards: A compilation for counselors.* Alexandria, VA: American Counseling Association.

Preston, J. (1999). *Integrative brief therapy: Cognitive, psychodynamic, humanistic, and neurobehavioral approaches.* New York: Impact.

Quick, E. K. (1996). *Doing what works in brief therapy.* San Diego: Academic Press.

Ramsey, M. (1996). Diversity identity development training: Theory informs practice. *Journal of Multicultural Counseling and Development, 24,* 229–240.

Remley, T. P., Jr., Herlihy, B. (2001). *Ethical, legal, and professional issues in counseling.* Upper Saddle River, NJ: Prentice-Hall.

Riemer-Reiss, M. L. (2000). Utilizing distance technology for mental health counseling. *Journal of Mental Health Counseling, 22*(3), 189–203.

Riordan, R. J., & Walsh, L. (1994). Guidelines for professional referral to alcoholics anonymous and other twelve step groups. *Journal of Counseling and Development, 72,* 351–355.

Ritchie, M. H. (1994). Cultural and gender biases in definitions of mental and emotional healthiness. *Counselor Education and Supervision, 33,* 344–348.

Robertiello, R. C. (1978). The occupational disease of psychotherapists. *Journal of Contemporary Psychotherapy,* 123–129.

Robinson, T. E., & Howard-Hamilton, M. F. (2000). *The convergence of race, ethnicity, and gender: Multiple identities in counseling.* Upper Saddle River, NJ: Prentice-Hall.

Roe, A. (1957). Early determinants of vocational choice. *Journal of Counseling Psychology, 4,* 212–217.

Rogers, C. R. (1942). *Counseling and psychotherapy.* Boston: Houghton Mifflin.

Rogers, C. R. (1951). *Client-centered therapy.* Boston: Houghton Mifflin.

Rogers, C. R. (1957). The necessary and sufficient conditions of therapeutic personality change. *Journal of Consulting Psychology, 21,* 93–103.

Rogers, C. R. (1961). *On becoming a person.* Boston: Houghton Mifflin.

Rogers, C. R. (1969). *Freedom to learn.* Columbus, OH: Charles E. Merrill.

Rogers, C. R. (1970). *On encounter groups.* New York: Harper and Row.

Roland, C. B., & Neitzschman, L. (1996). Groups in schools: A model for training middle school teachers. *Journal for Specialists in Group Work, 21,* 18–25.

Rosenzweig, S. (1936). Some implicit common factors in diverse methods in psychotherapy. *American Journal of Orthopsychiatry, 6,* 412–415.

Rowley, W. J., & MacDonald, D. (2001). Counseling and the law: A cross-cultural perspective. *Journal of Counseling and Development, 79,* 422–429.

Rubenfeld, S. (2001). Group therapy and complexity theory. *International Journal of Group Psychotherapy, 51*(4), 449–471.

Rutter, P. (1989). *Sex in the forbidden zone.* Los Angeles: Jeremy Tarcher.

Sampson, J. P., Jr. (2000). Using the Internet to enhance testing in counseling. *Journal of Counseling and Development, 78,* 348–356.

Sandhu, D. S., & Aspy, C. B. (1997). *Counseling for prejudice prevention and reduction.* Alexandria, VA: American Counseling Association.

Sartre, J. P. (1957). *Existentialism and human emotions.* New York: The Wisdom Library.

Savickas, M. L. (1997). Constructivist career counseling: Models and methods. *Advances in Personal Construct Psychology, 4,* 149–182.

Schafer, C. (1990a, March 1). Ethics, dual relationships come under scrutiny. *Guidepost,* pp. 2–3.

Schlossberg, N. K. (1984). *Counseling adults in transition.* New York: Springer.

Schlossberg, N. K., & Kent, L. (1979). Effective helping in women. In S. Eisenberg & L. E. Patterson (Eds.), *Helping clients with special concerns* (pp. 263–286). Chicago: Rand McNally.

Schneider, K. J. (1998). Toward a science of the heart: Romanticism and the revival of psychology. *American Psychologist, 53,* 277–289.

Schofield, W. (1964). *Psychotherapy: The purchase of friendship.* Englewood Cliffs. NJ: Prentice-Hall.

Schwartz, J. (1997). Meaning vs. medical necessity: Can psychoanalytic treatments exist in a managed care world? *Psychotherapy, 34,* 115–123.

Schwiebert, V. L., Myers, J. E., & Dice, C. (2000). Ethical guidelines for counselors working with older adults. *Journal of Counseling and Development, 78*(2), 123–129.

Seligman, L. (1998). *Selecting effective treatments* (2nd ed.). San Francisco: Jossey-Bass.

Seligman, M. (1983). Sources of psychological disturbance among siblings of handicapped children. *Personnel and Guidance Journal, 61,* 529–531.

Sexton, T. L., & Whiston, S. C. (1994). The status of the counseling relationship. *Counseling Psychologist, 22*(1), 6–78.

Shapiro, F. (1995). *Eye movement desensitization and reprocessing.* New York: Guilford.

Sharf, R. S. (2002). *Applying career development theory to counseling* (3rd ed.). Pacific Grove, CA: Brooks/Cole.

Shaver, K. G. (1985). *The attribution of blame.* New York: Springer-Verlag.

Shedler, J., & Block, J. (1990). Adolescent drug use and psychological health: A longitudinal inquiry. *American Psychologist, 45,* 612–630.

Sheehy, G. (1995). *New passages: Mapping your life across time.* New York: Random House.

Shute, N. (1997, September 8). The drinking dilemma. *U.S. News and World Report,* 55–65.

Silverstein, J. L. (1997). Acting out in group therapy: Avoiding authority struggles. *International Journal of Group Psychotherapy, 47,* 31–45.

Simon, G. M. (1991). Theoretical eclecticism: A goal we are obligated to pursue. *Journal of Mental Health Counseling, 13,* 112–118.

Sinacore-Guinn, A. L. (1995). The diagnostic window: Culture- and gender-sensitive diagnosis and training. *Counselor Education and Supervision, 35,* 18–31.

Skinner, B. F. (1938). *The behavior of organisms: An experimental analysis.* New York: Appleton-Century-Crofts.

Skinner, B. F. (1953). *Science and human behavior.* New York: Macmillan.

Skinner, B. F. (1983). Intellectual self-management in old age. *American Psychologist, 38,* 239–244.

Sklare, G. (1997). *Brief counseling that works: A solution focused approach for school counselors.* Thousand Oaks, CA: Corwin Press.

Skovholt, T. M. (2001). *The resilient practitioner: Burnout prevention and self-care strategies for counselors, therapists, teachers, and health professionals.* Boston: Allyn & Bacon.

Smith, D. S. (1982). Trends in counseling and psychotherapy. *American Psychologist, 37,* 802–809.

Smith, M. A., & Senior, C. (2001). The Internet and clinical psychology: A general review of implications. *Clinical Psychology Review, 21*(1), 129–136.

Snowden, L. R., & Cheung, F. K. (1990). Use of inpatient mental health services by member ethnic minority groups. *American Psychologist, 45*(3), 347–355.

Solomon, G. (2001). *Reel therapy: How movies inspire you to overcome life's problems*. New York: Lebhar-Friedman.

Speight, S. L., Meyers, L. J., Cox, C. L., & Highlen, P. S. (1991). A redefinition of multicultural counseling. *Journal of Counseling and Development, 70*, 29–36.

Spiegler, M. D., & Guevremont, D. C. (1998). *Contemporary behavior therapy* (3rd ed.). Pacific Grove, CA: Brooks/Cole.

Spitzer, R. L., Skodol, A. E., Gibbon, M., & Williams, J. (1994). *DSM-III case book*. Washington, DC: American Psychiatric Association.

Standard, R., & Hazler, R. (1995). Legal and ethical implications of HIV and duty to warn for counselors. *Journal of Counseling and Development, 73*, 397–400.

Stanley, J. (1999). *Reading to heal: How to use bibliotherapy to improve your life*. Boston: Houghton Mifflin.

Stanley, S., Bradbury, T., & Markman, H. (2000). Structural flaws in the bridge from basic research on marriage to intervention for couples. *Journal of Marriage and the Family, 62*(1), 256–264.

Steinman, S. O., Richardson, N. F., & McEnroe, T. (1998). *The ethical decision making manual for helping professionals*. Pacific Grove, CA: Brooks/Cole.

Stevens, M. J., & Morris, S. J. (1995). A format for case conceptualization. *Counselor Education and Supervision, 35*, 35–93.

Strasser, F., & Strasser, A. (1997). *Existential time-limited therapy: The wheel of existence*. New York: Wiley.

Straus, M. B. (1999). *No-talk therapy for children and adolescents*. New York: W. W. Norton.

Strong, S. R., & Claiborn, C. D. (1982). *Change through interaction*. New York: Wiley Interscience.

Strupp, H. (1989). Can the practitioner learn from the researcher? *American Psychologist, 44*(4), 717–724.

Strupp, H. H., & Binder, J. L. (1984). *Psychotherapy in a new key*. New York: Basic Books.

Sue, S., Ivey, A., & Pederson, P. (1996). *A theory of multicultural counseling and therapy*. Pacific Grove, CA: Brooks/Cole.

Sullivan, B. S. (1989). *Psychotherapy grounded in the feminine principle*. Wilmette, IL: Chiron.

Super, D. E. (1953). A theory of vocational development. *American Psychologist, 8*, 185–190.

Super, D. E. (1957). *The psychology of careers*. New York: Harper and Row.

Super, D. E. (1990). A life span, life space approach to career development. In D. Brown & L. Brooks (Eds.), *Career choice and development* (2nd ed.). San Francisco: Jossey-Bass.

Sweeney, T. J. (1998). *Adlerian counseling: A practitioner's guide* (4th ed.). New York: Brunner/Routledge.

Swenson, L. C. (1997). *Psychology and the law* (2nd ed.). Pacific Grove, CA: Brooks/Cole.

Swift, R. M. (1999). Drug therapy for alcohol dependence. *New England Journal of Medicine, 340*(19), 1482–1490.

Tallman, K, & Bohart, A. C. (1999). The client as a common factor: Clients as self-healers. In M. A. Hubble, B. L. Duncan, & S. D. Miller (Eds.), *The Heart and Soul of Change*. Washington, DC: American Psychological Association.

Talmon, M. (1990). *Single session therapy*. San Francisco: Jossey-Bass.

Taylor, B., & Wagner, M. (1976). Sex between therapist and clients: A review and analysis. *Professional Psychology, 7*, 593–601.

H., & Affleck, G. (1990). Blaming others for threatening events. *Psychological Bulletin*, ?09–232.

1972). *Working*. New York: Avon.

, C. E. (1969). The counselor as an applied behavioral scientist. *Personnel and Guidance Journal, 47*, 841–848.

Thorne, F. C. (1950). *The principles of personal counseling.* Brandon, VT: Clinical Psychology Publishing.

Tiedeman, D. V., & O'Hara, R. P. (1963). *Career development: Choice and adjustment.* New York: College Entrance Examination Board.

Tinsley, H. E., & Bradley, R. W. (1986). Test interpretation. *Journal of Counseling and Development, 64,* 462–466.

Tonigan, J. S., Toscova, R., & Miller, W. R. (1999). Meta-analysis of the literature on Alcoholics Anonymous: Sample and study characteristics moderate findings. *Journal of Studies in Alcohol, 57,* 65–72.

Truax, C. B., & Carkhuff, R. R. (1967). *Toward effective counseling and psychotherapy.* Chicago: Aldine.

Tryon, G. S. (2002). Engagement in counseling. In G. S. Tryon (Ed.), *Counseling based on process research.* Boston: Allyn & Bacon.

Tyler, L. (1970). Thoughts about theory. In W. H. Van Hoose & J. J. Pietrofesa (Eds.), *Counseling and guidance in the twentieth century* (pp. 298–305). Boston: Houghton Mifflin.

Vacc, N. A., & Juhnke, G. A. (1997). The use of structured clinical interviews for assessment in counseling. *Journal of Counseling and Development, 75,* 470–480.

Van der Walde, H., Urgenson, F. T., Weltz, S. H., & Hanna, F.J. (2002). Women and alcoholism: A biopsychosocial perspective and treatment approaches. *Journal of Counseling and Development, 80,* 145–153.

Van Hoose, W. H., & Kottler, J. A. (1985). *Ethical and legal issues in counseling and psychotherapy* (2nd ed.). San Francisco: Jossey-Bass.

Wachtel, P. (1977). *Psychoanalysis and behavior therapy: Toward an integration.* New York: Basic Books.

Wagner, E. E. (1987). A review of the 1985 standards for educational and psychological testing: User responsibility and social justice. *Journal of Counseling and Development, 66,* 202–203.

Wakefield, J. C. (1997). Diagnosing DSM-IV-Part I: DSM-IV and the concept of disorder. *Behavior Research and Therapy, 35,* 633–649.

Wasielewski, R. A., Scruggs, M. Y., & Scott, C. W. (1997). Student groups conducted by teachers. *Journal for Specialists in Group Work, 22,* 43–51.

Waters, E. B., & Goodman, J. (1990). *Empowering older adults.* San Francisco: Jossey-Bass.

Watkins, C. E. (1994). Thinking about tests and assessment and the Career Beliefs Inventory. *Journal of Counseling and Development, 72,* 421–428.

Watkins, C. E., Lopez, F. G., Campbell, V. L., & Himmell, C. D. (1986). Contemporary counseling psychology: Results of a national survey. *Journal of Counseling Psychology, 33,* 301–309.

Watson, J. C., & Bohart, A. (2001). Humanistic-existential therapies in the era of managed care. In K. J. Schneider, J. F. T. Bugental, & J. F. Pierson (Eds.), *The Handbook of Humanistic Psychology.* Thousand Oaks, CA: Sage.

Watzlawick, P., Weakland, J. H., & Fisch, R. (1974). *Change: Principles of problem formation and problem resolution.* New York: W. W. Norton.

Wedding, D., & Corsini, R. J. (2001). *Case studies in psychotherapy* (3rd ed.). Itasca, IL: F. E. Peacock.

Weigel, D. J., & Baker, B. G. (2002). Unique issues in rural couple and family counseling. *The Family Journal, 10*(1), 61–69.

Weil, A. (1972). *The natural mind.* Boston: Houghton Mifflin.

Weil, A., & Rosen, W. (1993). *From chocolate to morphine.* Boston: Houghton Mifflin.

Weinrach, S. G. (1996). Nine experts describe the essence of rational-emotive therapy while standing on one foot. *Journal of Counseling and Development, 74,* 326–331.

Welfel, E.R. (1998). *Ethics in counseling and psychotherapy: Standards, research, and emerging issues.* Pacific Grove, CA: Brooks/Cole.

Weltner, J. (1988, May/June). Different strokes: A pragmatist's guide to intervention. *Family Therapy Networker, 53–57.*

Wertz, F. J. (1998). The role of the humanistic movement in the history of psychology. *Journal of Humanistic Psychology, 38,* 42–70.

White, M., & Epston, D. (1990). *Narrative means to therapeutic ends.* New York: W. W. Norton.

Williams, P., & Davis, D. C. (2002). *Therapist as a life coach.* New York: W. W. Norton.

Wilson, F. R., & Owens, P. C. (2001). Group-based prevention programs for at-risk adolescents and adults. *Journal for Specialists in Group Work, 26*(3), 246–255.

Windle, M. (2001). Substance abuse among children and adolescents. In E. R. Welfel & R. E. Ingersoll (Eds.), *The mental health desk reference.* New York: Wiley.

Winslade, J., & Monk, G. (2000). *Narrative mediation: A new approach to conflict resolution.* San Francisco: Jossey-Bass.

Wise, R. A. (1988). The neurobiology of craving: Implications for the understanding and treatment of addiction. *Journal of Abnormal Psychology, 97,* 118–132.

Wolpe, J. (1958). *Psychotherapy by reciprocal inhibition.* Palo Alto, CA: Stanford University Press.

Wolpe, J. (1982). *The practice of behavior therapy* (2nd ed.). Elmsford, NY: Pergamon.

Worden, M., & Worden, B. D. (1998). *The gender dance in couples therapy.* Pacific Grove, CA: Brooks/Cole.

Worrell, J., & Papendrick-Remer, P. (2001). *Feminist perspectives in therapy.* New York: Wiley.

Wright, R. (1994). *The moral animal.* New York: Pantheon.

Wubbolding, R. (1990). *Expanding reality therapy.* Cincinnati: Real World.

Wubbolding, R. (2000). *Reality therapy for the 21st century.* New York: Brunner/Routledge.

Wylie, M. S. (1995, May/June). Diagnosing for dollars. *Family Therapy Networker, 22–33; 65–69.*

Yalom, I. (1980). *Existential psychotherapy.* New York: Basic Books.

Yalom, I. (1989). *Love's executioner and other tales of psychotherapy.* New York: Basic Books.

Yalom, I. (1995). *The theory and practice of group psychotherapy* (4th ed.). New York: Basic Books.

Young, M. E. (1992). *Counseling methods and techniques: An eclectic approach.* New York: Macmillan.

Young, M. E. (2001). *Learning the art of helping.* Upper Saddle River, NJ: Merrill.

Zayas, L. H., Torres, L. R., Malcolm, J., & DesRosiers, F. S. (1996). Clinicians' definitions of ethnically sensitive therapy. *Professional Psychology: Research and Practice, 27,* 78–82.

Zimmerman, T. S., (2002). *Balancing family and work: Special considerations in feminist therapy.* New York: Haworth Press.

Zuk, G. H. (1984). On the pathology of blaming. *International Journal of Family Therapy, 6,* 143–155.

Zunker, V. G. (2002). *Career counseling: Applied concepts of life planning* (6th ed.). Pacific Grove, CA: Brooks/Cole.

# INDEX